THE
NATURAL
REMEDIES
GUIDE

Thunder Bay Press
An imprint of Printers Row Publishing Group
9717 Pacific Heights Blvd, San Diego, CA 92121
www.thunderbaybooks.com • mail@thunderbaybooks.com

Printers Row Publishing Group is a division of Readerlink Distribution Services, LLC. Thunder Bay Press is a registered trademark of Readerlink Distribution Services, LLC.

Correspondence regarding the content of this book should be sent to Thunder Bay Press, Editorial Department, at the above address. Rights inquiries should be addressed to HarperCollins*Publishers*, 1 London Bridge Street, London SE1 9GF. www.harpercollins.co.uk.

Thunder Bay Press
Publisher: Peter Norton • Associate Publisher: Ana Parker
Editor: Dan Mansfield

Produced by HarperCollins*Publishers*
Editor: Sarah Vaughan • Designer: Rosamund Saunders
Authors: Rachel Newcombe, Claudia Martin, C. Norman Shealy, Julia Lawless, David Hoffman
General Editor: Rachel Newcombe
Cover and interior images © Shutterstock

Library of Congress Cataloging-in-Publication data available on request.

ISBN: 978-1-6672-0083-5

Printed in Bosnia-Herzegovina

26 25 24 23 22   1 2 3 4 5

THE
NATURAL
REMEDIES
GUIDE

General Editor:

Rachel Newcombe

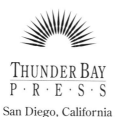

THUNDER BAY
P · R · E · S · S

San Diego, California

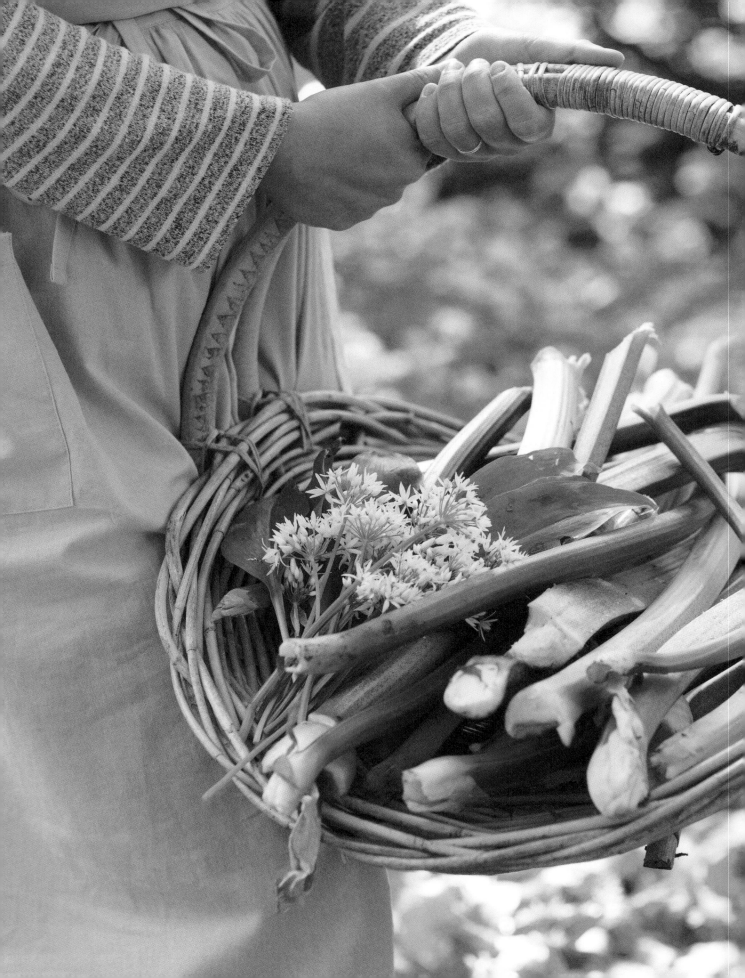

CONTENTS

Part Two: Aromatherapy and Essential Oils

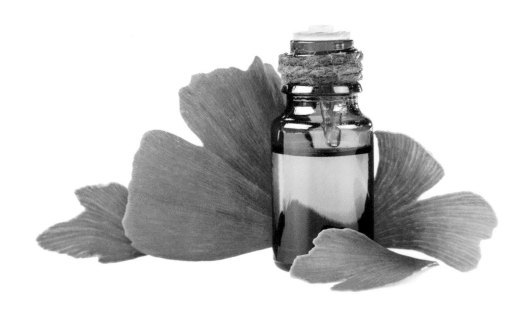

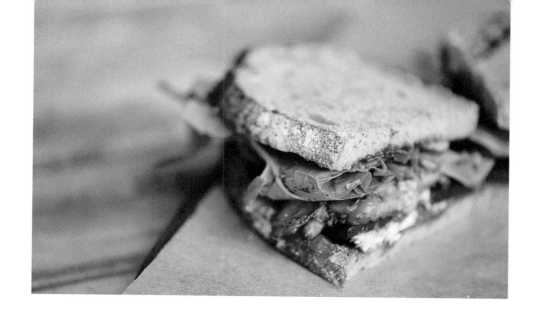

Part Three: Food and Drink

Part Four: Crystals

FOREWORD

Welcome to the world of natural remedies!

From tried and tested traditional herbal preparations and soothing and uplifting aroma blends, to ancient crystals and modern superfoods, *The Natural Remedies Guide* contains a plethora of ideas for intriguing remedies you could use for aiding basic body and mind care.

The book explores four main types of natural remedies—namely herbs, aromatherapy, food and drink, and crystals—and looks at the ways in which they could benefit basic health, beauty, home, and lifestyle needs. Each part includes an A to Z section of the key individual components, and then goes on to explain the ways in which they could be used for basic healing, health, and lifestyle issues. There's insight into the history and traditions of each approach, providing relevant context and analysis of how the approaches were relevant in both the past and present day.

When you're using this book and gaining inspiration for how to utilize the ideas, keep in mind that natural remedies should never be used as the first option for major illness, health problems, emergencies, or new symptoms of existing conditions—always see a medical professional first. Some herbal remedies may interact with any prescribed drugs you're taking, so consult with your doctor before making or taking them.

If you're in any doubt about how best to work with natural remedies, particularly herbs, aromatherapy, or crystals, seek help and advice from a trained holistic health practitioner.

Above all, though, enjoy your exploration of the world of natural remedies and discover the many ways you could incorporate them into your lifestyle today.

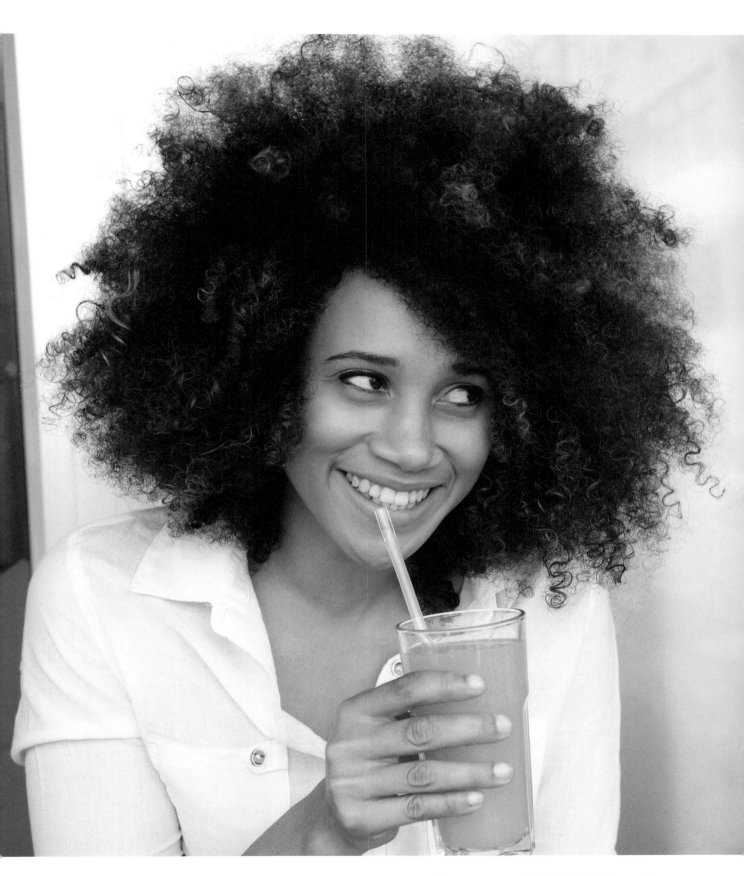

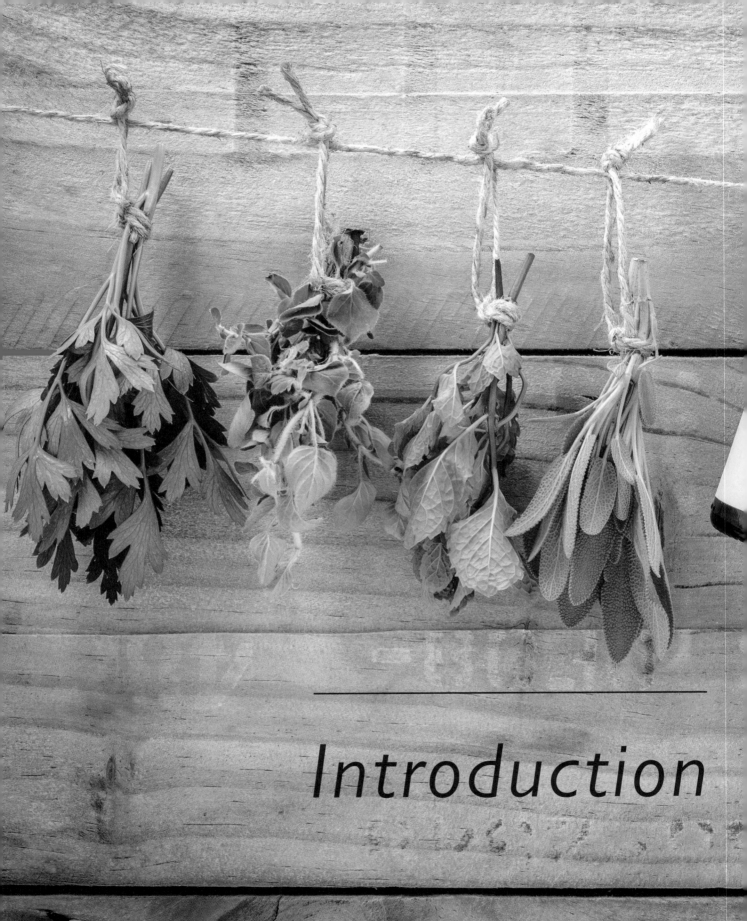

Introduction

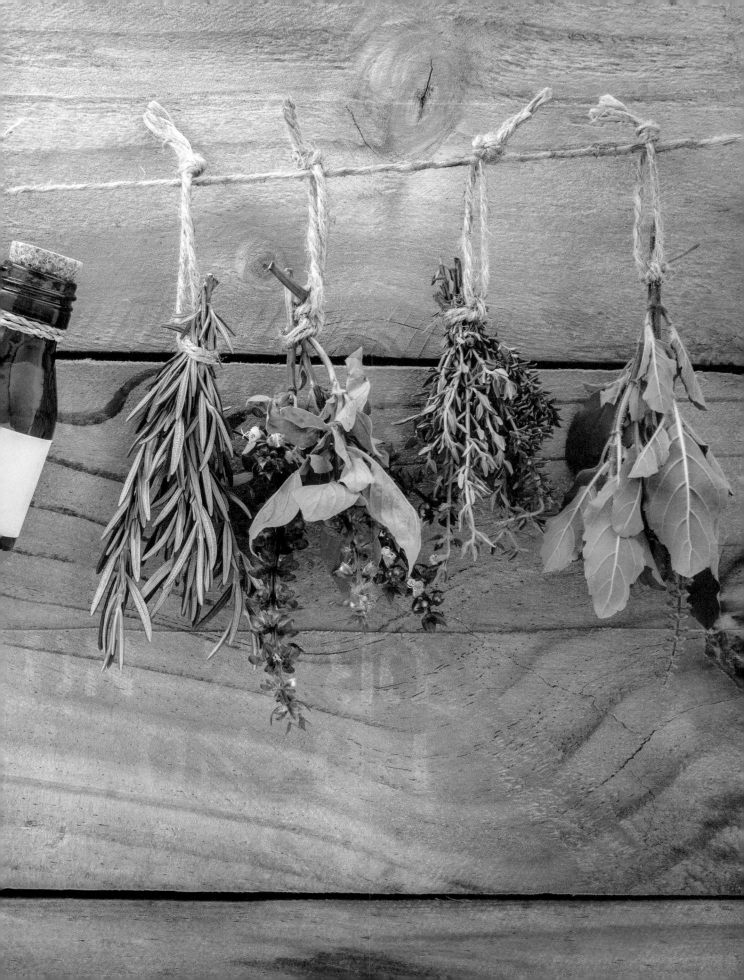

WHAT ARE
NATURAL REMEDIES?

Natural remedies have been used for centuries for curing and preventing minor ailments or injuries. Generations of our ancestors handed down knowledge of tried and tested solutions to common problems, such as treating nettle stings with dock leaves or using honey and lemon to ease a sore throat, and many are still as relevant today as they were in the past.

In fact, lots of natural remedies have numerous uses, and can even be used in combination in the home to help clean and purify your living environment or provide useful solutions to common problems, such as helping to eliminate strong cooking odors or remove stains from worktops. As the name suggests, natural remedies derive from natural ingredients or elements of the natural world. They utilize the power of Mother Nature to bring about health and healing, and focus on restoring equilibrium and wholeness to the body, mind, and spirit.

Natural remedies may also be referred to by some as alternative remedies, to describe how they're seen as standing apart from conventional medicine. This is often because the methods are based on belief systems that aren't fully recognized by scientists, or there's thought to be a lack of scientific evidence and medical studies to prove their worth.

Yet many forms of conventional medication are derived from plants and natural ingredients—aspirin, for example, is derived from willow bark—and many natural approaches are becoming more accepted by medical practitioners. So rather than viewing natural remedies as a standalone alternative to mainstream medicine, it's better to view them as complementary; they can work effectively when used hand-in-hand to help boost overall health and wellness.

This is especially so as natural remedies are part of a more holistic approach, focusing on dealing with the whole person, rather than just the individual physical or mental ailment. A holistic approach strives toward a state of balance, or homeostasis, and acknowledges that demands on one element can affect the whole of your well-being. For example, not being able to sleep can affect your mental health as well as leaving you physically drained and exhausted.

Optimum health and well-being is achieved when you look after all parts of your body and mind, which can include aspects such as eating a healthy diet, getting regular exercise, managing stress, looking after your mental health, living in a healthy environment, and getting the right amount of relaxation and sleep. It's not always easy to get this balance right while dealing with the demands of modern life, but by utilizing natural remedies and practicing methods of self-care, it can be made more achievable.

Natural remedies can take many different forms—from hands-on therapies such as aromatherapy massage, to the use of natural crystals for healing, superfoods for physical nourishment, and herbal remedies for minor injuries and skin-care needs.

Aromatherapy utilizes the benefits of essential oils, each of which have their own unique properties. Massage can be beneficial for many physical complaints, such as muscle strains or headaches, but there's much more to aromatherapy than just having a massage. Essential oils can be used in a myriad of different ways, from basic first-aid treatments and promoting a sense of calm for meditation and relaxation practice, to cosmetic and skin-care use and oils to use for maintaining furniture and wood.

Fresh and dried herbs can be used in a similar variety of ways, plus they can be grown and nurtured by your own hands, indoors on a windowsill or outside in a garden. Herbs can be added to foods and drinks to help minor ailments, made into compresses and oils, added to skin-care products such as scalp tonic or facial scrubs, and used in your home.

Food is typically viewed as fuel to give us energy and nutrition, yet the natural properties of plants, grains, meat, and dairy can all have a beneficial effect on health too, and food can be a form of natural medicine. The cloves of garlic you buy in the supermarket not only add flavor to your food but could also help ease the symptoms of a cold or boost your immunity when you're feeling under the weather.

Crystals formed deep in the crust of the earth over hundreds and thousands of years are believed by crystal therapists to have healing properties. They work on a more subtle energy level and, like other holistic therapies, can be used alongside traditional medicine to add an extra dimension to wellness and self-care. Plus, they can be used in the home too, helping to release negative energies and provide a sense of peace.

The more you get to know and use the different types of natural remedies in your everyday life, the more you'll learn about their benefits and discover how versatile and helpful they can be for any number of minor ailments and lifestyle issues.

Garlic-infused oil

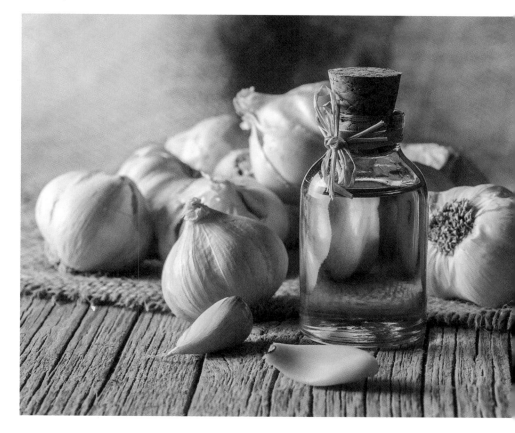

TRADITIONAL HOME AND FOLK REMEDIES

Every culture, across the centuries, has had its own understanding and ways of healing. Local plants, customs, and beliefs determined the form these took, which varied not only across countries but also between villages. Even today, away from the convenience of conventional physicians, local communities around the world practice their own form of medicinal healing using plants, age-old wisdom, and an instinctive and learned knowledge of their bodies as the tools.

A return to old ways

With the advent of technology and the growing dependence on the miracles of modern medicine, most of us have lost the art of looking after ourselves. We have become dependent on physicians, prescription drugs, store-bought preparations, and, through that, have lost an understanding of our bodies and how they work. Somewhere along the line we have put not only our faith but our independence in the hands of others. When we have a cold, a rash, even painful joints, we go straight to the medicine cabinet, or ring to arrange an appointment at the doctor's office. The use of natural preparations, and the number of people addressing minor complaints in their own homes, has hit an all-time low over the past decades, and only now are we experiencing a renaissance of natural healing and home remedies, as it becomes clear that conventional medicine, for all its wonders, is not the answer to everything.

Busy Western physicians have little time to spend diagnosing their patients, and our Western approach to pathology and anatomy is based on the theory that we are all the same. Individual personalities, lifestyles, emotions, spirituality, and even physical

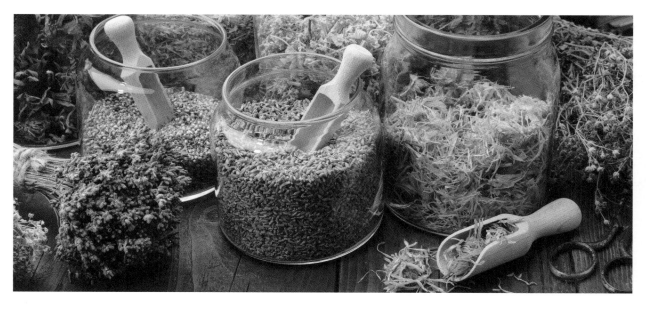

bodies are not taken into consideration for most conventional treatments, but we have now learned that it is the complex combination of these very things that can make us sick or well. When deciding on treatments, therefore, a wider picture needs to be examined.

In the past, many people had the knowledge and the wherewithal to treat themselves, using foodstuffs in their larders and plants growing in their yards and fields. There would have been a village healer or physician who could be called upon in times of emergency, but for day-to-day and common ailments, treatment was undertaken at home.

While the understanding of biochemistry could not match that of a modern physician, the knowledge of how plants and various substances work in the body, and, indeed, how the body responds in various situations and to different treatments, was much more profound. Women instinctively treated their children and their families—recognizing a bad temper as the onset of illness, perhaps, and being capable of addressing the cause of an illness according to a more general knowledge of the holistic being.

Today, most drugs on the market tend to deal with symptoms rather than the root cause of an illness. Conditions such as asthma, eczema, ME (chronic fatigue syndrome), headaches, and menstrual problems are controlled rather than cured. We take a tablet to ease the pain of a headache, but we do not stop and consider why we have a headache. We apply creams to stop the itching of eczema, but we do nothing to address the cause. In the past, we had a much greater general understanding of the causes and effects of illness, and a much more instinctive

approach to treatment. Folk medicine and home remedies kept the majority of people healthy, and it is that tradition to which many are increasingly returning today.

Preventing illness

Natural medicine in the home is more than just first aid for common and minor ailments. It can be preventive, using some of the most common items in the larder—onions, garlic, thyme, mint, sage, chamomile—to protect against many illnesses. Modern research—particularly over the last three decades—is now justifying the use of plants and household items, things that have been used for centuries in both folk medicine and traditional cooking. For example, mint calms the digestive system; lemon is a great detoxifier, helping the liver and kidneys to function effectively; rosemary has profound antiseptic powers and is a natural stimulant; and caraway seeds will prevent flatulence.

By incorporating some of these elements in your day-to-day meals, you not only add flavor and variety, but also provide the systems of your body with nourishment and support. These remedies have a beneficial effect on our general health, something that conventional drugs do not. Most available drugs work to address specific systems and do nothing for our overall health; many of them have side effects that are more dangerous than the symptoms they are addressing.

Traditional folk and home remedies tend to work *with* our bodies, allowing them to heal themselves by keeping them strong and healthy.

THE HISTORY OF NATURAL REMEDIES

Whenever possible, a system of folk medicine is best understood in a historical context. The Aztecs in Mexico provide a good example of how conventional medical systems can go hand in hand with folk medicine, allowing both to grow according to the needs of the population.

Aztec (as opposed to folk) medicine was highly organized and based on a complex theoretical structure and experimental research. Some segments of the population, however, had only limited access to this medicine, relying instead on traditional treatments. Aztec medicine was eliminated with the Spanish conquest, and their own treatment became the new medicine of the Aztecs. The system still offered limited access; however, some elements of the European approach were compatible with the folk medical practice of the Native Americans and were therefore incorporated into a new Mexican folk system that thrived and continued to incorporate elements of the new establishment medicine.

Similarly, Native North American systems, while not highly organized and academic, were the establishment medicine in their own societies before conquest. While Europeans brought their own medical systems, they also brought diseases that decimated populations and challenged indigenous medical systems. Again, this intrusive medicine became the establishment medicine, and Native American medicine, with some Euro-American elements, became folk medicine.

Discovering plant benefits

The history of using plants for medicine and healing goes back to the beginning of humankind. In their search for nourishment, primitive humans sampled many plants. Those that were palatable were used for food, while plants with toxic or unpleasant effects were avoided or used against enemies. Plants that caused physiological effects such as healing or hallucinations were saved for medicinal purposes and divination.

More than 4,000 years ago, the Chinese emperor Qien Nong (Chi'en Nung), also called Shennong, put together a book of medicinal plants called *Ben Zao* (*Pen Tsao*), or *Classic Materia Medica*. It contained descriptions of over 300 plants, several of which are still used in medicine today. At the same time, the Sumerians were recording prescriptions on clay tablets, and later the Egyptians wrote their medical systems on rolls of papyrus. The oldest such document, the Papyrus Kahun, dates from the time of King Amenemhat III and contains details about women's medical conditions.

The most famous of these medical papyri, the so-called Ebers Papyrus, reports on plants that are still used today—in both folk and conventional medicine. The Greeks and the Romans derived some of their herbal knowledge from these early civilizations. Their contributions are recorded in Dioscorides's *De Materia Medica* and the thirty-seven-volume natural history. Some of these works are known to us through translations into Arabic by Rhazes and Avicenna. The knowledge of medicinal plants was further nurtured by monks in Europe, who grew medicinal plants and translated the Arabic works. The first recognized apothecaries opened in Baghdad in the ninth century. By the thirteenth century, London had become a major trading center in herbs and spices.

In the Dark Ages, the belief of the Christian Church that disease was a punishment for sin caused a great setback in medical progress. Only in monasteries did herbals and other documented sources of natural medicine continue to be translated. However, the Renaissance provided a new forum for the development of the folk tradition. William Caxton printed dozens of medical manuals and Nicholas Culpeper translated the entire physicians' pharmacopeia, *The English Physician and Complete Herbal*, in 1653. It is still in print. The advent of alchemy, and the split between the "new philosophy" of reason and experiment, and the previous tradition of "science" (ancient medical doctrines, herbalism, astrology, and the occult) ended the golden age of herbals. Witch hunts disposed of village "healing women," women were forbidden to study, and all nonprofessional healers were declared heretics. The use of herbs became associated with magic and the occult, an uneasy alliance that has been difficult to shake. Herbalism was effectively dropped from mainstream medical training, though folk advice and treatment from the apothecary herbalist continued to be available, especially in less well-off areas.

Traditional folk medicine today

The term "folk medicine" refers to the traditional beliefs, practices, and materials that people use to maintain health and cope with disease, outside of an organized relationship with academic, professionally recognized, and established medical systems and treatments. Systems of folk medicine are very closely related to the history, traditions, and life of a recognizable social group, and the people who practice it often share the same belief system and approach to health as their patients.

As research into the active constituents of herbs continues, increasing numbers of ancient treatments and tonics are being rediscovered, recognized, and brought back into widespread use. The global transport network means that we now have access to treatments used in countries around the world, bringing us a variety of amazing plants such as tea tree oil, aloe vera, and ginkgo biloba. Today, more than 120 current prescription drugs are obtained from plants, and about 25 percent of all prescriptions contain one or more active ingredients from plants.

Comparison and evaluation of folk and academic medical systems and practices is difficult. While indiscriminate interpretation of folk medicine may result in inappropriate rejection of proven establishment methods—for example, drugs required to treat chronic and serious illness that may not have existed in the past. On the other hand, the dangerous aspects of folk medicine have often been emphasized, usually without recognizing their contributions to conventional medicine and the similarities between them.

Today, there is a greater understanding of the power of natural remedies, and their use is being slowly accepted and indeed encouraged, particularly for ailments that people can safely and appropriately treat at home, but severe illness and disorders should be referred to a professional practitioner. For more advice on when to self-treat, turn to pages 26–29.

TYPES OF NATURAL REMEDIES

Natural remedies can take many different forms, but all have the same characteristic at their heart: they derive from natural ingredients or natural elements.

In this book we're covering four main types of natural remedies that are easily accessible and can be used for mind and body self-care, enhancing health and well-being, namely: herbs and herbal remedies, aromatherapy and essential oils, food and drink, and crystals. They each have their own unique characteristics and can be used in a wide array of methods.

Herbs

Herbs have been used to make herbal remedies for centuries and are as relevant today for health and healing as they were in the past. A wide variety of herbs are used for healing purposes, and herbal remedies can be made from a number of different parts of the plants. For example, they can be made from:

- Leaves • Stems • Flowers • Fruits
- Roots • Seeds • Bark

Some herbal remedies are made from different types of seaweed and fungi. Herbal remedies can be made from common household plants and store-bought ingredients, making them an accessible tool. In a similar vein, flower essences are another form of natural remedy that can also be beneficial and tend to work on a more emotional level, helping you cope with trauma and emotional demands.

Aromatherapy and essential oils

Aromatherapy is an ancient holistic therapy that uses natural plant extracts to aid health and well-being, primarily through our sense of smell and skin absorption, via aromatherapy massage (oils should not be applied directly to the skin; a few drops should be added to a carrier oil in order to be diluted before massage). There are hundreds of essential oils made from plants and each has its own healing properties. The oils can be used individually or in combination with one another.

Some of the many different ways the power of aromatherapy can be used include:

- Diffusers • Hot and cold compresses
- Facial steamers • Massage • Inhalers • Masks
- Bathing • Body oils • Creams and lotions

Unlike some herbal remedies, it's not so easy to make your own essential oils, but they can be purchased from local health-food stores and other retailers. The good news is that a little goes a long way, so once purchased they should last you a while.

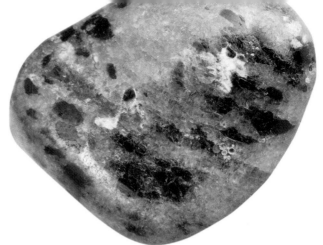

*Polished green zoisite
with red ruby corundum*

Food and drink

The adage "you are what you eat" is certainly true when it comes to diet and health. The foods and drinks you choose to consume can play a significant role in your health and well-being. This is one important area of your lifestyle that you can actively control and improve, as changes to your diet could help boost your overall health.

Natural foods and drinks can be regarded as a form of plant medicine. There's some overlap with herbal medicine, as ingredients such as garlic can be added to foods yet also made into herbal remedies.

Some foods are regarded as superfoods, as they have even more nutritional value and healing abilities than others, and are particularly valuable for including in your diet regularly. Superfoods can take many forms, including:

- Dairy products • Fruits • Vegetables
- Nuts and seeds • Fish • Grains

Simple changes to your diet, or switching ingredients to healthier options, can have health benefits, and a good diet can be a form of self-care for your body and mind. This includes being mindful of how you eat, taking time to enjoy the food you eat and digest it properly. The timing of your meals can also have an impact on your body.

Crystals

Crystals are another type of natural remedy and work on the chakras (see page 254) and aura to help rebalance the mind and spirit. Crystals are formed in the surface of the earth, often over hundreds and thousands of years, and built by nature into geometric forms. Even if you can't see it from the exterior of a crystal, the inner atoms are arranged into repeated lattices; they may be visible if you view a crystal under a microscope.

It's believed that all crystals have a unique energy or vibration, and it's this vibrational frequency that sets crystals apart from other stones. Each type of crystal has individual properties and can be used for different purposes, or simply as a decorative display in your home.

Crystals can be used in a number of different ways to help minor ailments and to aid in the rebalancing of the body's unseen energy points or chakras. For example, crystals can be:

- Used to cleanse and purify an indoor space
- Used to cleanse an aura
- Worn as jewelry
- Used in meditation
- Placed in a room to emit energy
- Placed on or around the body to aid minor ailments
- Made into elixirs and added to baths, creams, or lotions
- Used to purify other crystals

Crystals come in a rainbow of colors and are particularly beneficial for working with the mind and emotional issues, as well as some minor physical ailments.

NATURAL REMEDIES AS A FORM OF SELF-CARE

When you've got a busy and hectic life, it's easy to forget to look after yourself. But self-care is vitally important on a physical, mental, and emotional level. A buildup of stress, late nights, poor diet, and not getting enough exercise can take its toll on your health, often manifesting itself in unexpected symptoms and creeping up on you before you realize the damage is done.

A good life balance involves regular self-care, where you specifically focus on looking after yourself and your individual needs. Practicing self-care can help you learn more about your body's needs and how you react to stress and tiredness, plus it gives you time to indulge in the things you enjoy and that make you happy. For example, take time to yourself to read a good book, watch a film, do craft activities, go for a walk, do yoga, or have a massage. It's a time in which you can unwind, step back, and have a few moments to yourself.

Self-care should be something you practice regularly. It may be tricky to find time at first, but ideally you should try and integrate it into your daily life or weekly routine. It's not selfish to focus on self-care—it's empowering and self-respectful, helping you take control and give yourself the chance to live your life as the best version of yourself.

There are many elements involved in self-care practices, from improving your physical wellness and looking after your emotional health, to improving your work–life balance and social wellness. You don't have to work on everything at once, but small changes make a difference and are beneficial over time.

Natural remedies are an important part of a holistic self-care strategy and could help you gain optimum wellness physically, mentally, and emotionally, as well as acting as a form of preventive medicine too. The more you focus on yourself, the better you'll get to know your own individual needs and the ways in which you can help yourself. The use of natural remedies allows you to tune in to your body, mind, and spirit in new ways, adding an extra dimension to your self-care practice.

Physical self-care methods involve looking after your body to improve your physical wellness. You might want to give your body a boost by actively choosing to eat healthier foods or swapping unhealthy drinks for herbal teas and tisanes. Exercising can help your physical health in numerous ways, but sometimes it's hard to stick with exercises that you don't love doing. As part of your self-care, it's worth focusing on finding an exercise routine you enjoy, as it will make it more pleasurable to do and you will be more motivated to continue.

Mental self-care is often overlooked, but it's just as important. Natural remedies and holistic approaches can be used to aid development of emotional self-care practices to help deal with both current and preventive issues. For example, herbal remedies or aromatherapy could help you manage stress more effectively or boost your emotional resilience, whereas techniques such as meditation could provide you with new ways to calm an overactive mind, thus reducing the risk of burnout.

As you focus on your emotional self-care needs, you may begin to develop improved skills such as kindness, compassion, and communication, which enable you to cope better with challenging situations at home and at work.

Utilizing the power of natural remedies in a regular self-care routine can have numerous benefits on your health and well-being, transforming you for the better. Some of the benefits you could unlock include:

• Increased energy
• Better sleep
• A more nutritious, vitamin-rich diet
• A stronger body
• An improved ability to relax
• A reduction in stress and anxiety

• Improved productivity
• Better knowledge of your own needs
• Self-compassion

Whether you focus on giving your body a better balance of nutrition through eating healthy foods, use herbs and herbal remedies to help improve your sleep and boost your energy, or use crystals to help you work on your self-confidence and self-esteem, natural remedies can be key elements in helping you nurture and care for yourself.

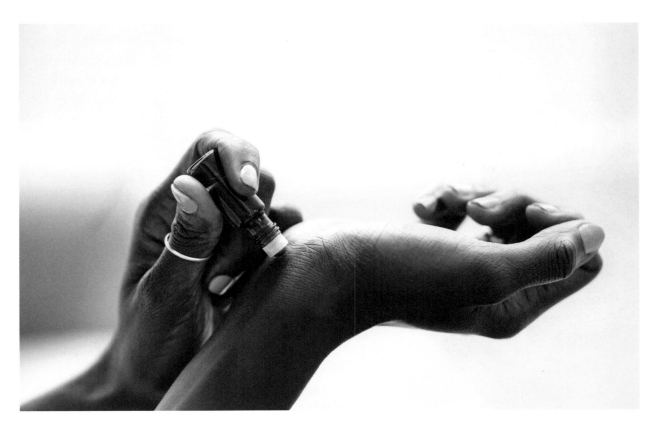

NATURAL REMEDIES FOR THE BODY

The body is one of the key areas that natural remedies can be useful for. Different types of natural remedies and therapies can help with a wide range of physical ailments and common minor complaints, as well as boost your general well-being.

Natural remedies can be used for ailments involving:

• The skin and hair
• Joints and muscles
• Headaches
• Colds and coughs
• Bruises and burns
• Indigestion
• Eyestrain and earache
• Constipation
• Bites and stings

The nature of natural and holistic therapies means that they work on many levels, so are often involved

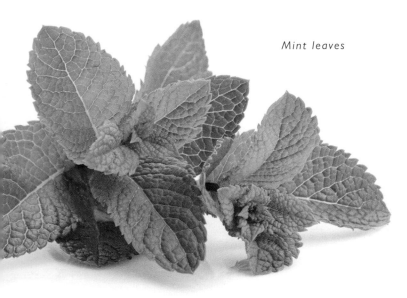

Mint leaves

in helping more than just the body; they work on the mind, emotions, and spirit too.

Therapies involving touch, such as aromatherapy massage, cause the body to respond on several levels. Changes may occur in your breathing and circulation; chemicals may be released in your nerves and body; there will be a sensory response to the touch and the scent of the oils being used; plus the pressure on your skin and muscles can help release areas of tension in your body.

There are many benefits that come with embracing natural remedies and holistic approaches in your life. While conventional medicine traditionally tends to focus on finding drugs to target specific symptoms once a medical problem has occurred, the overall aim of holistic remedies is to build up your ability to adapt and maintain health and well-being. When used alongside each other, as an integrated approach, you get the best of both worlds. For example, where a doctor would offer solutions to treat the symptoms of headaches, the holistic approach would explore the underlying causes, such as eyestrain, stress, or poor sleep habits.

Looking after your body through practical lifestyle changes, such as upping your daily nutritional intake, drinking more water, trying new forms of movement, or improving your posture, are also vital for the health of your body and integrate seamlessly into the holistic health approach alongside the use of natural remedies.

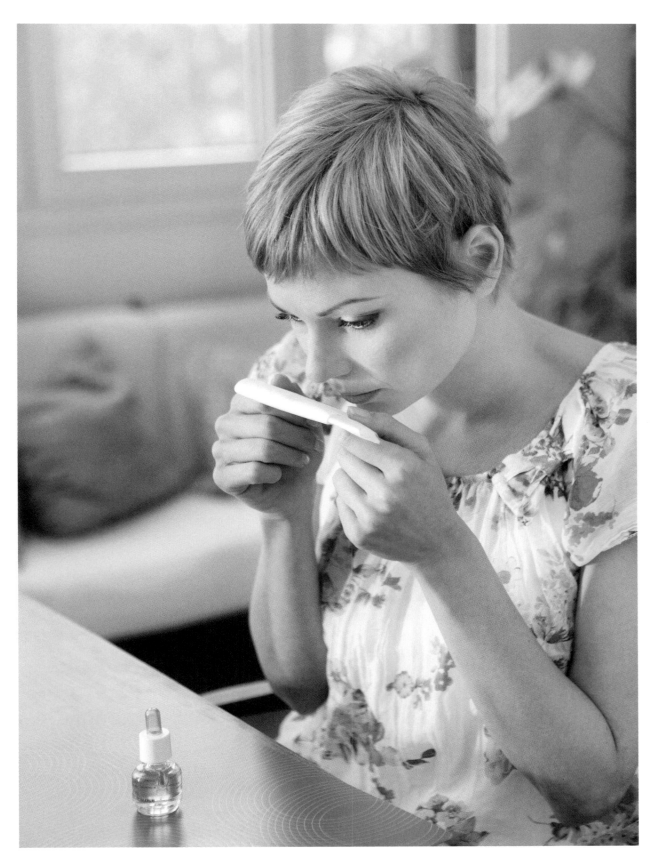

NATURAL REMEDIES FOR THE MIND

Mental health conditions are common, affecting around one in four people. In the past, there was often a stigma associated with mental health problems, but as more people are being diagnosed and openly talking about what it really means and feels like, that stigma is gradually receding. It's being recognized that conditions such as anxiety and depression are just as valid as broken bones or flu, even though the symptoms may not be visible. For those experiencing mental health problems, it makes a considerable difference to have the validity of their illness recognized, and helps open up wider discussions and knowledge of issues involving the mind.

While serious mental health conditions need to be dealt with by a medical professional and appropriate treatment regimes, there are many ways in which natural remedies could help with minor mind-related concerns. Symptoms such as mild anxiety, worrying, insomnia, stress, and an overactive mind may be calmed and eased with the use of natural approaches.

Scent

Aromatherapy uses essential oils that are extracted from the "essence" of plants. The oils are mixed with base or carrier oils to create blends that can be massaged into the skin, or various inhalation methods that allow you inhale the scent of the aromas.

When the aroma of the essential oils is inhaled, it stimulates your limbic system—the part of the brain that's involved with emotions and behaviors. Certain smells can unleash feelings of relaxation, help you feel more positive, or bring back happy memories.

Lavender oil, for example, is strongly associated with having a beneficial effect on sleep when sprayed on a pillow, used in massage, inhaled, or added to a bath before bed.

A similar effect occurs when oils are massaged into the skin, as the skin absorbs some of the plant chemicals. Both the scent of the oils and the action of massaging the skin can bring about positive changes and help you feel calmer or more uplifted.

Crystals

Crystals work on subtle energy levels and vibrations and may help to balance common conditions of the mind or help ground you back into reality. Crystals can be made into elixirs and added to spray bottles, so you can spritz your environment if you feel stressed. You can wear crystals as jewelry or talismans too, so you can keep them with you all day

if you're feeling anxious. Plus, they can be placed on or around your body to emit gentle vibrations. Some of the crystals that may be beneficial for healing the mind include black tourmaline, which can have a grounding effect; amethyst, which has a calm energy; lepidolite for mental exhaustion; and rose quartz for a comforting and healing energy.

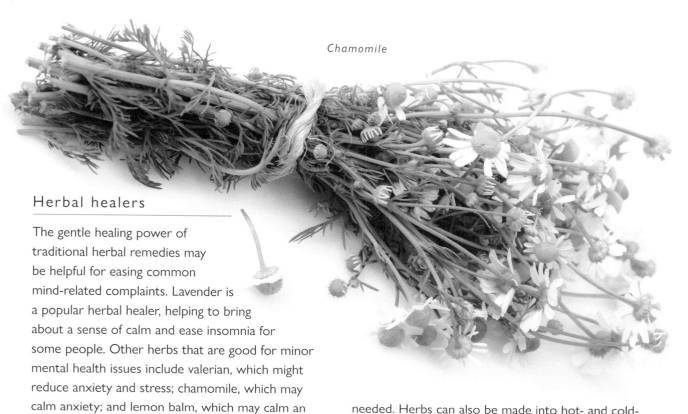

Chamomile

Herbal healers

The gentle healing power of traditional herbal remedies may be helpful for easing common mind-related complaints. Lavender is a popular herbal healer, helping to bring about a sense of calm and ease insomnia for some people. Other herbs that are good for minor mental health issues include valerian, which might reduce anxiety and stress; chamomile, which may calm anxiety; and lemon balm, which may calm an overactive mind or nervousness.

An easy way to access the potential benefits is by using dried herbs in teas or cordials, to sip when needed. Herbs can also be made into hot- and cold-pressed oils or balms and lotions that you can apply to your skin, or added to food for culinary purposes.

Flower power

Flower remedies work on a more emotional level and are designed to help balance emotions and the mind. The remedies contain the vibrational energy of different flowers, and each remedy works to improve certain negative thoughts and emotions, such as fear, uncertainty, loneliness, oversensitivity, despair, apathy, anger, worry, and loss.

Dr. Edward Bach, creator of the Bach Flower Remedies, developed the gentle, noninvasive remedies after noticing that diseases in the body can have underlying emotional causes. When the emotional symptoms were treated, people felt calmer and happier, allowing the body to heal and the physical symptoms to improve.

Natural remedies provide an additional avenue to explore if you experience minor mind complaints and, in some cases, could be used alongside traditional therapies for a complementary approach.

NOTE

If you're experiencing mental health problems that are frequent and interfering with your daily life, then always seek help from a medical professional and don't rely on natural remedies. If you're taking prescribed medication, then check first that additional herbal remedies won't cause any unwanted drug interactions.

DIAGNOSING AILMENTS AND PROFESSIONAL HELP

Before using healing remedies, you first need to know the ailment or health condition you are treating. While some issues might be obvious from the outset, such as a cough, feeling nauseous, or having a small cut on your arm, others can be harder to identify. As keen as you may be to treat everything yourself, it is important to recognize when you need to seek the advice of a trained and qualified medical practitioner for an accurate diagnosis.

How to diagnose minor ailments

Some health conditions are relatively easy to identify. Symptoms such as sneezing and coughing may be due to a cold, particularly if you know germs are going around or you have been in recent contact with someone else who has a cold. The sudden appearance of a rash or hives (urticaria) might be linked to an allergy you already know you have. If you develop bruises when you know you knocked your leg recently, then that is likely to be the cause. Sometimes your ailment might not be instantly obvious, or could be caused by one or more factors. Before you rush in and assume you know what the cause must be, it helps to carefully consider all your symptoms. This will help you make a more discerning diagnosis and reduce the risk of treating an ailment with the wrong remedy.

When making an assessment and diagnosing your minor ailments, it helps to consider factors such as:

• What symptoms you have
• When your symptoms started
• If anything makes your symptoms better
• If anything makes your symptoms worse
• What conditions you have had in the past
• How you are feeling
• If your symptoms could be linked to anything you have done, eaten, or experienced recently

• Any medication or herbal remedies you are currently taking
• Any allergies you have

These are the types of questions a health practitioner will ask you when you go to see them, so they are a good starting point for you to think about.

Some forms of healing therapies, such as traditional Chinese medicine (TCM), also look at your pulse rate and the state of your tongue to help with diagnosing ailments, but without professional training, these observations are unlikely to offer you much assistance in diagnosing your own minor ailments. If you are at all unsure about your personal diagnosis, or if your healing remedies do not have any effect, always consult a qualified medical practitioner.

When to see a qualified medical practitioner

As good as natural medicine is for many minor ailments, there are times when you should see a qualified medical practitioner for advice and treatment. Some health symptoms can be signs of underlying illness, and getting a diagnosis as soon as possible can often be crucial for treatment. Other symptoms might be linked to existing medical conditions, or even caused by prescription medicines that you are taking, so a proper medical review is helpful.

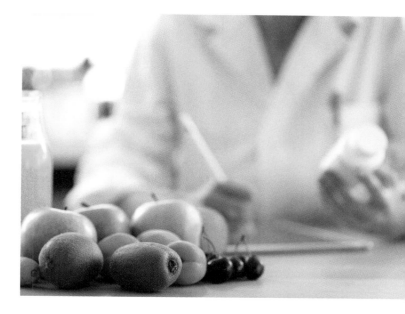

Some situations require medical treatment immediately. Call the emergency medical services if someone:

• Loses consciousness or is suddenly confused
• Has persistent chest pain
• Has seizures (fits)
• Has difficulty breathing
• Has severe bleeding that cannot be stopped
• Has a severe allergic reaction
• Has severe burns or scalds

There are many other symptoms that should be assessed by a medical practitioner, rather than trying to diagnose or treat them yourself. These include:

• A temperature or fever of 100.4°F (38°C) or above
• Coughing up blood
• A cough or hoarse voice that lasts for more than three weeks
• Severe pain that is increasing
• Unusual bruising for no apparent reason
• A severe headache or migraine that has lasted longer than 24 hours
• Blood in your stools
• Blood in your urine
• A rash that is worsening and spreading
• A rash that does not fade when you press a glass on it
• Sore, broken skin that has become red, inflamed, and oozing
• A mole that suddenly changes color, shape, or size or starts bleeding
• Diarrhea that lasts for three days or more
• Drowsiness or confusion
• Feeling generally unwell for no apparent reason

• Losing weight without trying
• Finding a new lump or bump somewhere on your body

Other situations where you should seek medical assistance include:

• If you have been involved in an accident
• If you have had a blow to the head
• If you think you could have broken bones
• If you have a large or deep burn, if a burn is very blistered and painful, or if the burn is on your hands or face
• If you have been bitten by a person or an animal

These lists do not cover every important symptom. If you feel unwell, or have any concerns about a medical condition, always see a health practitioner for advice. Even if it is a false alarm and nothing serious, it will offer reassurance that nothing major is wrong. Extra care should be taken with babies, children, the elderly, and pregnant women. Your family's health is important, so do not put yourself or others at risk by trying to diagnose or treat symptoms you do not fully understand.

USING NATURAL REMEDIES SAFELY

Herbal remedies are often regarded as natural and safe because they are derived from plants. However, in the same way that orthodox prescription medications and drugs are powerful and can have side effects, so too can herbal remedies, especially if taken at the same time as certain prescription medications.

For minor ailments and easily identifiable health concerns, treating yourself with natural healing remedies may make sense. If you are at all unsure what health ailment you are dealing with, or whether or not a particular remedy is suitable, it is best to be cautious and not try to treat yourself or others. There are also particular groups of people and circumstances in which you need to take particular care and not try to self-treat.

If you are pregnant or breastfeeding

In the same way that certain prescription medications are to be avoided while you are pregnant or breastfeeding, so too are natural healing remedies. During pregnancy, not only is your body going through huge changes, but you are also carrying your unborn baby. If you are tempted to try natural remedies to ease pregnancy ailments, it is best to avoid using anything without first checking with your medical team. In addition, always tell the medical team about any herbal remedies you have been taking.

The same note of caution applies when you are in labor, too. Herbal remedies could potentially interact with any drugs given to help you during birth. Certain herbal remedies are linked to blood thinning, which could pose problems if you need a Cesarean section, putting you at risk of extra bleeding.

If you breastfeed, it is wise to continue avoiding herbal remedies for a while, unless your medical team says it is safe, as what you consume can be passed on to your baby through your milk.

Babies and children

Babies and children can react differently to natural remedies than adults, due to their size and age. Remedies that may be safe for adults are not always suitable for use in infants and children, so it is best not to give them any herbal remedies without expert advice and checking with a medical practitioner.

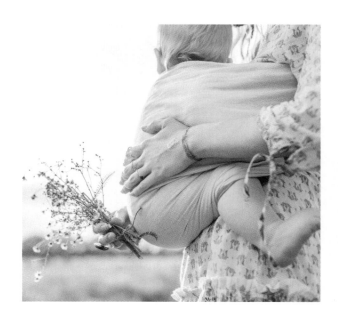

The elderly

As people get older, the way the body works undergoes changes, increasing the risk of side effects from taking herbal, prescribed, and over-the-counter medication.

The kidneys become less able to excrete medication into urine and the liver is less able to break down, or metabolize, medications. Due to this, any remedies taken may remain in the body for longer and affect people in different ways. Always consult a medical practitioner before taking an herbal remedy, especially if you are taking any other drugs.

If you are taking other medications

If you are already taking any over-the-counter or prescribed medications, check first with a medical practitioner or pharmacist before taking any herbal or natural remedies. Some ingredients can react badly with conventional medications, disrupting their effectiveness and causing unexpected side effects.

Even a seemingly innocuous ingredient such as grapefruit contains a chemical called furanocoumarin, which can affect drug metabolism, or the amount of time it takes for a medication to be broken down by the body. As a result, it can cause more of the active drug to be present in your body, leading to some very unpleasant and potentially serious side effects.

If you are having surgery or are undergoing treatment

If you have a planned surgical operation coming up, it is important to inform your medical practitioner in advance if you are taking any herbal remedies. They may need you to stop taking them in the weeks leading up to your operation.

Natural remedies, especially herbal, can also interact with conventional cancer treatments, such as radiotherapy, chemotherapy, biological therapy, or hormone treatment. They may make certain cancer drugs less effective or increase the risk of suffering from side effects. There is a lot to be learned about the interaction between cancer treatments and natural remedies, so before using any type of natural remedy, talk to your medical practitioner first.

People with cancer should also avoid deep massage, especially on any areas of the body where you are receiving radiotherapy. Always talk to your medical practitioner before massage.

NOTE

If you think you could be at risk of an herbal–drug interaction, contact your health-care provider. Always take prescribed medication as instructed. Do not stop taking a prescribed medication in favor of trying an alternative remedy unless advised to do so by a medical practitioner. Some herbal medicines can affect anesthetics and other medications used before, during, and after operations. Others can interfere with your blood clotting and blood pressure, and could increase the risk of bleeding during or after surgery.

NATURAL REMEDIES FOR A SUSTAINABLE HOME

If you're keen to have a more sustainable home and lifestyle, then the use of natural remedies fits in perfectly.

A sustainable home is a happy and healthy environment that makes the most of natural resources in the most efficient manner. It's about understanding how your lifestyle choices impact the world, meeting your needs without compromising the needs of future generations, and doing more to protect limited resources and have less of an impact on the environment.

When you consciously choose to use natural remedies to meet your basic home needs, you're taking a step toward embracing a more sustainable life.

Herbs and herbal remedies

The use of herbs and herbal remedies is a classic example of this. You can be forgiven for thinking that foraging in the wild and picking herbs to use at home could be bad for the planet. Yes, it could be detrimental if you pick too many and strip an area of vital resources, but picking some plants helps them continue to grow and thrive. You're also drawing on nature's resources, making use of what is already provided and available in your local area, which saves on traveling farther afield to acquire the ingredients you need or buying herbs that have a bigger carbon footprint.

You can add to your sustainability by growing herbs at home—a sunny kitchen windowsill is an ideal cultivation point and will ensure your herbs are on hand when you need them for culinary and remedy purposes. There are a multitude of ways you can use traditional herbal remedies in your home, from making infused oils and medicinal products, to creating your own skin-care and hair-care products.

Organic essential oils

When you're using essential oils in your home, opting to purchase organic versions is a more sustainable choice. There's less impact on the plants, no harsh chemicals involved in the growing process, and you can be sure that you're getting as natural and as pure a product as possible.

To cut down on the carbon footprint of the products, aim to source them from local suppliers who make the oils themselves.

Fennel plant, oil, and seeds

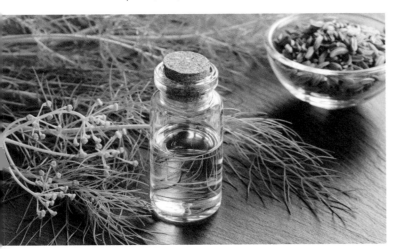

Food for a sustainable home

Actively choosing to eat more fresh produce such as fruits, vegetables, seeds, nuts, and beans in your home is not only good for you, but is also a positive sustainable step. Natural foods are all great sources of essential vitamins, minerals, fiber, and other nutrients, but they also tend to have a smaller carbon footprint and you can support local farmers and markets by choosing produce that's come from nearer your home instead of traveling halfway around the world before it reaches your plate.

Eating fresh produce rather than processed foods is more sustainable too. It's better for the environment, as processed foods tend to come with added packaging that creates waste, especially when it's made of plastic. Each time you eat a rainbow of freshly grown food, you're gaining more health benefits and also supporting the wide variety of foods grown by farmers.

Even better is choosing to grow your own fresh food at home. You can take small steps to be more sustainable by trying your hand at growing a few fruits or vegetables in a garden planter. Both strawberries and tomatoes are good plants to start with and both can be grown either in a pot or in hanging baskets, so the produce cascades down. You don't need a lot of space to get started with growing your own, and once you've tried it and enjoyed the taste of your own homegrown efforts, it can be addictive.

Growing your own produce means that you're in control of how you grow it, so you can be more mindful to the environment by avoiding chemicals and pesticides. Companion planting and permaculture gardening techniques involve planting

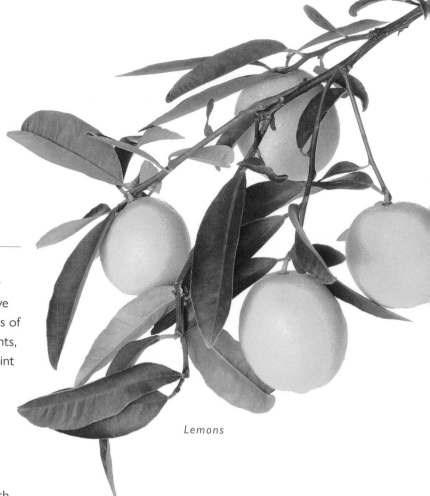

Lemons

flowers alongside vegetables. Insects such as bees will appreciate the chance for more pollinating flowers in your garden, and birds will enjoy pecking on the seeds of plants such as sunflowers at the end of their flowering period.

Sourcing ethical crystals

Not all crystals are obtained via ethical means and it can be hard to know exactly where they were originally from and whether the miners and the earth were treated with respect. But if you care strongly about your home being as sustainable as possible, it's worth working on sourcing ethical crystals. Good-quality, knowledgeable traders will be happy to provide you with details of where the crystals come from—at best, not just the country or general locale but the exact mine—and you can do your due diligence to find out if the locations mine ethically or not.

THE BENEFITS OF NATURAL REMEDIES

Choosing to use natural remedies brings with it many benefits. Some are hidden but reveal themselves as you use the remedies; others are more obvious from the outset. Here's an insight into some of the key benefits of these ancient healing practices.

Accessibility

Many forms of natural remedies, such as common superfoods, herbs, and other raw ingredients, are easily obtained, making them readily accessible. There are remedies you can access and make yourself from common cupboard items, without the need for expensive ingredients.

Affordability

Many natural remedies are an affordable option for basic health and well-being needs, and can be a more affordable method than buying prescription or over-the-counter drugs. This is especially so where you're able to grow or buy inexpensive ingredients yourself. With herbal remedies, a little often goes a long way, so you can store key ingredients to use another time. Learning to dry and harvest your own herbs also allows you to build up a cupboard of natural ingredients, ready to use whenever the need arises.

Natural properties

One of the key benefits of using natural remedies is that they consist of natural properties. You know exactly what you're using and what's going into your body and can be assured there are no harsh chemicals, unwanted additives, or harmful colorings.

Of course, just because ingredients are natural doesn't mean they can't be harmful, so take care in how you use natural remedies and always seek advice from a qualified practitioner, such as an herbalist or aromatherapist, if you have any doubts.

Supporting a healthy lifestyle

Using natural remedies can help support a healthy lifestyle and be part of a holistic healing approach. Used in conjunction with other healthy practices,

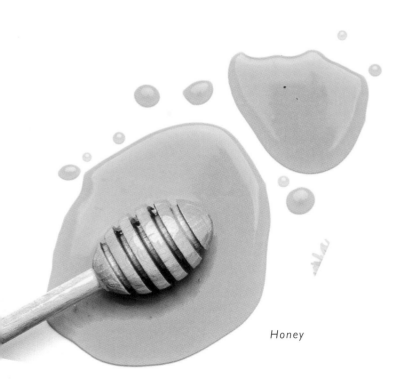

Honey

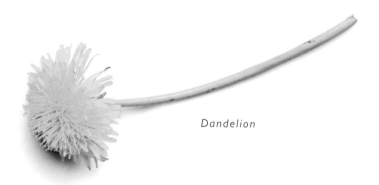

Dandelion

such as eating a nutritious diet, exercising regularly, and looking after your physical, emotional, and mental health, you could gain a more well-rounded approach to your overall health and well-being.

Based on ancient practices

When you explore the history of natural remedies, it becomes clear that many have been used for centuries to treat all manner of illnesses. It's reassuring to know that treatments used today are based on a long history of effective ancient practices, plus it may help you to feel a connection with past generations to still be using their tried and tested remedies.

Treats the cause, not just the symptoms

Natural remedies focus on treating the cause, not just the symptoms, giving you a more well-rounded approach to health and well-being. Instead of simply treating the symptoms you currently have, there's an emphasis on finding the root cause, which could reduce the chance of further problems and symptoms.

Empowering

The use of natural remedies can be empowering, helping you to gain a better understanding of your own health and well-being. As you learn more about how your body reacts to different forms of natural remedies, such as eating particular superfoods or inhaling the aroma of certain essential oils, you may begin to feel more in control of your own health.

Reduction in side effects

Using natural remedies to take care of minor symptoms could help reduce the risk of experiencing side effects from taking conventional drugs or medications. For example, if you swap popping a pill for a headache for consciously drinking more water and being better hydrated, or inhaling essential oils such as peppermint or eucalyptus, it could reduce the chances of you getting side effects from taking painkillers.

Of course, just because they're natural doesn't mean remedies won't be without their own side effects. Always follow the guidance for how much to use and avoid making your own herbal concoctions without professional advice.

Digestive and immune system friendly

Healthy bacteria are important as they help your body to break down food and maintain a strong immune system, so you ideally don't want to lose too many of them. Yet many prescription drugs can upset your digestive health, as they kill naturally present microbes and healthy bacteria that live in your gut, which is why you might experience side effects such as nausea, sickness, or diarrhea when taking some medications. Natural medicines tend not to have this effect.

There will inevitably be occasions when you'll need to take antibiotics for more serious illnesses. In such scenarios you can help your gut health by taking probiotic supplements or eating natural yogurt to help replenish healthy bacteria.

MAKING YOUR OWN NATURAL REMEDIES

One of the many benefits of natural remedies is that you can often make your own. Different remedies will require different methods and ingredients, but here's a general guide to some of the equipment you'll need to make your own remedies at home.

Colander or sieve

Any plants, leaves, stalks, berries, or produce that you've picked in the wild or at home in your garden needs a thorough wash before use. It's amazing how many tiny insects can be hiding on plants, leaves, or inside berries. A colander or sieve allows you to give everything a good wash and drain off before you use the items. Just take care if you're using particularly ripe berries, as they could become squishy when washed.

Hanging drying rack

A hanging drying rack is great to use for drying bunches of herbs. It's designed to be hung from the ceiling, so it won't take up room on a surface, and the bunches of herbs can be tied together and pegged or attached to the bars to dry. Aim to position your herb drying rack away from bright sunlight, as this could damage the potency, and in a location that has a good circulation of air. If you have room, it could be hung in a utility room, shed, garage, or even in an airing cupboard.

You might strike it lucky and find a hanging drying rack at a market or vintage store, or if you're good at DIY, you could have a go at making your own. If you're only just getting started with creating your own natural remedies, then a small drying rack should be suitable to get you going. You can always upgrade it to a larger rack in due course if required.

Crates

Shallow wooden fruit crates are useful for storing freshly harvested produce such as apples or pears. Keep them in a cool place, taking care to space out the fruits; you could also wrap them individually in newspaper until needed. Alternatively, prepare the fruit and freeze it until required.

Bottles, jars, and pots

You'll need a good supply of freshly cleaned and washed bottles, jars, and pots. In the interest of having a sustainable home, try and reuse as many vessels as you can, to save having to buy new. You could also ask friends to donate empty pots so that you can reuse them. Sterilize any bottles or jars if you're unsure what's been in them previously, especially where they may have been used for nonfood items. Brown or amber glass bottles may be of use for herbal or flower remedies, or crystal elixirs, as they will help protect the remedies from light.

Funnels

When you're straining liquids, it's easier to use funnels to ensure you get all the liquid into the receptacles. Stainless-steel funnels are more environmentally friendly than their plastic counterparts, won't taint the remedy with a plastic smell, will last well, are easy to clean, and come in a variety of sizes.

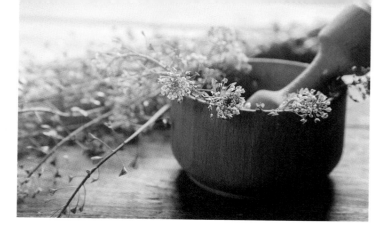

Mortar and pestle

Saucepans

For remedies that need cooking, saucepans are essential. For big batches, traditional preserving pots tend to be large and roomy. It's worth considering whether you need to use a different set of pans from your usual cooking paraphernalia, particularly if ingredients can be pungent or likely to stain.

Scales

Some natural remedies require ingredients to be properly measured out for accuracy, so make sure you have a pair of kitchen scales available to use.

Mortar and pestle

A mortar and pestle are always useful to have on hand to grind herbs and spices.

Potato ricer

A potato ricer may sound like an unusual piece of equipment for making natural remedies, but it can be incredibly useful. Professional herbalists use tincture presses to strain herbs and get all the moisture and goodness out of them, but a humble potato ricer will help you achieve the same results for a fraction of the cost.

Ball of string

String comes in useful for so many tasks involved with natural remedies, from tying back plants that you're growing in the garden, to securing bunches of herbs to dry.

French press

If you're making herbal teas or drinks, a French press is useful. It will allow you to make your beverage and serve it without a bundle of herbs also making it into your mug.

Tea strainer

A tea strainer can be handy to strain small amounts of remedies.

Muslin

Pieces of muslin cloth can be used to create DIY strainers, such as when making preserves, jams, or herbal remedies.

Labels

All remedies that you make need to be labeled—it's amazing how easy it is to forget what something is. Sticky labels are good as they can be used on bottles, jars, and pots. Add the date too, so you know when you made the remedy and can gauge how long it's likely to last.

> ### NOTE
> When you're picking plants, herbs, fruits, or vegetables from your own garden or in the wild, always make sure you know exactly what the ingredient is. If you are in any way uncertain, don't pick it or use it.

BUYING AND SOURCING NATURAL REMEDIES

There are plenty of options available to allow you to buy, grow, and source the ingredients for making natural remedies.

Herbs

The herbs needed for making herbal remedies can be sourced in the wild, from your own garden, or bought in dried form or as fresh plants. If you're picking herbs in the wild, then it's best to ensure they're located well away from the banks of roads or popular dog walking areas, so the plants aren't exposed to unwanted chemicals or fumes.

The prepacked or bottled dried herbs sold for cooking purposes are just as useful for making herbal remedies as they are for culinary needs, so offer an easy and accessible way to obtain the ingredients you need. Plus, they can double up as extra ingredients for cooking too!

Fresh herb plants can be purchased from grocery stores or markets. If you want the plants to be as natural as possible, look for organically grown herbs.

Nothing beats having your own fresh herbs to draw upon whenever you need them, and many basic herbs can easily be grown inside your home on a kitchen windowsill, as well as outside in pots and planters. Growing herbs gives you the chance to love and nurture your plants and be aware of everything that's gone into their care. You can control the growing environment and the soil, being careful to avoid adding any pesticides or chemicals.

Essential oils

In order to embrace the powers of aromatherapy, you'll need to equip yourself with some essential oils. A few bottles of your favorite scents will be fine to start with and you can gradually buy more over time. The price of essential oils does vary considerably depending on the method of extraction and the cost of growing and harvesting the plants. Oils such as rose otto or jasmine (where the flowers need to be hand-picked) are typically higher priced.

Take care to ensure the product you're purchasing is a pure essential oil—anything marked as a "fragrance oil" or "perfume oil" won't be pure. Essential oils usually come in sealed, dark-colored bottles, often amber or brown in color, and have dropper dispensers. Essential oils aren't regulated by any standards, so it's advisable to buy from a reputable brand to ensure you're getting the best quality. Organic essential oils are available too, and may be a more superior oil.

Store your essential oils in a cool, dark place or pop them into a box. Storing them away from sunlight will help them last longer.

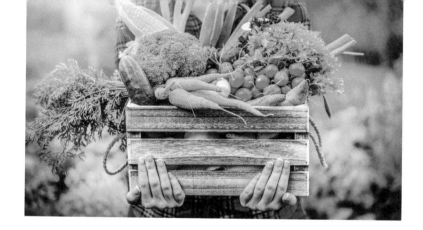

Food and drink

Superfoods and drinks can be purchased from local grocery stores, health stores, or markets. When buying fresh produce, you may want to look for organically grown fruits or vegetables to ensure you're getting chemical- and pesticide-free foods, and consider locally grown options if you're concerned about your carbon footprint.

Get into the habit of reading packaging, to ensure anything prepacked is exactly what you think it is and doesn't contain any additional or unexpected ingredients. This is also beneficial if there are ingredients you are allergic to or wish to avoid.

Like herbs, there are some foods that you can grow yourself if you wish. If you have outdoor space, setting up a small fruit or vegetable patch can be rewarding, or you could try growing produce such as strawberries in pots, planters, or a window box. As well as the ease of being able to pick fresh produce and eat seasonally grown food whenever you want, it also allows you full control of the growing conditions.

Crystals

If you want to work with crystals, then you will need to invest in some. Crystals vary in price—in some cases the price depends on the rarity of the crystal or how easy it is to obtain, while in other cases it depends on the size of the piece in question. From a practical point of view, you don't need to rush out and buy a large selection from the outset. You can get started perfectly well by sticking to a few basic crystals (see page 251 for an idea of those needed for an essential self-care kit).

Crystals tend to be sold by specialty gem and rock stores, or can be purchased online. Ideally, it's better to go to a shop to buy your crystals, as you can touch and feel the stones, to see whether the surface texture is glossy and smooth or left unpolished and natural. There's also the argument that by touching the stones you can use your intuition and get a sense of which crystals resonate most with you. The stones with vibrations that feel most in tune with you are likely to be better to work with.

Crystals aren't regulated by any governing body, so there's no way of telling exactly how or where they've been sourced, beyond the information provided by the seller.

As you learn more about natural remedies and discover the types of preventive methods that you could adopt, you can gradually build up your own cupboard of different ingredients.

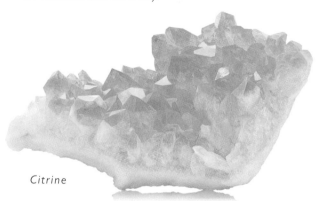

Citrine

HOW TO USE THIS BOOK

In the pages of this book you'll discover an informative guide to four popular areas of natural remedies—herbs, aromatherapy and essential oils, food and drink, and crystals—and practical ideas for a variety of ways in which you could use them in your life.

There are helpful resources and tips, inspiring techniques, and remedy ideas for minor health complaints, skin care, lifestyle needs, and in your home.

How you use the book is up to you. You can take it at your own pace and dip in and out as the need arises, or read from cover to cover and devour it all in one go. Above all, be open to new ideas, have fun exploring nature's remedies, and enjoy discovering how they could be used alongside traditional medicine.

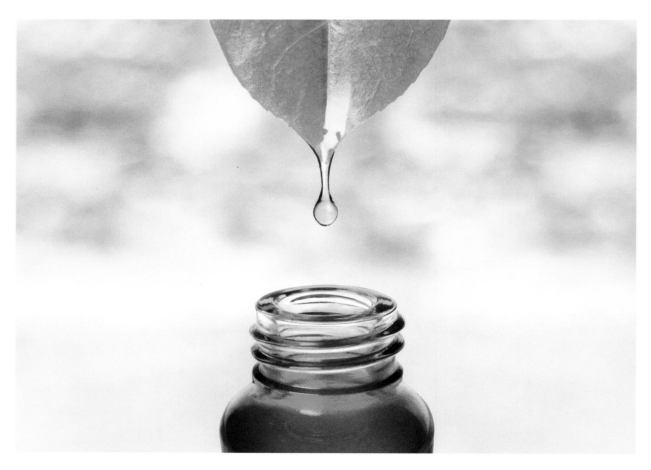

Part one: Herbs

Part one focuses on herbs and includes an A to Z guide to some of the most popular and commonly used herbs. There's an insight into the world of herbalism and a look at how you can use, prepare, grow, harvest, and store herbs safely at home. You'll also find plenty of ideas as to how you can use herbs for minor first-aid treatments and common ailments, as well as ways to use them in your home and to make your own natural beauty treatments. It also touches on flower essences and the benefits they might have for emotional health complaints.

Part two: Aromatherapy and Essential Oils

The focus of part two is the art of aromatherapy and essential oils. There's an overview of what aromatherapy is and how you can use the therapy and essential oils in your life. The A to Z of essential oils covers some of the most well-known and loved oils and their benefits. You'll discover advice and information on utilizing the benefits of aromatherapy massage, using inhalation techniques, the power of touch and smell, skin-care solutions, and minor health conditions that could be helped by essential oils and aromatherapy.

Part three: Food and Drink

Nutrition is a vital part of maintaining health, so part three covers food and drink, with a particular focus on superfoods. The A to Z is arranged by different types of foods, such as fruits, vegetables, nuts and seeds, grains, and oils, making it easy to find the foods you'd like to learn about. There's information on eating for health and wellness, such as the importance of mindful eating and getting the timing of meals right, plus lots of ideas for including more superfoods in your diet. There are quick and easy ideas for superfood favorite meals, such as healthy soups, stir-fries, and salads, as well as delicious smoothies and juices. Plus, there are even some tips on having a go at growing your own fresh and nutritional produce.

Part four: Crystals

Part four explores the wonderful world of crystals and how they could be used to help heal minor ailments. You can read about what crystals are, why they're a natural remedy, and how to understand crystal vibrations, then check out an informative A to Z guide to some of the more popular crystals in a rainbow of colors. There are ideas and inspiration for how you could use crystals in your life, from making elixirs and balancing the chakras, to using crystal layouts and meditating with crystals. You'll discover the key crystals involved in aiding common ailments and learn how you could create your very own crystal charging and purifying station in your home.

If the book inspires you to explore more deeply into the realm of natural remedies, you'll find some useful resources and further reading ideas at the end of the book.

Happy reading, and we hope you find plenty of ways to use natural remedies for your physical and mental well-being, in your home and as part of your lifestyle.

GLOSSARY OF TERMS

Here's a useful guide to some of the terminology you may come across when learning about different types of natural therapies.

ANTIOXIDANTS
Antioxidants are compounds found in foods, such as fruits, vegetables, nuts, and seeds, that help to protect your cells from free radicals (substances found in processed foods or environmental toxins, for example) and boost your immunity. Some examples of antioxidants include vitamins A, C, and E, beta-carotene, lycopene, and selenium.

AROMATHERAPY
Aromatherapy is a holistic healing technique that uses natural plant extracts—essential oils—to aid health and well-being. Aromatherapy can be achieved using various methods, including inhalation of aromatic oils and massage.

AURA
The aura is an invisible energy field that surrounds all living things. Some people are able to see auras, and their colors can be used to interpret health and vitality.

CARRIER OILS
Carrier oils are used as the base for essential oil massage blends, so that they can be used on the body (the majority of essential oils can't be used directly on the skin, as they are too harsh). Typically, oils such as sweet almond, olive, cold-pressed coconut, and jojoba are used as carrier oils.

CHAKRA
A chakra is an invisible spiritual energy center that's located within your body. The word chakra comes from ancient Sanskrit, and means "wheel" or "disk," and chakras can be thought of as being like a spinning wheel of energy.

COMPRESS
A compress is a clean piece of cotton or muslin fabric that is soaked in warm water or an herbal remedy and then applied to the skin. It may be used to treat a minor wound, ease a swollen joint, or aid muscle soreness.

DECOCTION
A decoction is an herbal liquid that is made by simmering fresh or dried herbs, berries, bark, or roots in water. When completed, it can be strained and drunk, a bit like an herbal tea.

ELECTROMAGNETIC FIELD
An electromagnetic field is an invisible field of radiation produced by electric or magnetic devices such as mobile phones, radar systems, electric trolleys, power lines, microwave ovens, pylons, and X-ray machines.

ESSENTIAL FATTY ACIDS
Essential fatty acids are fatty acids that the body can't make itself, so they have to be obtained from the diet. They aid the normal functioning of cells and body processes, such as helping to regulate blood cholesterol levels, keeping skin and hair healthy, and aiding heart health. There are two main types: linoleic acid (an omega-6) and alpha-linolenic acid (an omega-3).

ESSENTIAL OILS
Essential oils are natural oils that are extracted from plants through distillation methods. They contain the true essence, or distinctive aroma, of the plants and are believed to have their own individual properties for health and well-being.

FLOWER ESSENCES

Flower essences are liquid extract infusions that are made from plants and are said to contain the essence of flowers. The essences are particularly aimed at helping with emotional issues such as worry, anxiety, grief, and loneliness.

GRIDDING

Gridding is the art of laying out crystals in a pattern or grid formation to create a more focused and potentially more powerful healing technique.

GROUNDING

Grounding is a technique where you consciously connect yourself to the earth. It's particularly useful during times of stress or anxiety, but can also help provide a firm foundation for meditation and other holistic therapies.

HERBAL REMEDIES

Herbal remedies are natural remedies that are made from the roots, leaves, stalks, flowers, bark, or seeds of plants.

HOLISTIC THERAPIES

Holistic therapies are healing methods that tend to view the person as a whole and treat both the underlying causes of illness as well as the symptoms. The word holistic originates from the Greek word holos, which means "whole."

MACERATION

In herbal medicine, a maceration is the process by which herbs, especially roots or tougher parts of plants, are chopped and broken down. Some plants respond better to being made into cold macerations, to help preserve the potency of the active ingredients, whereas others can be heated to make warm macerations. The eventual product is a liquid that can be strained and drunk.

POULTICE

A poultice is a soft paste made from herbs or plants. The paste is typically spread onto a piece of cloth, sometimes while still warm, then placed on the body to help an inflamed or aching limb.

QI

Qi—pronounced "chee"—is a vital form of life energy. The idea of qi originates from traditional Chinese medicine, where it's believed that blockages or deficiencies in qi relate to physical, mental, and emotional health issues.

SELF-CARE

Self-care is the act of consciously looking after yourself, whether physically, mentally, or emotionally.

SUBTLE ENERGY FIELD

A subtle energy field is the term used to describe an invisible layer of energy that surrounds all living things.

SUPERFOODS

Superfoods are healthy foods that offer excellent nutritional benefits and are packed with vitamins, minerals, and antioxidants. Many superfoods are plant-based.

TINCTURE

A tincture is a concentrated form of liquid remedy typically made from soaking one or more herbs, including the leaves or roots, in oil, alcohol, or a mixture of alcohol and water. A tincture is taken orally.

TONIC WINE

A tonic wine is a form of herbal wine that is made using extracts of various herbs, berries, roots, or even flowers. Depending on the ingredients, tonic wine can help certain ailments.

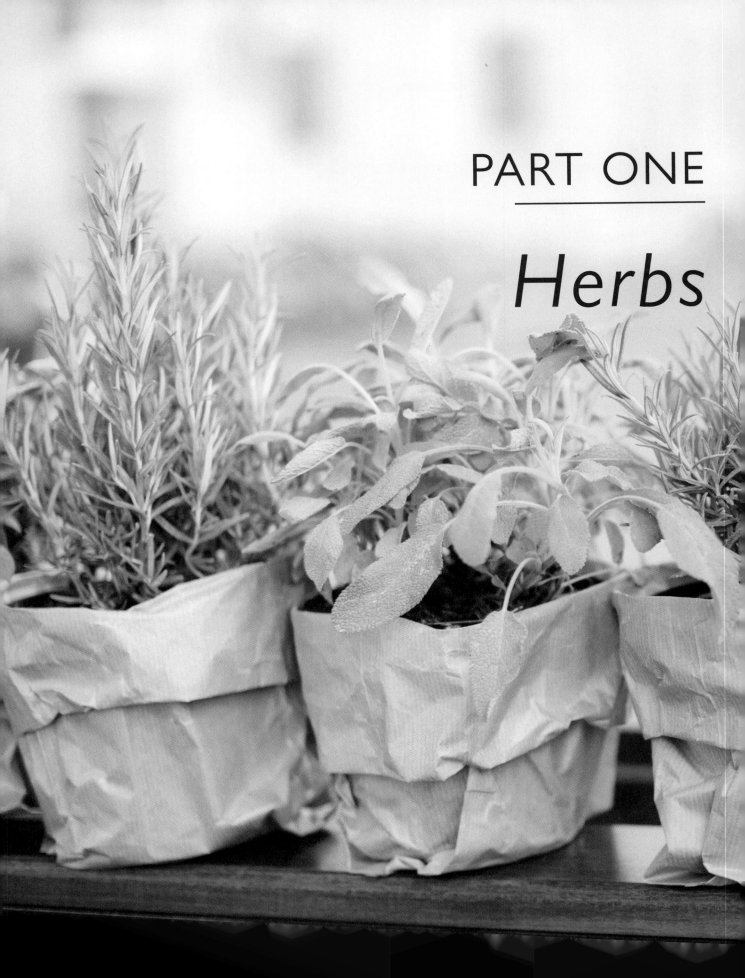

PART ONE

Herbs

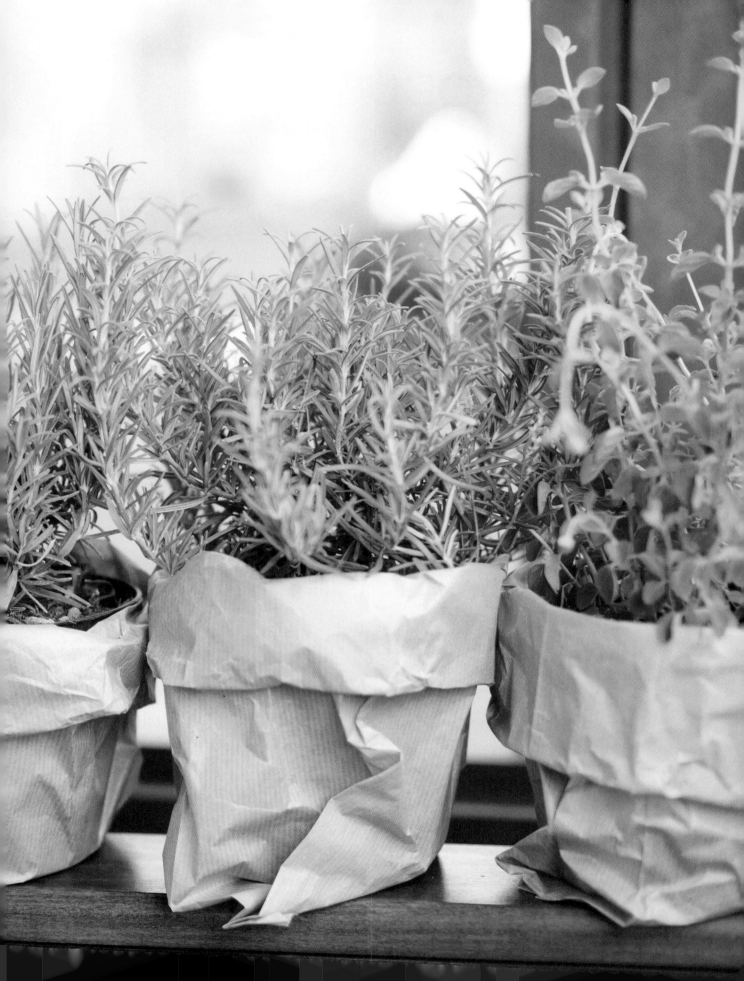

AN INTRODUCTION TO HERBALISM

Since before recorded history, humans have used plants for food, medicines, shelter, clothing, dyes, weapons, and musical instruments. The cultural development of different countries and the rise and fall of empires have often been linked to the understanding and exploitation of plants. Herbalism, the use of plants for medicinal purposes, has been common to all peoples, and our understanding of herbalism has been passed down by word of mouth from generation to generation.

History of herbalism

It is the most natural thing in the world to use local flora for food and medicine, and to list this knowledge for posterity. All native cultures have a well-developed understanding of local plants, and most of the world, even today, relies on herbal expertise for its primary health care. Shamans, wise women, bush doctors, traditional healers, and native medicine workers carry on a tradition thousands of years old.

Herbalism is the oldest, most tested, and proven form of medicine in the world. The Ebers Papyrus of the ancient Egyptians lists eighty-five herbs, some of which, like mint, are used in a similar way today. The Chinese herbal called *Ben Zao (Pen Tsao)* contains over a thousand herbal remedies. The Assyrian and Babylonian scribes wrote herbal recipes on clay tablets.

The Greek Hippocrates (477–360 BCE), known as the "father of medicine," mentions herbs, remedies, and treatment stratagems that are still valid today. Indeed, there is much practical and theoretical knowledge to be rediscovered. Globally, herbal lore is a treasure chest beyond price.

In the West, the Saxons wrote *Bald's Leechbook*, a mixture of remedies and ritual. Their nine sacred herbs included yarrow, marigold, and hawthorn.

A modern practitioner of herbal medicine would rate them equally highly. The golden age of herbals was precipitated by the development of the printing press. Nicholas Culpeper (1616–54) printed the *London Dispensatory* (1649) in English (it had previously been printed in Latin), and later published his *Complete Herbal*—a book, he boasted, from which any man (or woman) could find out how to cure themselves for less than three pennies! Culpeper's *Complete Herbal* was immensely popular and is still available today.

Botanical medicine was regarded as fringe medicine for many years. It was valued as a starting place for modern research, but thought to have nothing to offer Western society as a therapy in itself. Pharmaceutical companies identified the active therapeutic principles of many plants, synthesized commercial analogues, and patented new drugs. But in doing so they often missed the major principles of using natural sources for therapeutic purposes.

Herbalism, when practiced properly, is marked by a completely different attitude from orthodox medicine. It is a holistic system that uses plants, or plant parts, in a nonintrusive way. Herbalists believe that the constituents of a plant work synergistically to stimulate the natural healing process.

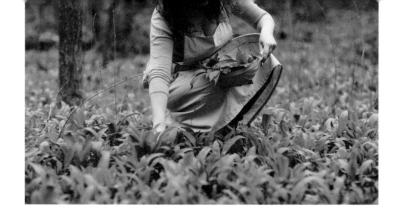

As a self-help system

Modern herbalism can be practiced on two levels: as a self-help system, and by a professional herbalist. These levels differ in the range of herbs that can be used, the results that can be achieved, and the amount of responsibility taken for treatment. As a self-help system, herbs are ideal as a simple system of home care for first aid, everyday ailments, the management of chronic conditions, strengthening of the body, and preventive treatment. Herbs can be taken safely as long as a few simple rules are adhered to (see pages 46–47).

Seeing a professional

An herbalist is simply defined as someone who uses plants for healing, yet each country has different requirements or standards in order for practitioners to be able to call themselves an herbalist, or to be recognized as one by a professional board or guild. While in the United States an herbalist is a self-defined professional—for which there isn't one common training program but many—the American Herbalists Guild recommends that to be a practicing herbalist you must have completed at least 800 hours of formal study and a 400-hour clinical placement; have a working knowledge of at least 150 medicinal herbs; and a practical understanding of human anatomy. Furthermore, to become a registered herbalist and one of their members, other strict requirements are to be met as part of their application process. For a list of organizations that keep a register of qualified herbal practitioners, see Resources and Further Reading on pages 298–299.

A consultation with an herbalist will take about an hour and consider all aspects of health, diet, exercise, and lifestyle. Your herbalist will take a "holistic" view, which means taking into consideration everything that affects your health on a physical, mental, emotional, and spiritual level. You will be asked questions about: age, career, concerns, appetite, sleeping patterns, previous medicines and illnesses, bowel movements, family, symptoms, personality and what is important to you, and any other aspect that is relevant.

As well as listening to what you say, your therapist will want to know how you feel and will note your appearance. The condition of your hair and skin, your facial expression, your posture, and how you move all provide important clues that will aid a diagnosis. There may also be a physical examination. Before a first visit, it is worth spending some time considering your health and your expectations. It is useful to make a list of relevant points in your medical history and questions you want to ask, as these can easily be missed or forgotten in the stress of a first meeting. If for any reason you do not get on with the practitioner, try another one. It is important that there is a relationship of mutual trust and respect

After a consultation, an herbalist will provide you with an herbal program that addresses your specific wellness goals and concerns. Many herbs prescribed will be familiar to you, but some will be unknown. In the United States, the Food and Drug Administration (FDA) regulates the manufacture and labeling of herbal products, and has legal authority to ensure all herbal products follow current good manufacturing processes with respect to ingredients and claims.

USING HERBS SAFELY AT HOME

The tenets of herbalism

To be able to care for yourself and your family by making natural remedies is a pleasure, and the benefits are legion. The organic chemistry of remedy-making is an extension of cooking, and the same principles and skills apply. For success, use the best-quality ingredients, practice absolute cleanliness, and follow the instructions carefully.

It is important to remember that several herbs may be recommended for a particular ailment; all are slightly different. For example, would rose, lavender, rosemary, or chamomile be best for your headache?

Would a cool compress be best, or a long soak in a rosemary bath? Knowledge of the herb, the individual, and the different methods must be combined to prescribe remedies that will be really effective. Remember these basic tenets of herbalism:

• The whole plant is better than an isolated extract
• Treat the whole person, not just the symptoms
• Practice minimum effective treatment and minimum intervention
• Strengthen the body and encourage it to heal itself

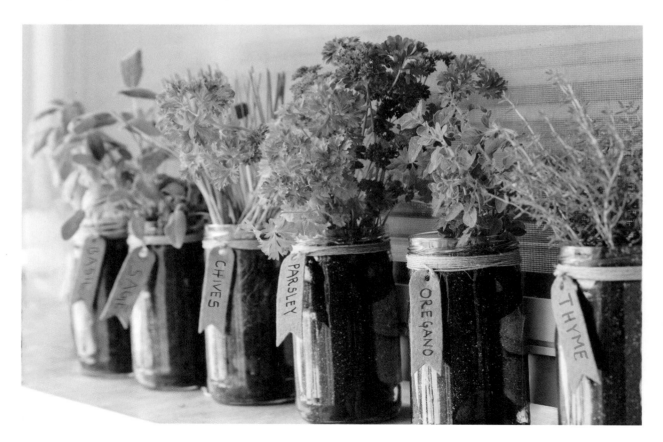

As a self-help system, herbs are ideal as a simple system of home care.

Where to get herbs

Many herbs and herbal products are freely available. Plants or seeds can be bought from garden centers (always check the Latin name) and online, then grown in the garden or in a window box. Dried herbs are available from herb stores and some health-food stores, as well as online. Always specify the herb (the Latin name if possible) and the part of the plant to be used—root, bark, leaf, or flower.

Herbal products, remedies, tinctures, tablets, etc. are available from health-food stores, and some pharmacies and grocery stores. Always read the label and the instructions carefully.

Regarding plants picked from the wild, different countries have different rules and some plants are protected by law. Check the legal situation and get permission from the landowner. Check identification carefully and pick the minimum required, with proper regard for conservation. Never gather roots from the side of the road, by recently sprayed crops or foliage, or from sick-looking plants.

Using the fresh plant

The easiest way to take an herb is to pick it directly from the plant. Leaves can be used in salads, sandwiches, or soups. Chickweed, chicory, dandelion, and marigold make excellent salad additions. Nettle is traditional for green soup. Elderflower fritters are fun. Chewing a few fresh leaves of marjoram will help clear the head. Horseradish leaves will clear sinuses. Sage eases mouth sores and sore throats.

For cuts, grazes, and stings, pick four or five leaves (dock is traditional when stung on countryside walks as it is so readily available) and rub the leaves together between the hands to bruise them and release the juices. When damp, apply to the affected area and hold in place. Poultices can be made in the same way.

Fresh leaves can also be used to make water infusions (teas), decoctions, tinctures, infused oils, and creams. Most recipes give the amounts for dried herbs. When using fresh material, add one-third more, as fresh plants contain a considerable amount of water.

Preparations

Most herbs are sold in dried form, which can simply be powdered and sprinkled onto food (half a flat teaspoon twice daily), but most are prepared further. Herbs are prepared for:
• Availability and preservation, so that seasonal plants are available to use all year round
• Convenience, as compressed tablets are often more convenient to take than a cup of tea
• To aid the action of the herb—for example, infused oils for rubs, or with added honey to give a soothing and demulcent quality to thyme

USING AND PREPARING HERBS FOR INTERNAL USE

Common internal preparations

For internal use, herbal remedies can be bought or made in a variety of forms:

TINCTURES. Tinctures are the most common type of internal remedy prescribed by herbalists. They are made by soaking the flowers, leaves, or roots of the herbs in alcohol to extract and preserve their properties. Tinctures keep well and are easy to store. Because they are highly concentrated, you need only take a small amount at a time. Tinctures can be made with fresh or dried herbs. The absolute strength of the alcohol needed varies slightly depending on the herb, but the method given opposite is sufficient for standard home use. A tincture can also be diluted with water: 2 teaspoons tincture to 1 cup of water can be used as skin lotion, a wash, foot bath, gargle, or compress.

INFUSIONS. Infusions are less concentrated than tinctures and are an easy way to take herbs at home. The herbalist prescribes fresh or dried flowers, leaves, or green stems of the herbs, which you make into a "tea"—a rather misleading word as it suggests a pleasant drink, which is rarely the case with prescription herbs. Sweeten with honey if you find the taste unpalatable. The properties of some herbs—for example, comfrey, marshmallow, and valerian root—are destroyed by heat, so they should be infused or "macerated" in cold water for up to 12 hours. As well as "teas," water infusions are used as gargles, lotions for the skin, compresses, and for:

• FOMENTATIONS. Dilute with an equal amount of water for hand or foot baths.

• DECOCTIONS. Decoctions are similar to infusions, but are made from tougher materials such as roots, bark, nuts, and seeds. They can also be used in the same ways as water infusions, for hand baths, gargles, etc.

• SYRUPS AND HONEYS. These are ideal for administering to children because they are sweet. They can also be used to sweeten other herbal preparations, or be added to food and drink.

• TABLETS AND CAPSULES. These are taken in the same way as a conventional drug, and are useful for people who would rather not taste the remedy.

Carriers

Two main carriers for herbs when taken internally:

• WATER. Used for infusions (teas) of flowers, leaves, some seeds, and fruit. Infusions are quickly assimilated and utilized by the body, and are gentle for children, convalescents, and those with a delicate digestion. They are ideal for diuretic, diaphoretic, cooling, and cleaning regimes. Decoctions are used for stronger preparations.

• ALCOHOL. The carrier for tinctures and spiced wines, made from all plant parts, especially hard parts. Alcohol adds some temporary heat and stimulation and spiced wines make good aperitifs, to stimulate and improve digestion. It is convenient, although not for those intolerant of alcohol, or for babies. Preparations made from alcohol will keep indefinitely.

Methods and dosages

INFUSION (TEA)

1 teaspoon of herb to 1 cup water

Brewing Times

To some extent this depends on personal taste, but the following is a good guide:

- Up to 3 minutes for flowers and soft leaves
- Up to 5 minutes for seeds and leaves

Dose

For children, reduce proportionally. Give a child of seven half the standard adult dose. At six months, use 1 teaspoon of the standard tea. For breastfeeding infants, give the remedy to the mother. Adults may drink:

- 1 cup three times a day for normal conditions
- 1 cup up to six times a day for acute conditions
- 1 cup twice a day as a long-term strengthening tonic

DECOCTION

3 tablespons herb to 3⅔ cups water

Method

Put herb in saucepan and add the water. Cover, bring to a boil, and then turn the heat down to simmer for 10–15 minutes. Strain thoroughly, discard the herb, and pour into a clean bottle. The decoction will keep in a refrigerator for two to three days.

Dose

Adults may take:

- ⅓ cup twice a day for normal conditions, and as a tonic
- ⅓ cup three to six times a day for acute conditions

SYRUP AND HONEY

Method

Make a standard decoction, as detailed above. Return to heat, remove lid, and simmer gently until liquid is reduced to 1¼ cups, which may take a few hours. Add 2 cups honey or 2½ cups sugar, stirring until completely dissolved. Pour into a bottle, label, and date.

Dose

Adults may take 2 teaspoons three to six times a day. Children under five may take 1 teaspoon three times a day.

TINCTURE

Method

To make 1¼ cups tincture, chop ½ cup dried or 1 cup fresh herb. Put in a large glass jar and cover with ¾ cup alcohol, such as vodka or brandy, and ⅓ cup water. Put on a lid and leave for two weeks, shaking occasionally. Strain well through a muslin bag and pour into an amber glass bottle. Label and date, then keep indefinitely in a cool place away from children.

Dose

Adults may take:

- 1 teaspoon three times a day, standard
- 5 drops to 1 teaspoon a day as a tonic
- 1 teaspoon six times a day for acute conditions

ALCOHOL-SPICED OR TONIC WINE

Method

Place 1 cup herb(s) or ¼–½ cup spices (depending on taste) in a clean bowl, bottle, or other container. Cover with 10½ cups wine. Stand for two weeks, strain, and bottle.

Dose

Adults may take ½ cup twice a day before meals (warm water can be added).

USING AND PREPARING HERBS FOR EXTERNAL USE

Common external preparations

Herbs may be prepared or bought in a variety of forms for external use:

• CREAMS AND OINTMENTS. These are applied externally to soothe irritated or inflamed skin conditions, or to ease the pain of sprains or bruises. Creams moisten dry or cracked skin, and massaging ointments into bruises helps to ease the pain. In both cases the active ingredients of the herb pass through the pores of the skin into the bloodstream to encourage healing. Creams can be made from infused oils (see recipe in "Methods and dosages," opposite).

• LINIMENTS AND RUBS. These oil-based preparations may be used in massage to ease joints or to soothe skin conditions.

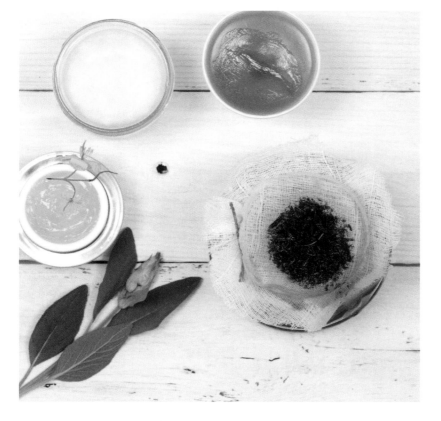

• COMPRESSES. Either hot or cold, compresses help with aches, pains, and swollen joints. Fold a clean piece of cotton into an infusion of the prescribed herb and apply to the point of pain. Repeat as the compress cools or, in the case of cold compresses, until the pain eases.

• POULTICES. Made from bruised fresh herbs or dried herbs moistened into a paste with hot water, compresses are also good for painful joints or for drawing out infection from boils, spots, or wounds. Place the herb on a clean piece of cotton and bandage onto the affected area. Leave in place for around 2 hours or until the symptoms ease.

• HERBAL BATHS. Perhaps the most pleasant of the herbal remedies, baths are a useful supplement to other forms of treatment. The heat of the water activates the properties of the volatile oils so that they are absorbed through the pores of the skin and inhaled through the nose. In both cases they pass into the bloodstream, and when inhaled they also pass through the nervous system to the brain.

Methods and Dosages

LINIMENT

A liniment is a soothing rub to relieve fatigued and stiff muscles and joints.

Method

• Put the fresh herb in a jar and cover with olive oil.
• Leave for up to six weeks.
• Strain the mixture through a cloth.
• Stand until the oil separates off; use this ointment as your liniment.

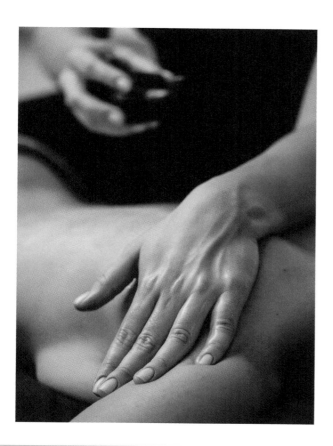

INFUSED OIL

Oil is soothing and nourishing for the skin, and acts as a lubricant to carry the active principles of the herbs in rubs, massage oils, and salves. All parts of the plant can be infused in oil. There are two methods of infusion: hot and cold. Hot is used for thyme, rosemary, comfrey root, and spices such as cayenne, mustard, and ginger. Cold is used for flowers, such as St. John's wort.

Method

This double method makes a strong infused oil that can be used as it is, mixed with tincture for a liniment, or thickened with beeswax (for a thin cream, use 1 part beeswax to 10 parts infused oil; for a thick salve, use 1 part beeswax to 5 parts infused oil). To make 1¼ cups:

• Chop 2–3¼ cups dried herbs or spices, or 3–4 cups fresh herbs.
• Put half into a clean pan with a lid and cover with 2 cups pure vegetable oil (a light vegetable oil is best).
• Put in a water bath and simmer gently for 2 hours (it is important that direct heat is not used, as this might burn the oil).
• Strain, and then throw away the used herbs.
• Put the remaining unused herbs in the pan.
• Cover these with the oil (it will have changed color, having picked up some of the quality of the herbs).
• Replace the lid and return the pan to the water bath for another couple of hours.
• Strain, then pour the oil into clean bottles, label, and add the date.

A TO Z OF HERBS

ALOE *Aloe vera*
Family: Liliaceae

PART USED: Fresh or dehydrated juice from the leaves.

CONSTITUENTS: Aloins, anthraquinones, resin.

ACTIONS: Cathartic, vulnerary, emmenagogue, vermifuge. External demulcent, vulnerary.

INDICATIONS: May be used internally where a powerful cathartic is needed. In a small dosage it increases the menstrual flow. Externally the juice is used fresh for minor burns, sunburn, insect bites, etc.

PREPARATION AND DOSAGE: For internal use, take up to 2–3 drops of the juice. For external use, put some of the fresh juice onto the afflicted area.

CAUTION: As aloe stimulates uterine contractions, it should be avoided during pregnancy. As it is excreted in the mother's milk, it should be avoided during breastfeeding, or it may be purgative to the child.

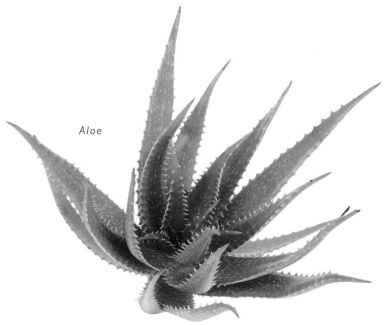

Aloe

ANGELICA *Angelica archangelica*
Family: Umbelliferae

PART USED: Roots and leaves are used medicinally; the stems and seeds are used in confectionery.

COLLECTION: The root is collected in the fall of its first year. If it is very thick, it can be cut longitudinally to speed its drying. The leaves should be collected in June.

CONSTITUENTS: Essential oils, including phellandrene and pinene, angelica acid, coumarin compounds, bitter principle, tannins.

ACTIONS: Carminative, antispasmodic, expectorant, diuretic, diaphoretic.

INDICATIONS: This herb is a useful expectorant for coughs, bronchitis, and pleurisy, especially when they are accompanied by fever, colds, or influenza. The leaf can be used as a compress in inflammations of the chest. Its content of carminative essential oil explains its use in easing intestinal colic and flatulence. As a digestive agent, it stimulates appetite. It has been shown to help ease rheumatic inflammations. In cystitis, it acts as a urinary antiseptic.

PREPARATION AND DOSAGE: Decoction: put a teaspoonful of the cut root in a cup of water, bring it to a boil, and simmer for 2 minutes. Take it off the heat and let it stand for 15 minutes. Take one cup three times a day. Tincture: take ½–1 teaspoon of the tincture three times a day.

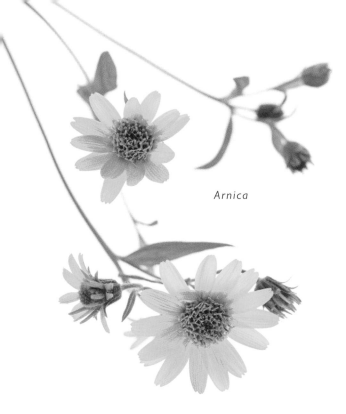

Arnica

ANISEED *Pimpinella anisum*
Family: Umbelliferae

PART USED: Dried fruit.

COLLECTION: The ripe dry fruit should be gathered between July and September.

CONSTITUENTS: Up to 6 percent volatile oils, which include anethole, 30 percent fatty oils, choline.

ACTIONS: Expectorant, antispasmodic, carminative, parasiticide, aromatic.

INDICATIONS: The volatile oil in aniseed provides the basis for its internal use to ease griping, intestinal colic, and flatulence. It also has a marked expectorant and antispasmodic action and may be used in bronchitis, in tracheitis where there is persistent irritable coughing, and in whooping cough. Externally, the oil may be used in an ointment base for the treatment of scabies. The oil by itself will help in the control of lice.

PREPARATION AND DOSAGE: Infusion: the seeds should be gently crushed just before use to release the volatile oils. Pour a cup of boiling water over 1–2 teaspoonfuls of the seeds and let it stand covered for 5–10 minutes. Take one cup three times daily. To treat flatulence, the tea should be drunk slowly before meals. Oil: one drop of the oil may be taken internally by mixing it into half a teaspoonful of honey.

ARNICA *Arnica montana*
Family: Asteraceae

PART USED: Flower heads.

COLLECTION: The flowers are collected between June and August.

CONSTITUENTS: Essential oils, sesquiterpene lactones, bitter glycosides, alkaloid, polyacetylenes, flavonoids, tannins.

ACTIONS: Anti-inflammatory, vulnerary.

INDICATIONS: While this herb should not be taken internally as it is potentially toxic, it provides us with one of the best remedies for external local healing and may be considered a specific when it comes to the treatment of bruises and sprains. The homeopathic preparation is safe to take externally, especially when taken according to homeopathic directions. The herb itself, used externally, will help in the relief of rheumatic pain and the pain and inflammation of phlebitis and similar conditions. It may, in fact, be used wherever there is pain or inflammation on the skin, as long as the skin is not broken.

PREPARATION AND DOSAGE: You can prepare your own tincture of this herb as follows: pour 2⅓ cups 70 percent alcohol over 3¼ cups freshly picked flowers. Seal it tightly in a clear glass container and let it stand for at least a week in the sun or in a warm place. Filter it and it is ready for use. To store it, put the tincture in a sealed container and keep it out of direct sunlight.

CAUTION: Do not use internally.

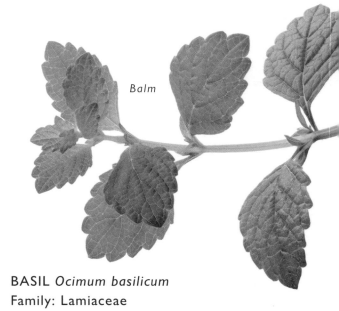

Balm

BALM *Melissa officinalis*
Family: Lamiaceae

PART USED: Dried aerial parts or fresh in season.

COLLECTION: The leaves may be harvested two or three times a year between June and September. They are gathered by cutting off the young shoots when they are approximately 12 inches long. They should be dried in the shade at a temperature not above 95°F (35°C).

CONSTITUENTS: Rich in essential oil containing citral, citronellal, geraniol, and linalool; bitter principles, flavones, resin.

ACTIONS: Carminative, antispasmodic, antidepressive, diaphoretic, hypotensive.

INDICATIONS: An excellent carminative herb that relieves spasms in the digestive tract and is used in flatulent dyspepsia. Because of its antidepressive properties, it is primarily indicated where there is dyspepsia associated with anxiety or depression, as the gently sedative oils relieve tension and stress reactions, thus acting to lighten depression. Balm has a tonic effect on the heart and circulatory system, causing mild vasodilation of the peripheral vessels, thus acting to lower blood pressure. It can be used in feverish conditions, such as influenza.

PREPARATION AND DOSAGE: Infusion: pour a cup of boiling water onto 2–3 teaspoonfuls of the dried herb or 4–6 fresh leaves and leave to infuse for 10–15 minutes, well covered until drunk. A cup of this tea should be taken in the morning and the evening, or when needed. Tincture: take ½–1¼ teaspoons of the tincture three times a day.

BASIL *Ocimum basilicum*
Family: Lamiaceae

PART USED: Leaves and as an oil.

COLLECTION: Basil can be grown on a windowsill if kept in a sunny position.

CONSTITUENTS: Rich in essential oil containing estragol, eugenol, lineol, linalool; caffeic acid, tannins, beta carotene, and vitamin C.

ACTIONS: Expectorant, antiseptic, antibacterial, antifungal, stimulating, antidepressant, antispasmodic, carminative, tonic, diaphoretic, fever-reducing.

INDICATIONS: Basil oil relieves mental fatigue, clears the mind, and improves concentration. It has a strong effect on the emotions and can ease fear or sadness. The oil is good for chest infections, congested sinuses, chronic colds, and head colds. Basil relieves abdominal pains, indigestion, and vomiting. Massage with basil oil works well on tired muscles; it also eases arthritis, rheumatism, and gout. Wipe with basil tea to treat acne.

PREPARATION AND DOSAGE: Infusion: Steep 3 teaspoons of dried leaves in a cup of boiling water for 20 minutes. Apply with a cotton ball to freshly washed skin to help acne, or drink up to 3 cups of the tea per day as an internal antibacterial treatment.

CAUTION: Do not use during pregnancy, as basil has been used as a menstruation-promoter and labor-inducer. Basil oil may irritate people with sensitive skin. Do not use the oil from exotic basil, which is slightly toxic.

Blue cohosh is a plant that comes to us from the Native Americans.

BLACK COHOSH *Cimicifuga racemosa*
Family: Ranunculaceae

PART USED: Root and rhizome; dried, not fresh.

COLLECTION: The roots are unearthed with the rhizome in the fall after the fruits have ripened. They should be cut lengthwise and dried carefully.

CONSTITUENTS: Resin, bitter glycosides, ranunculin (which changes to anemonin upon drying), salicylic acid, tannins, estrogenic principle.

ACTIONS: Emmenagogue, antispasmodic, alterative, sedative.

INDICATIONS: Black cohosh is an herb from the Native Americans and is a powerful relaxant and a normalizer of the female reproductive system. It may be used to relieve ovarian cramps, cramping pain in the womb, or in painful or delayed menstruation. It has a normalizing action on the balance of female sex hormones and may be used to regain normal hormonal activity. It is very active in the treatment of rheumatic conditions. It may be used in cases of rheumatic pains, but also in rheumatoid arthritis, osteoarthritis, and in muscular and neurological pain. It finds use in sciatica and neuralgia. As a relaxing nervine, it may be used in situations where such an agent is needed. It will be useful in labor to aid uterine activity while allaying nervousness. It will reduce spasm and so aid in the treatment of pulmonary complaints such as whooping cough. It has been found beneficial in cases of tinnitus.

PREPARATION AND DOSAGE: Decoction: pour a cup of water onto ½–1 teaspoonful of the dried root and bring to a boil. Let it simmer for 10–15 minutes. This should be drunk three times a day. Tincture: take ½–¾ teaspoon three times a day.

BLUE COHOSH *Caulophyllum thalictroides*
Family: Berberidaceae

PART USED: Rhizome and root.

COLLECTION: The roots and rhizomes are collected in the fall, as at the end of the growing season they are richest in natural chemicals.

CONSTITUENTS: Steroidal saponins, alkaloids.

ACTIONS: Uterine tonic, emmenagogue, antispasmodic, antirheumatic.

INDICATIONS: A plant that comes to us from the Native Americans, which shows in its other names of partridge vine (aka squaw vine) and papoose root. It is an excellent uterine tonic that may be used in any situation where there is a weakness or loss of tone. It may be used at any time during pregnancy if there is a threat of miscarriage. Similarly, because of its antispasmodic action, it will ease false labor pains. However, when labor does ensue, the use of blue cohosh just before birth will help ensure an easy delivery. In all these cases it is a safe herb to use. As an emmenagogue, it can be used to bring on a delayed or suppressed menstruation while ensuring that the pain that sometimes accompanies it is relieved. It may be used in cases where an antispasmodic is needed, such as in colic, asthma, or nervous coughs. It has a reputation for easing rheumatic pain.

PREPARATION AND DOSAGE: Decoction: put 1 teaspoonful of the dried root in a cup of water, bring to a boil, and simmer for 10 minutes. This should be drunk three times a day. Tincture: take ¼–½ teaspoon of the tincture three times a day.

BORAGE *Borago officinalis*
Family: Boraginaceae

PART USED: Dried leaves.

COLLECTION: The leaves should be gathered when the plant is coming into flower in the early summer. Strip each leaf off singly and reject any that are marked in any way. Do not collect when wet with rain or dew.

CONSTITUENTS: Saponins, mucilage, tannins, essential oil.

ACTIONS: Diaphoretic, expectorant, tonic, anti-inflammatory, galactagogue.

INDICATIONS: Borage acts as a restorative agent on the adrenal cortex, which means that it will revive and renew the adrenal glands after a medical treatment with cortisone or steroids. There is a growing need for remedies that will aid this gland with the stress it is exposed to, both externally and internally. Borage may be used as a tonic for the adrenals over a period of time. It may be used during fevers and especially during convalescence. It has a reputation as an anti-inflammatory herb used in conditions such as pleurisy. The leaves and seeds stimulate the flow of milk in nursing mothers.

PREPARATION AND DOSAGE: Infusion: pour a cup of boiling water onto 2 teaspoonfuls of the dried herb and leave to infuse for 10–15 minutes. This should be drunk three times a day. Tincture: take ¼–¾ teaspoon of the tincture three times a day.

BROOM TOPS *Sarothamnus scoparius*
Family: Papilionaceae

PART USED: Flowering tops.

COLLECTION: May be gathered throughout the spring, summer, and fall. The tops may be dried in the sun or by heat.

CONSTITUENTS: Alkaloids, including sparteine and cystisine; flavonoid glycosides, tannins, bitter principle, volatile oil.

ACTIONS: Cardioactive diuretic, hypertensive, peripheral vasoconstrictor, astringent.

INDICATIONS: Broom is a valuable remedy where there is a weak heart and low blood pressure. Since it is also a diuretic and produces peripheral constriction of the blood vessels while increasing the efficiency of each stroke of the heart, it can be used where water retention occurs due to heart weakness. Broom is used in cases of overly profuse menstruation.

PREPARATION AND DOSAGE: Infusion: pour a cup of boiling water onto 1 teaspoonful of the dried herb and let it infuse for 10–15 minutes. This should be drunk three times a day. Tincture: take ¼–½ teaspoon of the tincture three times a day.

CAUTION: Do not use broom in pregnancy or hypertension.

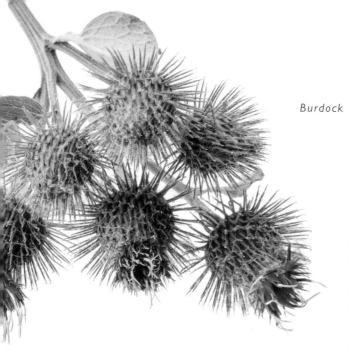

Burdock

BUCKTHORN *Rhamnus cathartica*
Family: Rhamnaceae

PART USED: Fresh or dried fruit.

COLLECTION: The fruit should be collected in September and October.

CONSTITUENTS: Anthraquinone derivates, including rhamnocarthrin; vitamin C.

ACTIONS: Laxative, diuretic, alterative.

INDICATIONS: Buckthorn is an effective and safe laxative.

PREPARATION AND DOSAGE: Infusion: pour a cup of boiling water onto 2 teaspoonfuls of the fruit and leave to infuse for 10–15 minutes. This should be drunk in the morning or evening, as it takes about 12 hours to be effective. The seeds (about 10) may also be chewed before eating in the morning. If the dose is too high, buckthorn might cause extreme diarrhea and possibly vomiting. Tincture: take ¼–½ teaspoon of the tincture night and morning.

BURDOCK *Arctium lappa*
Family: Asteraceae

PART USED: Roots and rhizome.

COLLECTION: The roots and rhizome should be unearthed in September or October.

CONSTITUENTS: Flavonoid glycosides, bitter glycosides, alkaloid, antimicrobial substance, inulin.

ACTIONS: Alterative, diuretic, bitter.

INDICATIONS: Burdock is a most valuable remedy for the treatment of skin conditions that result in dry and scaly skin. It may be most effective for psoriasis if used over a long period of time. Similarly, all types of eczema (though primarily the dry kinds) may be treated effectively if burdock is used over a period of time. It will be useful as part of a wider treatment for rheumatic complaints, especially where they are associated with psoriasis. Part of the action of this herb is through the bitter stimulation of the digestive juices and especially of bile secretion. Thus it will aid digestion and appetite. It may also help cystitis. In general, burdock will move the body to a state of integration and health, removing such indicators of systemic imbalance as skin problems and dandruff. Externally, it may be used as a compress or poultice to speed up the healing of wounds and ulcers. Eczema and psoriasis may also be treated this way externally.

PREPARATION AND DOSAGE: Decoction: put 1 teaspoonful of the root into a cup of water, bring to a boil, and simmer for 10–15 minutes. This should be drunk three times a day. Tincture: take ½–¾ teaspoon of the tincture three times a day.

Cardamom

CARAWAY *Carum carvi*
Family: Umbelliferae

PART USED: Seeds.
COLLECTION: The flowering heads (umbels) are collected in July and left to ripen. The seeds are then easily collected as they can be shaken off.
CONSTITUENTS: Up to 6 percent volatile oil, including carvone and limonene; fatty oil and tannins.
ACTIONS: Carminative, antispasmodic, expectorant, emmenagogue, galactagogue, astringent, aromatic.
INDICATIONS: Caraway is used as a calming herb to ease flatulent dyspepsia and intestinal colic, especially in children. It will stimulate the appetite. Its astringency will help in the treatment of diarrhea as well as in laryngitis as a gargle. It can be used in bronchitis and bronchial asthma. Its antispasmodic actions help in the relief of period pains. It has been used to increase milk flow in nursing mothers.
PREPARATION AND DOSAGE: Infusion: pour a cup of boiling water onto 1 teaspoonful of freshly crushed seeds and leave to infuse for 10–15 minutes. This should be drunk three times a day. Tincture: take ¼–¾ teaspoon of the tincture three times a day.

CARDAMOM *Elattaria cardamomum*
Family: Zingiberaceae

PART USED: Seeds.
COLLECTION: The seeds are mainly obtained from commercial plants in Sri Lanka or southern India. The crop is gathered between October and December.
CONSTITUENTS: Up to 4 percent volatile oil, including terpineol, cineole, limonene, sabinene, and pinene.

ACTIONS: Carminative, sialagogue, orexigenic, aromatic.
INDICATIONS: This valuable culinary herb may be used to treat flatulent dyspepsia and to relieve griping pains. It will stimulate the appetite and the flow of saliva. It is often used as a carminative flavoring agent when purgatives are given.
PREPARATION AND DOSAGE: Infusion: pour a cup of boiling water onto 1 teaspoonful of the freshly crushed seeds and leave to infuse for 10–15 minutes. This should be drunk three times a day. If treating flatulence or loss of appetite, drink half an hour before meals.

CAYENNE *Capsicum minimum*
Family: Solanaceae

PART USED: Fruit.
COLLECTION: The fruit should be harvested when fully ripe, and dried in the shade.
CONSTITUENTS: Capsaicin, carotenoids, flavonoids, essential oil, vitamin C.
ACTIONS: Stimulant, carminative, tonic, sialagogue, rubefacient, antiseptic.
INDICATIONS: Cayenne is the most useful of the systemic stimulants. It regulates the blood flow, equalizing and strengthening the heart, arteries, capillaries, and nerves. It is a general tonic and is

specific for the circulatory and digestive system. It may be used in flatulent dyspepsia and colic. If there is insufficient peripheral circulation, leading to cold hands and feet and possibly chilblains, cayenne may be used. It is used for treating debility and for warding off colds. Externally, it is used as a rubefacient in problems like lumbago and rheumatic pains. As an ointment, it helps unbroken chilblains, as long as it is used in moderation! As a gargle in laryngitis, it combines well with myrrh. This combination is also a good antiseptic wash.

PREPARATION AND DOSAGE: Infusion: pour a cup of boiling water onto ½–1 teaspoonful of cayenne and leave to infuse for 10 minutes. A tablespoon of this infusion should be mixed with hot water and drunk when needed. Tincture: take up to ¼ teaspoon of the tincture three times a day or when needed.

CHAMOMILE, GERMAN *Matricaria chamomilla*
Family: Asteraceae

PART USED: Flowers.

COLLECTION: The flowers should be gathered between May and August when they are not wet with dew or rain. They should be dried with care at not too high a temperature.

CONSTITUENTS: Volatile oil that includes chamazulene and isadol; mucilage, coumarin, flavone glycosides.

ACTIONS: Antispasmodic, carminative, anti-inflammatory, analgesic, antiseptic, vulnerary.

INDICATIONS: Chamomile is renowned for its medical and household uses. The apparently endless list of conditions it can help all fall into areas that the relaxing, carminative, and anti-inflammatory actions can aid. It is an excellent, gentle sedative, useful and safe for use with children. It will contribute its relaxing actions in any combination and is thus used in anxiety and insomnia. Indigestion and inflammations such as gastritis are often eased with chamomile. Similarly, it can be used as a mouthwash for inflammations of the mouth, such as gingivitis, and for bathing inflamed and sore eyes. As a gargle, it will help sore throats. As an inhalation over a steam bath, it will speed recovery from nasal catarrh. Externally, it will speed wound healing and reduce the swelling due to inflammation. As a carminative with relaxing properties, it will ease flatulence and dyspeptic pain.

PREPARATION AND DOSAGE: Infusion: pour a cup of boiling water onto 2 teaspoonfuls of the dried leaves and leave to infuse for 5–10 minutes. For digestive problems, this tea should be drunk after meals. A stronger infusion should be used as a mouthwash for conditions such as gingivitis. Half a cup of flowers boiled in 9½ cups of water makes a steam bath. Cover your head with a towel and inhale the steam. Tincture: take ½–¾ teaspoon of the tincture three times a day.

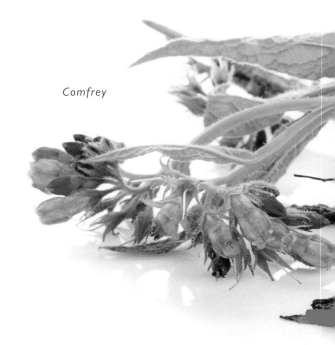

Comfrey

CINNAMON *Cinnamomum zeylanicum*
Family: Lauraceae

PART USED: Dried inner bark of the shoots.

COLLECTION: The bark is collected commercially throughout the tropics.

CONSTITUENTS: Volatile oils.

ACTIONS: Carminative, astringent, aromatic, stimulant.

INDICATIONS: Cinnamon is usually used as a carminative addition to other herbs. It relieves nausea and vomiting. Because of its mild astringency, it is used against diarrhea.

PREPARATION AND DOSAGE: The bark, usually powdered, may be freely used in mixtures or by itself to flavor teas.

CLOVES *Eugenia caryophyllus*
Family: Myrtaceae

PART USED: Dried flowers and oil.

COLLECTION: The flower buds are collected from this tree when their lower parts turn from green to purple. It grows all around the Indian Ocean.

CONSTITUENTS: Up to 20 percent of volatile oil.

ACTIONS: Stimulant, carminative, aromatic.

INDICATIONS: Cloves may be used to allay nausea, vomiting, and flatulence and to stimulate the digestive system. It is a powerful local antiseptic and mild anesthetic, which may be used externally in toothache.

PREPARATION AND DOSAGE: Cloves may be used as a spice in foods or in teas by putting some cloves into a cup with boiling water and infusing them for 10 minutes. For toothache, put a clove near the tooth and keep in the mouth.

Alternatively, pour some clove oil on a cotton ball and put this near the tooth.

COMFREY *Symphytum officinale*
Family: Boraginaceae

PART USED: Root and rhizome, leaf.

COLLECTION: The roots should be unearthed in the spring or fall, when the allantoin levels are the highest. Split the roots down the middle and dry in moderate temperatures of about 100–140°F (38–60°C).

CONSTITUENTS: Mucilage, gum, allantoin, tannins, alkaloids, resin, volatile oil.

ACTIONS: Vulnerary, demulcent, astringent, expectorant.

INDICATIONS: The impressive wound-healing properties of comfrey are partially due to the presence of allantoin. This chemical stimulates cell proliferation and so augments wound-healing both inside and out. A high quantity of demulcent mucilage makes comfrey a powerful healing agent in gastric and duodenal ulcers, hiatus hernia, and ulcerative colitis. It has been used with benefit in cases of bronchitis and irritable cough, where it will soothe and reduce irritation while helping expectoration. Comfrey may be used externally to speed wound-healing and guard against scar tissue developing incorrectly. Care

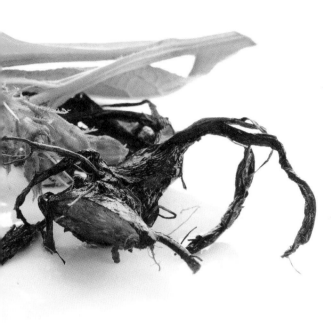

should be taken with very deep wounds, however, as the external application of comfrey can lead to tissue forming over the wound before it has healed deeper down, possibly leading to abscesses. It may be used for any external ulcer, for wounds and fractures, as a compress or poultice. It is excellent in chronic varicose ulcers.

PREPARATION AND DOSAGE: Decoction: put 1–3 teaspoonfuls of the dried herb in a cup of water, bring to a boil, and let simmer for 10–15 minutes. This should be drunk three times a day. Tincture: take ½–¾ teaspoon of the tincture three times a day.

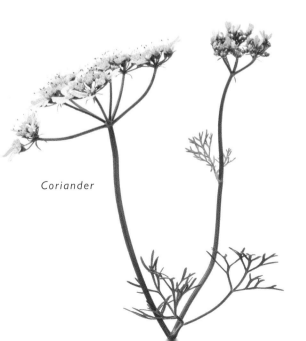

Coriander

CORIANDER *Coriandrum sativum*
Family: Umbelliferae

PART USED: Ripe seeds.

COLLECTION: The flowering heads (umbels) are collected in the late summer and left to ripen. The seeds are then easily collected as they can be shaken off.

CONSTITUENTS: Essential oil, including coriandrol; fatty oil, tannins, sugar.

ACTIONS: Carminative, aromatic.

INDICATIONS: This exquisite spice is used medicinally as an herb that helps the digestive system get rid of wind and eases the spasm pain (colic) that sometimes accompanies it. Coriander will also ease diarrhea, especially in children. It may be used as an equivalent to "gripe water," which is usually made from dill seeds. The oil acts as a stimulant to the stomach, increasing secretion of digestive juices and thus also stimulating the appetite.

PREPARATION AND DOSAGE: Infusion: pour a cup of boiling water onto 1 teaspoonful of the bruised seeds and leave to infuse for 5 minutes in a closed pot. This should be drunk before meals.

DAISY *Bellis perenis*
Family: Asteraceae

PART USED: Fresh or dried flower heads.

COLLECTION: The flowers may be picked between March and October.

CONSTITUENTS: Saponins, tannins, essential oil, flavones, bitter principle, mucilage.

ACTIONS: Expectorant, astringent.

INDICATIONS: Daisy, one of our most common plants, is useful for coughs and catarrh. For all conditions that manifest in these forms, daisy may be used freely and safely. It has a reputation of value in arthritis and rheumatism, as well as in liver and kidney problems. Due to its astringency, it is also useful for diarrhea.

PREPARATION AND DOSAGE: Infusion: pour a cup of boiling water onto 1 teaspoonful of the dried herb and leave to infuse for 10 minutes. This should be drunk three or four times a day. Tincture: take ½–¾ teaspoon of the tincture three times a day.

DANDELION *Taraxacum officinale*
Family: Asteraceae

PART USED: Root or leaf.

COLLECTION: The roots are best collected between June and August when they are at their most bitter. Split longitudinally before drying. The leaves may be collected at any time.

CONSTITUENTS: Glycosides, triterpenoids, choline, up to 5 percent potassium.

ACTIONS: Diuretic, cholagogue, antirheumatic, laxative, tonic.

INDICATIONS: Dandelion is a very powerful diuretic, its action comparable to that of the drug Frusemide.

The usual effect of a drug stimulating the kidney function is a loss of vital potassium from the body, which aggravates any cardiovascular problem present. With dandelion, however, we have one of the best natural sources of potassium. It thus makes an ideally balanced diuretic that may be used safely wherever such an action is needed, including in cases of water retention due to heart problems. It is specific in cases of congestive jaundice. As part of a wider treatment for muscular rheumatism, it can be most effective. This herb is a most valuable general tonic and perhaps the best widely applicable diuretic and liver tonic.

PREPARATION AND DOSAGE: Decoction: put 2–3 teaspoonfuls of the root into a cup of water, bring to a boil, and gently simmer for 10–15 minutes. This should be drunk three times a day. The leaves may be eaten raw in salads. Tincture: take 1–2 teaspoons of the tincture three times a day.

DILL *Anethum graveolens*
Family: Umbelliferae

PART USED: Seeds.

COLLECTION: The seeds should be collected when fully ripe; that is when they have turned brown. They should be spread out to dry, but not in artificial heat.

CONSTITUENTS: 4 percent volatile oil, which includes carvone and limonene.

ACTIONS: Carminative, aromatic, antispasmodic, galactagogue.

INDICATIONS: Dill is an excellent remedy for flatulence and the colic that is sometimes associated with it. This is the herb of choice in the colic of children. It will stimulate the flow of milk in nursing

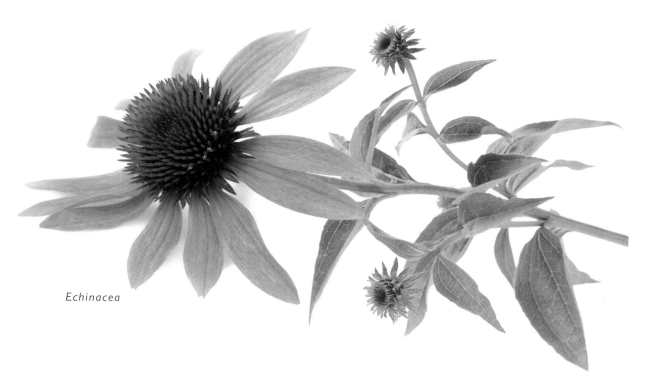

Echinacea

mothers. Chewing the seeds will clear up bad breath (halitosis).

PREPARATION AND DOSAGE: Infusion: pour a cup of boiling water onto 1–2 teaspoonfuls of the gently crushed seeds and leave to infuse for 10–15 minutes. For the treatment of flatulence, take a cup before meals. Tincture: take ¼–½ teaspoon of the tincture three times a day.

ECHINACEA *Echinacea angustifolia*
Family: Asteraceae

PART USED: Root.

COLLECTION: The roots should be unearthed in the fall. It is suggested that the fresh extract is more effective than the dried root.

CONSTITUENTS: Volatile oil, glycoside, echinaceine, phenolics.

ACTIONS: Antimicrobial, alterative.

INDICATIONS: Echinacea is the prime remedy to help the body rid itself of microbial infections. It is effective against both bacterial and viral attacks. It may be used in conditions such as boils, and other infections of that sort. In conjunction with other herbs, it may be used for any infection anywhere in the body. For example, in combination with yarrow or bearberry, it will effectively stop cystitis. It is especially useful for infections of the upper respiratory tract, such as laryngitis, tonsillitis, and for catarrhal conditions of the nose and sinus. In general, it may be used widely and safely. The tincture or decoction may be used as a mouthwash in the treatment of pyorrhea and gingivitis. It may be used as an external lotion to help septic sores and cuts.

PREPARATION AND DOSAGE: Decoction: put 1–2 teaspoonfuls of the root in a cup of water and bring it slowly to a boil. Let it simmer for 10–15 minutes. This should be drunk three times a day. Tincture: take ¼–¾ teaspoon of the tincture three times a day.

Echinacea root

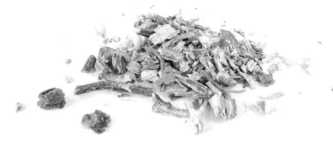

Elderberry flowers are ideal for the treatment of colds and influenza.

ELDERBERRY *Sambucus nigra*
Family: Caprifoliaceae

PART USED: Bark, flowers, berries, leaves.

COLLECTION: The flowers are collected in the spring and early summer and dried as rapidly as possible in the shade. The bark and berries are best collected in August and September.

CONSTITUENTS: Flowers: flavonoids, including rutin, isoquercitrine, and kampherol; the hydrocyanic glycoside sambunigrine; tannins; essential oil. Berries: invert sugar; fruit acids; tannin; vitamin C and P; anthrocyanic pigments; traces of essential oil.

ACTIONS: Bark: purgative, emetic, diuretic. Leaves: externally emollient and vulnerary, internally as purgative, expectorant, diuretic, and diaphoretic. Flowers: diaphoretic, anticatarrhal. Berries: diaphoretic, diuretic, laxative.

INDICATIONS: The elderberry tree is a veritable medicine chest by itself. The leaves are used primarily for bruises, sprains, wounds, and chilblains. It has been reported that elderberry leaves may be useful in an ointment for tumors. Elderberry flowers are ideal for the treatment of colds and influenza. They are indicated in any catarrhal inflammation of the upper respiratory tract such as hay fever and sinusitis. Catarrhal deafness responds well to elderberry flowers. Elderberries have similar properties to elderberry flowers, with the addition of their usefulness in rheumatism.

PREPARATION AND DOSAGE: Infusion: pour a cup of boiling water onto 2 teaspoonfuls of the dried or fresh blossoms and leave to infuse for 10 minutes. This should be drunk hot three times a day. Juice: boil fresh berries in water for 2–3 minutes, then express the juice. To preserve, bring the juice to a boil with one part honey to ten parts juice. Take one glass diluted with hot water twice a day. Ointment: take three parts fresh elderberry leaves and heat them with six parts melted petroleum jelly until the leaves are crisp. Strain and store.

EYEBRIGHT *Euphrasia officinalis*
Family: Scrophulariaceae

PART USED: Dried aerial parts.

COLLECTION: Gather the whole plant while in bloom in the late summer or fall and dry it in an airy place.

CONSTITUENTS: Glycosides, including aucubin, tannins, resins, volatile oil.

ACTIONS: Anticatarrhal, astringent, anti-inflammatory.

INDICATIONS: Eyebright is an excellent remedy for the problems of mucous membranes. The combination of anti-inflammatory and astringent properties makes it relevant in many conditions. Used internally, it is a powerful anticatarrhal and thus may be used in nasal catarrh, sinusitis, and other congestive states. It is best known for its use in conditions of the eye, where it is helpful in acute or chronic inflammations, stinging and weeping eyes, as well as oversensitivity to light. Used as a compress and taken internally, it is used in conjunctivitis and blepharitis.

PREPARATION AND DOSAGE: Infusion: pour a cup of boiling water onto 1 teaspoonful of the dried herb and leave to infuse for 5–10 minutes. This should be drunk three times a day. Compress: place a teaspoonful of the dried herb in 2⅓ cups water

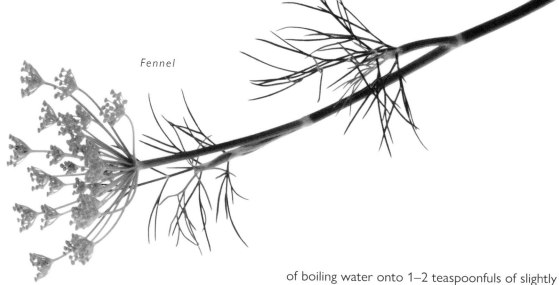

Fennel

and boil for 10 minutes, then let cool slightly. Moisten a compress (cotton ball, gauze, or muslin) in the lukewarm liquid, wring out slightly, and place over the eyes. Leave the compress in place for 15 minutes. Repeat several times a day. Tincture: take ¼–¾ teaspoon of the tincture three times a day.

FENNEL *Foeniculum vulgare*
Family: Umbelliferae

PART USED: Seeds.

COLLECTION: The seeds should be harvested when ripe and split in the fall. The brown umbel should be cut off. Comb the seeds to clean them. Dry slightly in the shade.

CONSTITUENTS: Up to 6 percent volatile oil, which includes anethole and fenchone; fatty oil 10 percent.

ACTIONS: Carminative, aromatic, antispasmodic, stimulant, galactagogue, rubefacient, expectorant.

INDICATIONS: Fennel is an excellent stomach and intestinal remedy that relieves flatulence and colic while also stimulating the digestion and appetite. It is similar to aniseed in its calming effect on bronchitis and coughs. It may be used to flavor cough remedies. Fennel will increase the flow of milk in nursing mothers. Externally, the oil eases muscular and rheumatic pains. The infusion may be used to treat conjunctivitis and inflammation of the eyelids (blepharitis) as a compress.

PREPARATION AND DOSAGE: Infusion: pour a cup of boiling water onto 1–2 teaspoonfuls of slightly crushed seeds and leave to infuse for 10 minutes. This should be drunk three times a day. To ease flatulence, take a cup half an hour before meals. Tincture: take ½–¾ teaspoon of the tincture three times a day.

FENUGREEK *Trigonella foenum-graecum*
Family: Papilionaceae

PART USED: Seeds.

CONSTITUENTS: Steroidal saponins including diosgenin, alkaloid, 30 percent mucilage, bitter principle, volatile and fixed oil.

ACTIONS: Expectorant, demulcent, tonic, galactagogue.

INDICATIONS: Fenugreek is an herb that has an ancient history. It has great use in local healing and reducing inflammation for conditions such as wounds, boils, and sores. It can be taken to help bronchitis and gargled to ease sore throats. Its bitterness explains its role in soothing disturbed digestion. It is a strong stimulator of milk production in mothers, for which it is perfectly safe, and has a reputation of stimulating development of the breasts.

PREPARATION AND DOSAGE: Poultice: for external use, the seeds should be pulverized to make a poultice. Decoction: to increase milk production, gently simmer 1½ teaspoonfuls of the seeds in a cup of water for 10 minutes. Drink a cup three times a day. To make a more pleasant drink, add 1 teaspoonful of aniseed to this mixture. Tincture: take ¼–½ teaspoon of the tincture three times a day.

Garlic is among the few herbs that have a universal usage and recognition.

FEVERFEW *Tanacetum parthenium*
Family: Asteraceae

PART USED: Leaves.

COLLECTION: The leaves may be picked throughout the spring and summer, although just before flowering is best.

CONSTITUENTS: Rich in sesquiterpene lactones including parthenolide, as well as volatile oil, tannins, and sesquiterpenes.

ACTIONS: Anti-inflammatory, vasodilatory, relaxant, digestive bitter, uterine stimulant.

INDICATIONS: Feverfew has regained its deserved reputation as a primary remedy in the treatment of migraine headaches, especially those that are relieved by applying warmth to the head. It may also help arthritis when it is in the painfully active inflammatory stage. Dizziness and tinnitus may be eased, especially if it is used in conjunction with other remedies. Painful periods and sluggish menstrual flow will be relieved by feverfew.

PREPARATION AND DOSAGE: It is best to use the equivalent of one fresh leaf one to three times a day. It is best used fresh or frozen.

CAUTION: Feverfew should not be used during pregnancy because of the stimulant action on the womb. The fresh leaves may cause mouth ulcers in sensitive people.

FLAX *Linum usitatissimum*
Family: Linaceae

PART USED: Ripe seeds.

COLLECTION: The seed pods are gathered when fully ripe in September.

CONSTITUENTS: 30–40 percent of fixed oil, which includes linoleic, linolenic, and oleic acids; mucilage, protein, the glycoside linamarin.

ACTIONS: Demulcent, antitussive, laxative, emollient.

INDICATIONS: Flax may be used in all pulmonary infections, especially in bronchitis with much catarrh formed. It is often used as a poultice in pleurisy and other pulmonary conditions. As a poultice, it can be used for boils and carbuncles, shingles, and psoriasis. As a purgative, it relieves constipation.

PREPARATION AND DOSAGE: Infusion: pour a cup of boiling water onto 2–3 teaspoonfuls of the dried herb and leave to infuse for 10–15 minutes. This should be drunk morning and evening. Tincture: take ½–1¼ teaspoons of the tincture three times a day.

GARLIC *Allium sativum*
Family: Liliaceae

PART USED: Bulb.

COLLECTION: The bulb with its numerous cloves should be unearthed when the leaves begin to wither in September. They should be stored in a cool, dry place.

CONSTITUENTS: Volatile oil, mucilage, glucokinins, germanium.

ACTIONS: Antiseptic, antiviral, diaphoretic, cholagogue, hypotensive, antispasmodic.

INDICATIONS: Garlic is among the few herbs that have a universal usage and recognition. Its daily usage aids and supports the body in ways that no other herb does. It is one of the most effective antimicrobial plants available, acting on bacteria, viruses, and alimentary parasites. The volatile oil is an effective agent, as it is largely excreted via the lungs.

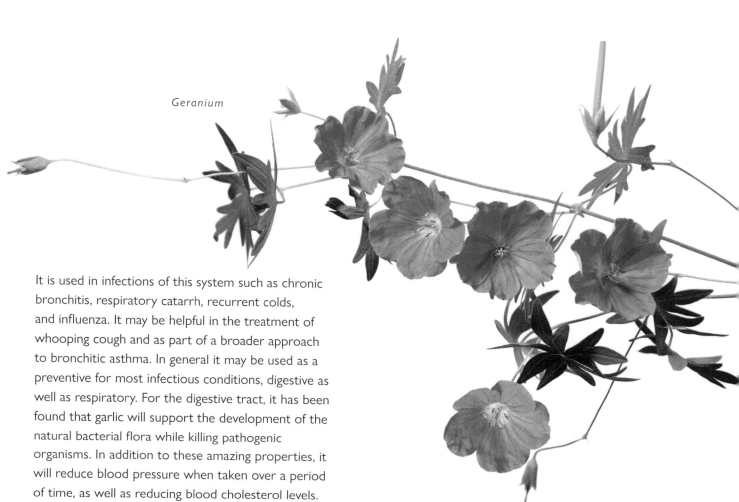

Geranium

It is used in infections of this system such as chronic bronchitis, respiratory catarrh, recurrent colds, and influenza. It may be helpful in the treatment of whooping cough and as part of a broader approach to bronchitic asthma. In general it may be used as a preventive for most infectious conditions, digestive as well as respiratory. For the digestive tract, it has been found that garlic will support the development of the natural bacterial flora while killing pathogenic organisms. In addition to these amazing properties, it will reduce blood pressure when taken over a period of time, as well as reducing blood cholesterol levels. Garlic should be thought of as a basic food that will augment the body's health and protect it in general. It has been used externally for the treatment of ringworm and threadworm.

PREPARATION AND DOSAGE: A clove should be eaten three times a day. If the smell becomes a problem, use garlic oil capsules; take three a day as a prophylactic or three times a day when an infection occurs.

GERANIUM (aka American cranesbill)
Geranium maculatum
Family: Geraniaceae

PART USED: Rhizome.
COLLECTION: The rhizome is unearthed in September and October, cut into pieces, and dried.
CONSTITUENTS: 12–25 percent tannins, with the level being highest just before flowering.
ACTIONS: Astringent, antihemorrhagic, anti-inflammatory, vulnerary.

INDICATIONS: Geranium, or American cranesbill, is an effective astringent used in diarrhea, dysentery, and hemorrhoids. When bleeding accompanies duodenal or gastric ulceration, this remedy is used in combination with other relevant herbs. Where blood is lost in the feces, this herb will help, though careful diagnosis is vital. It may be used where excessive blood loss during menstruation (menorrhagia) occurs.
PREPARATION AND DOSAGE: Decoction: put 1–2 teaspoonfuls of the rhizome in a cup of cold water and bring to a boil. Let simmer for 10–15 minutes. This should be drunk three times a day. Tincture: take ½–¾ teaspoon of the tincture three times a day.

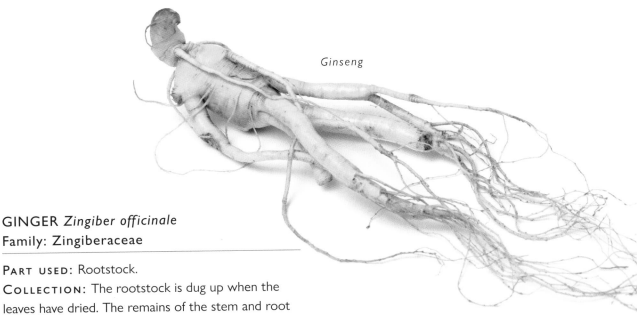

Ginseng

GINGER *Zingiber officinale*
Family: Zingiberaceae

PART USED: Rootstock.

COLLECTION: The rootstock is dug up when the leaves have dried. The remains of the stem and root fibers should be removed. Wash thoroughly and dry in the sun.

CONSTITUENTS: Rich in volatile oil, which includes zingiberene, zingiberole, phellandrene, borneol, cineole, citral; starch, mucilage, resin.

ACTIONS: Stimulant, carminative, rubefacient, diaphoretic.

INDICATIONS: Ginger may be used as a stimulant of the peripheral circulation in cases of bad circulation, chilblains, and cramps. In feverish conditions, ginger acts as a useful diaphoretic, promoting perspiration. As a carminative, it promotes gastric secretion and is used in dyspepsia, flatulence, and colic. As a gargle, it may be effective in the relief of sore throats. Externally, it is the base of many fibrositis and muscle sprain treatments.

PREPARATION AND DOSAGE: Infusion: pour a cup of boiling water onto 1 teaspoonful of the fresh root and let it infuse for 5 minutes. Drink whenever needed. Decoction: if you are using the dried root in powdered or finely chopped form, make a decoction by putting 1½ teaspoonfuls into a cup of water. Bring to a boil and simmer for 5–10 minutes. This can be drunk whenever needed. Tincture: take ¼–½ teaspoon of the tincture three times a day.

GINSENG *Panax ginseng*
Family: Araliaceae

PART USED: Root.

COLLECTION: Ginseng is cultivated in China, Korea, and the northeastern United States.

CONSTITUENTS: Steroidal glycosides called panaxoside, sterols, vitamins of D group.

ACTIONS: Antidepressive, strengthens the immune system, and improves physical and mental performance.

INDICATIONS: Ginseng has an ancient history and as such has accumulated much folklore about its actions and uses. Many of the claims that surround it are inflated, but it is clear that this is a unique plant. It has the power to move a person to their physical peak, generally increasing vitality and physical performance. Specifically, it will raise lowered blood pressure to a normal level. It affects depression, especially where this is due to debility and exhaustion. It can be used in general for exhaustion states and weakness. It has a reputation as an aphrodisiac. Occasionally, the use of this herb may produce headaches.

PREPARATION AND DOSAGE: The root is chewed or a decoction may be made. Put ½ teaspoonful of the powdered root in a cup of water, bring to a boil, and simmer gently for 10 minutes. This should be drunk three times a day.

GOLDEN RAGWORT (aka life root)
Senecio aureus
Family: Asteraceae

PART USED: Dried aerial parts.

COLLECTION: The herb should be collected just before the small flowers open in the summer.

CONSTITUENTS: Alkaloids, including senecifoline, senecine, resins.

ACTIONS: Uterine tonic, diuretic, expectorant, emmenagogue.

INDICATIONS: As a uterine tonic, golden ragwort (aka life root) may be used safely wherever strengthening and aid are called for. It is especially useful in cases of menopausal disturbances of any kind. Where there is delayed or suppressed menstruation, golden ragwort may be used. It also has a reputation as a general tonic.

PREPARATION AND DOSAGE: Infusion: pour a cup of boiling water onto 1–3 teaspoonfuls of the dried herb and leave to infuse for 10–15 minutes. This should be drunk three times a day. Tincture: take ¼–¾ teaspoon three times a day.

GOLDEN SEAL *Hydrastis canadensis*
Family: Ranunculaceae

PART USED: Root and rhizome.

COLLECTION: Unearth root and rhizome from three-year-old plants in the fall, after the ripening of the seeds. Clean carefully and dry slowly in the air.

CONSTITUENTS: 5 percent of the root consists of the alkaloids hydrastine, berberine, and canadine; traces of essential oil; resin; fatty oil.

ACTIONS: Tonic, astringent, anticatarrhal, laxative, muscular stimulant, oxytocic, bitter.

INDICATIONS: Golden seal is one of the most useful herbs available to us. It owes most of its specific uses to the powerful tonic qualities shown toward the mucous membranes of the body. It is thus of service in all digestive problems—for example, in gastritis, septic ulceration, and colitis. Its bitter stimulation gives it a role in loss of appetite. All catarrhal states benefit from golden seal, especially upper respiratory tract catarrh. The tonic and astringency contribute to its use in uterine conditions such as menorrhagia (excessive menstruation). With the additional stimulation of involuntary muscles, it is an excellent aid during childbirth, but for just this reason it should be avoided during pregnancy. Externally, it is used for the treatment of eczema, ringworm, pruritus (itching), earache, and conjunctivitis.

PREPARATION AND DOSAGE: Infusion: pour a cup of boiling water onto ½–1 teaspoonful of the powdered herb and leave to infuse for 10–15 minutes. This should be drunk three times a day. Tincture: take ½–¾ teaspoon of the tincture three times a day.

CAUTION: As golden seal stimulates the involuntary muscles of the uterus, it should be avoided during pregnancy.

Ripe chestnuts should be gathered as they fall from the trees.

HAWTHORN BERRIES *Crataegus oxyacanthoides*
Family: Rosaceae

PART USED: Ripe fruit.

COLLECTION: The berries are collected in September and October.

CONSTITUENTS: Saponins, glycosides, flavonoids, acids, including ascorbic acid, tannins.

ACTIONS: Cardiac tonic, hypotensive.

INDICATIONS: Hawthorn berries provide us with one of the best tonic remedies for the heart and circulatory system. They act in a normalizing way upon the heart by either stimulating or depressing its activity depending upon the need. In other words, hawthorn berries will move the heart to normal function in a gentle way. As a long-term treatment, they may safely be used in heart failure or weakness and can be a good general tonic for the circulatory system.

PREPARATION AND DOSAGE: Infusion: pour a cup of boiling water onto 2 teaspoonfuls of the berries and leave to infuse for 20 minutes. This should be drunk three times a day over a long period. Tincture: take ½–¾ teaspoon of the tincture three times a day.

HOPS *Humulus lupulus*
Family: Cannabinaceae

PART USED: Flower inflorescence.

COLLECTION: The hops cones are gathered before they are fully ripe in August and September. They should be dried with care in the shade.

CONSTITUENTS: Lupulin, bitters, resin, volatile oil, tannins, estrogenic substance.

ACTIONS: Sedative, hypnotic, antiseptic, astringent.

INDICATIONS: Hops is a remedy that has a marked relaxing effect upon the central nervous system. It is used extensively for the treatment of insomnia. It will ease tension and anxiety and may be used where this tension leads to restlessness, headaches, and possibly indigestion. As an astringent with these relaxing properties, it can be used in conditions such as mucous colitis. It should, however, be avoided where there is a marked degree of depression, as this may be accentuated. Externally, the antiseptic action is utilized for the treatment of ulcers.

PREPARATION AND DOSAGE: Infusion: pour a cup of boiling water onto 1 teaspoonful of the dried flowers and leave to infuse for 10–15 minutes. A cup should be drunk at night to induce sleep. This dose may be strengthened if needed. Tincture: take ¼–¾ teaspoon of the tincture three times a day.

CAUTION: Do not use in cases with marked depression.

HORSE CHESTNUT *Aesculus hippocastanum*
Family: Hippocastanaceae

PART USED: The fruit that is the horse chestnut itself.

COLLECTION: The ripe chestnuts should be gathered as they fall from the trees in September and October.

CONSTITUENTS: Saponins, tannins, flavones, starch, fatty oil, the glycosides aesculin and fraxin.

ACTIONS: Astringent, circulatory tonic.

INDICATIONS: The unique actions of horse chestnut are on the vessels of the circulatory system. It seems to increase the strength and tone of the veins in particular. It may be used internally to aid

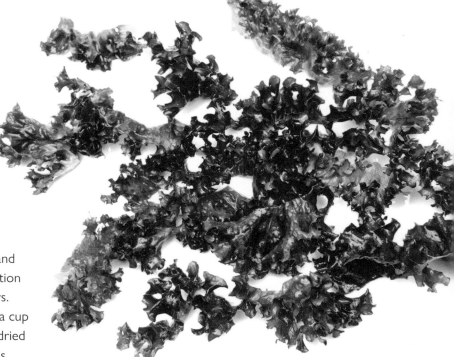

Irish moss

the body in the treatment of problems such as phlebitis, inflammation in the veins, varicosity, and hemorrhoids. Externally, it may be used as a lotion for the same conditions, as well as for leg ulcers.

PREPARATION AND DOSAGE: Infusion: pour a cup of boiling water onto 1–2 teaspoonfuls of the dried fruit and leave to infuse for 10–15 minutes. This should be drunk three times a day or used as a lotion. Tincture: take ¼–¾ teaspoon of the tincture three times a day.

HORSERADISH *Armoracia rusticana*
Family: Cruciferae

PART USED: Taproot.

COLLECTION: The roots are collected in the winter and stored in sand.

CONSTITUENTS: Essential oil that contains mustard oil glycosides; sinigrin.

ACTIONS: Stimulant, carminative, rubefacient, mild laxative, diuretic.

INDICATIONS: Horseradish is an old household remedy useful wherever a stimulating herb is called for. It can be used in influenza and fevers and it stimulates the digestive process while easing wind and griping pains. It has been used in cases of urinary infection. Externally, it has a stimulating action similar to mustard seed. It can be used for rheumatism and as a poultice in bronchitis.

PREPARATION AND DOSAGE: The fresh root is often used as a vegetable. Infusion: pour a cup of boiling water onto 1 teaspoonful of the powdered or chopped root. Leave to infuse for 5 minutes. This should be drunk three times a day or more often when being used to treat influenza or fevers.

IRISH MOSS (aka carragheen) *Chondrus crispus*
Family: Rhodophyta

PART USED: The dried thallus. It is a seaweed.

COLLECTION: It is collected from the rocky coastlines of northwestern Europe, especially Ireland, all year round at low tide.

CONSTITUENTS: Up to 80 percent mucilage, carrageenans, iodine, bromine, iron, other mineral salts, vitamins A and B1.

ACTIONS: Expectorant, demulcent.

INDICATIONS: The mucilage present in this plant is used in large quantities by the food industry to make jellies or aspic and as a smooth binder. This very property is the basis of its use in digestive conditions where a demulcent is called for, such as gastritis and ulcers. However, its main use is in respiratory problems such as bronchitis. It finds a use in cosmetics as a skin softener.

PREPARATION AND DOSAGE: Infusion: pour a cup of boiling water onto 1–1½ teaspoonfuls of the dried herb and leave to infuse for 10 minutes. This should be drunk three times a day. Tincture: take ¼–½ teaspoon of the tincture three times a day.

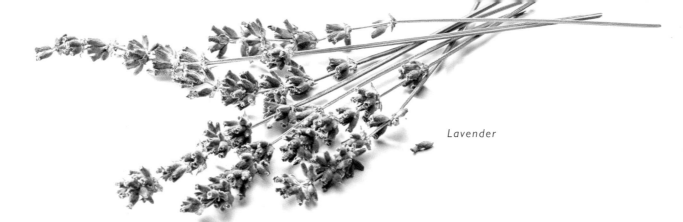

Lavender

JUNIPER BERRIES *Juniperus communis*
Family: Cupressaceae

PART USED: Dried ripe berries.

COLLECTION: The ripe, unshriveled berries should be collected in the fall and dried slowly in the shade, to avoid losing the oil present.

CONSTITUENTS: Rich in essential oil that contains monoterpenes and sesquiterpenes; invert sugar, flavone glycosides, resin, tannins, organic acids.

ACTIONS: Diuretic, antiseptic, carminative, antirheumatic.

INDICATIONS: Juniper berries make an excellent antiseptic in conditions such as cystitis. The essential oil present is quite stimulating to the kidney nephrons, and so this herb should be avoided in kidney disease. The bitter action aids digestion and eases flatulent colic. It is used in rheumatism and arthritis. Externally, it eases pain in the joints or muscles.

PREPARATION AND DOSAGE: Infusion: pour a cup of boiling water onto 1 teaspoonful of lightly crushed berries and leave to infuse for 20 minutes. A cup should be drunk night and morning. For the treatment of chronic rheumatism, this treatment should be continued for 4–6 weeks in the spring and fall.

CAUTION: Should be avoided in kidney disease and in pregnancy.

LAVENDER *Lavendula officinalis*
Family: Lamiaceae

PART USED: Flowers.

COLLECTION: Gather just before opening between June and September. They should be dried gently at a temperature not above 95°F (35°C).

CONSTITUENTS: Fresh flowers contain up to 0.5 percent volatile oil, among other constituents, linalyl acetate, linalool, geraniol, cineole, limonene, and sesquiterpenes.

ACTIONS: Carminative, antispasmodic, antidepressant, rubefacient.

INDICATIONS: An effective herb for headaches, especially when they are related to stress. Lavender can be quite effective in the clearing of depression, especially if used in conjunction with other remedies. As a gentle strengthening tonic of the nervous system, it may be used in states of nervous debility and exhaustion. It can be used to soothe and promote natural sleep. Externally, the oil may be used as a stimulating liniment to help ease rheumatism.

PREPARATION AND DOSAGE: Infusion: pour a cup of boiling water onto 1 teaspoonful of the dried herb and leave to infuse for 10 minutes. This can be drunk three times a day. External use: the oil can be inhaled, rubbed on the skin, or used in baths.

LICORICE *Glycyrrhiza glabra*
Family: Leguminosae

PART USED: Dried root.

COLLECTION: The roots are unearthed in the late fall. Clean thoroughly and dry.

CONSTITUENTS: Glycosides called glycyrrhizin and glycyrrhizinic acid; saponins, flavonoids, bitter, volatile oil, coumarins, asparagine, estrogenic substances.

ACTIONS: Expectorant, demulcent, mild laxative, anti-inflammatory, adrenal agent, antispasmodic.

INDICATIONS: One of a group of plants that have a marked effect upon the endocrine system. The glycosides present have a structure that is similar to the natural steroids of the body. They explain the

Marigold is one of the best herbs for treating local skin problems.

beneficial action that licorice has in the treatment of adrenal gland problems such as Addison's disease. It has a wide usage in bronchial problems such as catarrh, bronchitis, and coughs in general. Licorice is used in allopathic medicine as a treatment for peptic ulceration, a similar use to its herbal use in gastritis and ulcers. It can be used in the relief of abdominal colic.

PREPARATION AND DOSAGE: Decoction: put ½–1 teaspoonful of the root in a cup of water, bring to a boil, and simmer for 10–15 minutes. This should be drunk three times a day. Tincture: take ¼–⅔ teaspoon three times a day.

MALLOW *Malva sylvestris*
Family: Malvaceae

PART USED: Flowers and leaves.
COLLECTION: The flowers and leaves are collected and dried with care between July and September.
CONSTITUENTS: Mucilage, essential oil, trace of tannin.
ACTIONS: Demulcent, anti-inflammatory, expectorant, astringent.
INDICATIONS: Internally, it may be used to aid recovery from gastritis and stomach ulcers, laryngitis and pharyngitis, upper respiratory catarrh, and bronchitis. Externally, it may be used as an addition to bathwater or as a compress against abscesses, boils, and minor burns.
PREPARATION AND DOSAGE: Infusion: pour a cup of boiling water onto 2 teaspoonfuls of the dried herb and leave to infuse for 10–15 minutes. This should be drunk three times a day. Compress: put 1 teaspoonful of the herb in a cup of water, bring to

a boil, and simmer gently for 10–15 minutes. This decoction can be used for a compress. Tincture: take ½–¾ teaspoon three times a day.

MARIGOLD *Calendula officinalis*
Family: Asteraceae

PART USED: Yellow petal (florets).
COLLECTION: Collect the whole flower tops or just the petals between June and September. Dry with great care to avoid discoloration.
CONSTITUENTS: Saponins, carotenoids, bitter principle, essential oil, sterols, flavonoids, mucilage.
ACTIONS: Anti-inflammatory, astringent, vulnerary, antifungal, cholagogue, emmenagogue.
INDICATIONS: It may be used safely wherever there is an inflammation on the skin, whether due to infection or physical damage. It may be used for any external bleeding or wound, bruising, or strains. It will also be of benefit in slow-healing wounds and skin ulcers. It is ideal for first-aid treatment of minor burns and scalds. Local treatments may be with a lotion, a poultice, or compress, whichever is most appropriate. Internally, it acts as a valuable herb for digestive inflammations or ulcers. Thus it may be used in the treatment of gastric and duodenal ulcers. Marigold has marked antifungal activity and may be used both internally and externally to combat such infections. As an emmenagogue, it has a reputation of helping delayed menstruation and painful periods. It is in general a normalizer of the menstrual process.
PREPARATION AND DOSAGE: Infusion: pour a cup of boiling water onto 1–2 teaspoonfuls of the florets and infuse for 10–15 minutes. Drink three times a day. Tincture: take ¼–¾ teaspoon three times a day.

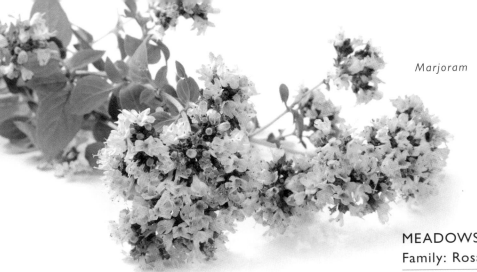

Marjoram

MARJORAM, WILD *Origanum vulgare*
Family: Lamiaceae

PART USED: Aerial parts.

COLLECTION: The herb is gathered as soon as it flowers, avoiding the larger, thicker stalks.

CONSTITUENTS: Essential oil with thymol, carvacrol; acids, tannins, bitter principle.

ACTIONS: Stimulant, diaphoretic, antiseptic, expectorant, emmenagogue, rubefacient.

INDICATIONS: As a diaphoretic, it is often used in the treatment of colds and flu. The antiseptic properties give it a use in the treatment of mouth conditions as a mouthwash for inflammations of the mouth and throat. It may also be used externally for infected cuts and wounds. The infusion is used in coughs and whooping cough. Headaches, especially when due to tension, may be relieved by a tea of marjoram or by rubbing the forehead and temples with the oil. The oil may also be used for rubbing into areas of muscular and rheumatic pain. A lotion may be made that will soothe stings and bites.

PREPARATION AND DOSAGE: Infusion: pour a cup of boiling water onto 1 teaspoonful of the herb and leave to infuse for 10–15 minutes. This should be drunk three times a day. Mouthwash: pour 2⅓ cups of boiling water onto 2 tablespoonfuls of the herb. Let stand in a covered container for 10 minutes. Reheat to use as a gargle. Gargle for 5–10 minutes, up to four times a day.
Tincture: take ¼–½ teaspoon three times a day.

MEADOWSWEET *Filipendula ulmaria*
Family: Rosaceae

PART USED: Aerial parts.

COLLECTION: The fully opened flowers and leaves are picked at the time of flowering, which is between June and August. They should be dried gently at a temperature not exceeding 100°F (38°C).

CONSTITUENTS: Essential oil with salicylic acid compounds called spiraeine and gaultherin; salicylic acid, tannins, citric acid.

ACTIONS: Antirheumatic, anti-inflammatory, stomachic, antacid, antiemetic, astringent.

INDICATIONS: Meadowsweet is one of the best digestive remedies available. It acts to protect and soothe the mucous membranes of the digestive tract, reducing excess acidity and easing nausea. It is used in the treatment of heartburn, hyperacidity, gastritis, and peptic ulceration. Its gentle astringency is useful in treating diarrhea in children. The presence of aspirin-like chemicals explains meadowsweet's action in reducing fever and relieving the pain of rheumatism in muscles and joints.

PREPARATION AND DOSAGE: Infusion: pour a cup of boiling water onto 1–2 teaspoonfuls of the dried herb and leave to infuse for 10–15 minutes. Drink three times a day or as needed. Tincture: take ¼–¾ teaspoon of the tincture three times a day.

NETTLE *Urtica dioica*
Family: Urticaceea

PART USED: Aerial parts.

COLLECTION: The herb should be collected when the flowers are in bloom.

CONSTITUENTS: Histamine, formic acid, chlorophyll, glucoquinine, iron, vitamin C.

ACTIONS: Astringent, diuretic, tonic.

INDICATIONS: Nettles are one of the most widely applicable plants we have. They strengthen and support the whole body. They are beneficial in all the varieties of eczema, especially in nervous eczema. As an astringent, they may be used for nosebleeds or to relieve the symptoms wherever there is hemorrhage in the body—for example, in uterine hemorrhage.

PREPARATION AND DOSAGE: Infusion: pour a cup of boiling water onto 1–3 teaspoonfuls of the dried herb and leave to infuse for 10–15 minutes. Drink three times a day. Tincture: take ¼–¾ teaspoon three times a day.

OREGANO *Origanum vulgare*
Family: Lamiaceae

PART USED: Leaves, flowers.

COLLECTION: Can be gathered when it flowers.

CONSTITUENTS: Essential oil, including thymol and carvacrol.

ACTIONS: Stimulant, antiseptic, expectorant.

INDICATIONS: Its stimulating nature makes it popular to use for colds and flu, and its antiseptic properties mean it's helpful for treating mouth conditions; it can be made into a mouthwash. A cup of oregano may help to relieve a tension headache. Oil of oregano can be applied to muscle pain or an infusion can be added to a warm bath.

PREPARATION AND DOSAGE: Infusion: infuse 1 teaspoon of oregano in a cup of boiling water for 10 minutes. Drink 2–3 times a day. Mouthwash: pour two cups of boiling water onto 2 tablespoons of oregano. Cover and leave to stand for 10 minutes. Gargle for 5–10 minutes, 3–4 times a day. Tincture: take ¼–½ teaspoon three times a day.

CAUTION: Avoid high doses during pregnancy.

PARSLEY *Petroselinum crispum*
Family: Umbelliferae

PART USED: Taproot, leaves, and seeds.

COLLECTION: The root is collected in the fall from two-year-old plants. The leaves can be used any time during the growing season.

CONSTITUENTS: Essential oil, including apiol and myristicin; vitamin C, glycoside apiin, starch.

ACTIONS: Diuretic, expectorant, emmenagogue, carminative, supposed aphrodisiac.

INDICATIONS: The fresh herb is one of our richest sources of vitamin C. Medicinally, parsley has three main areas of usage. Firstly, it is an effective diuretic, helping the body get rid of excess water, and so may be used wherever such an effect is desired. Remember, however, that the cause of the problem must be sought and treated—don't just treat symptoms. The second area of use is as an emmenagogue stimulating the menstrual process. The third use is as a carminative, easing flatulence and the colic pains that may accompany it.

PREPARATION AND DOSAGE: Infusion: pour a cup of boiling water onto 1–2 teaspoonfuls of the leaves or root and leave to infuse for 5–10 minutes in a closed container. Drink three times a day. Tincture: take ½–¾ teaspoon of the tincture three times a day.

CAUTION: Do not use during pregnancy in medicinal dosage as there may be excessive stimulation of the womb.

PEPPERMINT *Mentha piperita*
Family: Lamiaceae

PART USED: Aerial parts.

COLLECTION: The aerial parts are collected just before the flowers open.

CONSTITUENTS: Up to 2 percent volatile oil containing menthol, menthone, and jasmone; tannins, bitter principle.

ACTIONS: Carminative, antispasmodic, aromatic, diaphoretic, antiemetic, nervine, antiseptic, analgesic.

INDICATIONS: Peppermint is one of the best carminative agents available. It has a relaxing effect on the visceral muscles, antiflatulent properties, and stimulates bile and digestive juice secretion, all of which help explain its value in relieving intestinal colic, flatulent dyspepsia, and other associated conditions. The volatile oil acts as a mild anesthetic to the stomach wall, which allays feelings of nausea and the desire to vomit. Peppermint plays a role in the treatment of ulcerative colitis and Crohn's disease. It is most valuable in the treatment of fevers and especially colds and influenza. As an inhalant, it can be used as a temporary treatment for nasal catarrh. Where migraine headaches are associated with the digestion, this herb may be used. As a nervine it acts as a tonic, easing anxiety, tension, hysteria, etc. In painful periods (dysmenorrhea), it relieves the pain and eases associated tension. Externally it may be used to relieve itching and inflammations.

PREPARATION AND DOSAGE: Infusion: pour a cup of boiling water onto a heaping teaspoonful of the dried herb and leave to infuse for 10 minutes. This may be drunk as often as desired. Tincture: take ¼–½ teaspoon of the tincture three times a day.

RASPBERRY *Rubus idaeus*
Family: Rosaceae

PART USED: Leaves and fruit.

COLLECTION: Collect the leaves throughout the growing season. Dry slowly in a well-ventilated area to ensure preservation of properties.

CONSTITUENTS: Leaves: fruit sugar, volatile oil, pectin, citric acid, malic acid.

ACTIONS: Astringent, tonic, refrigerant, parturient.

INDICATIONS: Raspberry leaves have a long tradition of use in pregnancy to strengthen and tone the tissue of the womb, assisting contractions and checking any hemorrhage during labor. This action will occur if the herb is drunk regularly throughout pregnancy and also taken during labor. As an astringent, it may be used in a wide range of cases, including diarrhea, leukorrhea, and other loose conditions. It is valuable in the easing of mouth problems such as mouth ulcers, bleeding gums, and inflammations. As a gargle, it will help sore throats.

PREPARATION AND DOSAGE: Infusion: pour a cup of boiling water onto 2 teaspoonfuls of the dried herb and leave to infuse for 10–15 minutes. This may be drunk freely. Tincture: take ½–¾ teaspoon of the tincture three times a day.

RED CLOVER *Trifolium pratense*
Family: Papilionaceae

PART USED: Flower heads.

COLLECTION: The flower heads are gathered between May and September.

CONSTITUENTS: Phenolic glycosides, flavonoids, coumarins, cyanogenic glycosides.

ACTIONS: Alterative, expectorant, antispasmodic.

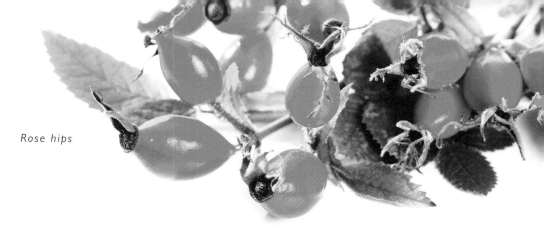

Rose hips

INDICATIONS: Red clover is one of the most useful remedies for children with skin problems. It may be used with complete safety in any case of childhood eczema. It may also be of value in other chronic skin conditions such as psoriasis. While being most useful with children, it can also be of value for adults. The expectorant and antispasmodic action gives this remedy a role in the treatment of coughs and bronchitis, but especially in whooping cough. As an alterative it is indicated in a wide range of problems when approached in a holistic sense.

PREPARATION AND DOSAGE: Infusion: pour a cup of boiling water onto 1–3 teaspoonfuls of the dried herb and leave to infuse for 10–15 minutes. This should be drunk three times a day. Tincture: take ½–1¼ teaspoons of the tincture three times a day.

ROSE HIPS *Rosa canina*
Family: Rosaceae

PART USED: The fruit (hips) and seeds of the dog rose.

COLLECTION: The hips are collected in the fall.

CONSTITUENTS: Vitamin C, tannins, pectin, carotene, fruit acids, fatty oil.

ACTIONS: Nutrient, mild laxative, mild diuretic, mild astringent.

INDICATIONS: Rose hips provide one of the best natural and freely available sources of vitamin C. They will help the body's defenses against infections and especially the development of colds. They make an excellent spring tonic and aid in general debility and exhaustion. They will help in cases of constipation and mild gallbladder problems as well as conditions of the kidney and bladder.

PREPARATION AND DOSAGE: The decoction or syrup may be taken freely. Decoction: put 2½ teaspoonfuls of the cut hips in a cup of water, bring to a boil, and simmer gently for 10 minutes. Syrup: to make a syrup, see the preparation of herbs (page 49). For this or any other culinary preparation, it is important to remove the seeds from the hips as well as the fine, brittle hairs found at one end. Tincture: take ½–¾ teaspoon three times a day.

ROSEMARY *Rosmarinus officinalis*
Family: Lamiaceae

PART USED: Leaves and twigs.

COLLECTION: Gather leaves throughout summer, but they are at their best during flowering time.

CONSTITUENTS: 1 percent volatile oil, including borneol, linalool, camphene, cineole, and camphor; tannins, bitter principle, resins.

ACTIONS: Carminative, aromatic, antispasmodic, antidepressive, antiseptic, rubefacient, parasiticide.

INDICATIONS: Rosemary acts as a circulatory and nervine stimulant, which in addition to the toning and calming effect on digestion makes it a remedy suitable for psychological tension. This may show, for instance, as flatulent dyspepsia, headache, or depression associated with debility. Externally, it may be used to ease muscular pain, sciatica, and neuralgia. It acts as a stimulant to the hair follicles and the oil may be used in premature baldness.

PREPARATION AND DOSAGE: Infusion: pour a cup of boiling water onto 1–2 teaspoonfuls of the dried herb and leave to infuse for 10–15 minutes. This should be drunk three times a day. Tincture: take ¼–½ teaspoon of the tincture three times a day.

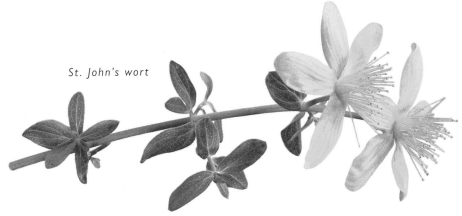

St. John's wort

SAGE *Salvia officinalis*
Family: Lamiaceae

PART USED: Leaves.

COLLECTION: Sage can be grown on a windowsill if kept in a sunny position.

ACTIONS: Astringent, stimulant, antiseptic, carminative, antispasmodic, nervine, strengthening tonic for women.

INDICATIONS: Take for depression and nervous exhaustion, post-viral fatigue, and general debility. Use for anxiety and confusion in elderly people, or accompanying exhaustion and weakened states. Drink sage tea for indigestion, wind, loss of appetite, and mucus on the stomach. Take cold tincture for excessive sweating and night sweats, or weak lungs with persistent and recurrent coughs and allergies. Use as a tea or compress for menopausal hot flashes, menstrual cramps, and premenstrual painful breasts. Cold sage tea taken every few hours will usually dry up breast milk. Use as a gargle and mouthwash for sore throats, laryngitis, tonsillitis, mouth ulcers, and inflamed and tender gums. Use as an antiseptic wash for dirty wounds that are slow to heal.

PREPARATION AND DOSAGE: Traditionally, one cup a day maintains health in old age. Gargling: for an extra-strength gargle, add 5 drops of tincture of myrrh (from pharmacies or herb stores) to a cup of sage tea. Tincture: 4 teaspoons daily, in a little water.

ST. JOHN'S WORT *Hypericum perforatum*
Family: Hypericaceae

PART USED: Aerial parts.

COLLECTION: The entire plant above ground should be collected when in flower and dried.

CONSTITUENTS: Glycosides, including rutin; volatile oil, tannins, resin, pectin.

ACTIONS: Anti-inflammatory, astringent, vulnerary, sedative.

INDICATIONS: Taken internally, St. John's wort has a sedative and pain-reducing effect, which gives it a place in the treatment of neuralgia, anxiety, tension, and similar problems. It is especially regarded as an herb to use where there are menopausal changes triggering irritability and anxiety. It is recommended, however, that it not be used when there is marked depression. In addition to neuralgic pain, it will ease fibrositis, sciatica, and rheumatic pain. Externally, it is a valuable healing and anti-inflammatory remedy. As a lotion, it will speed the healing of wounds and bruises, varicose veins, and mild burns. The oil is especially useful for the healing of sunburn.

PREPARATION AND DOSAGE: Infusion: pour a cup of boiling water onto 1–2 teaspoonfuls of the dried herb and infuse for 10–15 minutes. Drink three times a day. Tincture: take ¼–¾ teaspoon three times a day.

TARRAGON *Artemisia dracunculus*
Family: Asteraceae

PART USED: Leaves.

COLLECTION: Tarragon can be grown on a windowsill if kept in a sunny position.

CONSTITUENTS: Eugenol.

ACTIONS: Anti-inflammatory.

INDICATIONS: Tarragon is rich in immune-boosting antioxidants, and minerals such as calcium, iron, and manganese, contributing to healthy bones, blood, and skin. Also known as dragon wort, in folk traditions its cooling properties make it a popular remedy for

In folk traditions tarragon's cooling properties make it a popular remedy for premenstrual syndrome.

premenstrual syndrome and menopausal hot flashes, as well as for a variety of ailments from hiccups to carpal tunnel syndrome, and to aid sleep. The leaves may also help relieve toothache.

PREPARATION AND DOSAGE: Infusion: pour a cup of boiling water onto 1 teaspoonful of the herb and infuse for 10–15 minutes. Drink one cup to relieve hiccups or at bedtime to aid healthy sleep. For toothache, chew a leaf or drink a cup of infusion.

THUJA *Thuja occidentalis*
Family: Cupressaceae

PART USED: Young twigs.

COLLECTION: The twigs of this evergreen conifer can be gathered all year round, but are best during the summer.

CONSTITUENTS: 1 percent volatile oil, including thujone; flavonoid glycoside, mucilage, tannins.

ACTIONS: Expectorant, stimulant to smooth muscles, diuretic, astringent, alterative.

INDICATIONS: Thuja's main action is due to its stimulating and alterative volatile oil. In bronchial catarrh, thuja combines expectoration with a systemic stimulation beneficial if there is also heart weakness. Thuja should be avoided where the cough is due to overstimulation, as in dry, irritable coughs. Thuja has a specific reflex action on the uterus and may help in delayed menstruation. Where urinary incontinence occurs due to loss of muscle tone, thuja may be used. It has a role to play in the treatment of psoriasis and rheumatism. Externally, it may be used to treat warts. It is reported to counteract the ill effects of smallpox vaccination. A marked antifungal effect is found if used externally for ringworm and thrush.

PREPARATION AND DOSAGE: Infusion: pour a cup of boiling water onto 1 teaspoonful of the dried herb and infuse for 10–15 minutes. Drink three times a day. Tincture: take ¼–½ teaspoon three times a day.

CAUTION: Avoid during pregnancy.

THYME *Thymus vulgaris*
Family: Lamiaceae

PART USED: Leaves and flowering tops.

COLLECTION: The flowering branches should be collected between June and August on a dry, sunny day. The leaves are stripped off the dried branches.

CONSTITUENTS: More than 1 percent volatile oil, which includes thymol, carvacrol, cymol, linalool, borneol; bitter principles, tannins, flavonoids, triterpenoids.

ACTIONS: Carminative, antimicrobial, antispasmodic, expectorant, astringent, anthelmintic.

INDICATIONS: With its high content of volatile oil, thyme makes a good carminative for use in dyspepsia and sluggish digestion. This oil is also a strongly antiseptic substance, which explains many of thyme's uses. It can be used externally as a lotion for infected wounds, but also internally for respiratory and digestive infections. It may be used as a gargle in laryngitis and tonsillitis, easing sore throats and soothing irritable coughs. It is an excellent cough remedy, producing expectoration and reducing unnecessary spasm. It may be used in bronchitis, whooping cough, and asthma. As a gentle astringent, use for childhood diarrhea and bed-wetting.

PREPARATION AND DOSAGE: Infusion: pour a cup of boiling water onto 2 teaspoonfuls of the dried herb and infuse for 10 minutes. Drink three times a day. Tincture: take ½–¾ teaspoon three times a day.

VALERIAN *Valeriana officinalis*
Family: Valerianaceae

PART USED: Rhizome and roots.

COLLECTION: The roots are unearthed in the late fall. Clean thoroughly and dry in the shade.

CONSTITUENTS: Volatile oil, including valerianic acid, isovalerianic acid, borneol, pinene, camphene; volatile alkaloids.

ACTIONS: Sedative, hypnotic, antispasmodic, hypotensive, carminative.

INDICATIONS: Valerian is one of the most useful relaxing nervines that is available to us. This fact is recognized by orthodox medicine as is shown by its inclusion in many pharmacopoeias as a sedative. It may safely be used to reduce tension and anxiety, overexcitability, and hysterical states. It is an effective aid in insomnia, producing a natural healing sleep. As an antispasmodic herb, it will aid in the relief of cramps and intestinal colic and will also be useful for the cramps and pain of periods. As a pain reliever, it is most indicated where that pain is associated with tension. Valerian can also also help in migraine and rheumatic pain.

PREPARATION AND DOSAGE: Infusion: pour a cup of boiling water onto 1–2 teaspoonfuls of the root and leave to infuse for 10–15 minutes. This should be drunk when needed. Tincture: take ½–¾ teaspoon of the tincture three times a day.

VERVAIN *Verbena officinalis*
Family: Labiatae

PART USED: Aerial parts.

COLLECTION: The herb should be collected just before the flowers open, usually in July. Dry quickly.

CONSTITUENTS: Bitter glycosides called verbenalin; essential oil, mucilage, tannins.

ACTIONS: Nervine tonic, sedative, antispasmodic, diaphoretic, possible galactagogue, hepatic.

INDICATIONS: Vervain will strengthen the nervous system while relaxing any tension and stress. It can be used to ease depression and melancholia, especially when this follows illness such as influenza. Vervain may be used to help in seizure and hysteria. As a diaphoretic, it can be used in the early stages of fevers. As a hepatic remedy, it will be of help in inflammation of the gallbladder and jaundice. It may be used as a mouthwash against tooth decay and gum disease.

PREPARATION AND DOSAGE: Infusion: pour a cup of boiling water onto 1–3 teaspoonfuls of the dried herb and leave to infuse for 10–15 minutes. This should be drunk three times a day. Tincture: take ½–¾ teaspoon of the tincture three times a day.

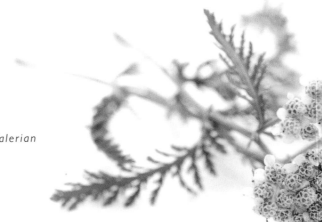

Valerian

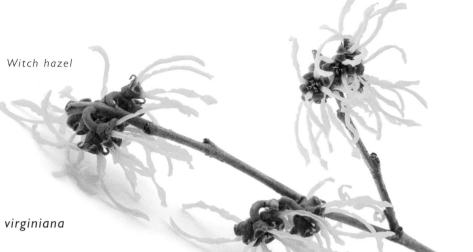

Witch hazel

WITCH HAZEL *Hamamelis virginiana*
Family: Hamamelidaceae

PART USED: Bark or leaves.

COLLECTION: The leaves can be gathered throughout the summer and dried quickly to ensure that they do not become discolored. The bark is gathered in the spring after sprouting.

CONSTITUENTS: Rich in tannins and gallic acid, bitters, traces of volatile oil.

ACTIONS: Astringent.

INDICATIONS: This herb can be found in most households in the form of distilled witch hazel. It is the most applicable and easy-to-use astringent for common usage. As with all astringents, this herb may be used wherever there has been bleeding, both internally or externally. It is especially useful in the easing of hemorrhoids. It has a deserved reputation in the treatment of bruises and inflamed swellings, also with varicose veins. Witch hazel will control diarrhea and aid in the easing of dysentery.

PREPARATION AND DOSAGE: Infusion: pour a cup of boiling water onto 1 teaspoonful of the dried leaves and leave to infuse for 10–15 minutes. This should be drunk three times a day. Ointment: witch hazel can be made into an excellent ointment. Tincture: take ¼–½ teaspoon of the tincture three times a day.

YARROW *Achillea millefolium*
Family: Asteraceae

PART USED: Aerial parts.

COLLECTION: The whole of the plant above ground should be gathered when in flower between June and September.

CONSTITUENTS: Up to 0.5 percent volatile oil, flavonoids, tannins, bitter alkaloid.

ACTIONS: Diaphoretic, hypotensive, astringent, diuretic, antiseptic.

INDICATIONS: Yarrow is one of the best diaphoretic herbs and is a standard remedy for aiding the body to deal with fevers. It lowers blood pressure due to a dilation of the peripheral vessels. It stimulates the digestion and tones the blood vessels. As a urinary antiseptic, it is indicated in infections such as cystitis. Used externally, it will aid in the healing of wounds. It is considered to be a specific in thrombotic conditions associated with high blood pressure.

PREPARATION AND DOSAGE: Infusion: pour 1 cup of boiling water onto 1–2 teaspoonfuls of the dried herb and leave to infuse for 10–15 minutes. This should be drunk hot three times a day. When feverish, it should be drunk hourly. Tincture: take ½–¾ teaspoon of the tincture three times a day.

HOME HERBAL MEDICINE ESSENTIALS

In the same way that you have a traditional first-aid kit at home, it's also good to have some herbal medicine essentials on hand when needs arise. In some cases you might have the raw ingredients or dried herbs available to create a remedy, but it's also useful to have some ready-made herbal products in your home herbal medicine box.

Aloe vera gel

The discomfort of burns, sunburn, and stings can be eased by applying aloe vera to the skin. If you have a plant, you can simply cut a leaf off and squeeze out the gel-like goodness, but for times when you've no plant available, packaged aloe vera gel is a good staple to have.

Arnica

Arnica is great for helping to encourage healing, whether from bumps, knocks, or sprains, and to speed up the progress of bruises, swellings, and muscular aches. You do have to be careful not to apply it to broken skin though, as it can cause irritation, so specially formulated tubes of arnica cream are useful to keep in your herbal medicine box. You could also consider arnica balm, which can be massaged into the skin, or homeopathic arnica tablets in doses such as 6x and 30x, which can be safely taken internally.

Calendula cream

Calendula cream is made from marigold plants and is useful to have in stock if you frequently suffer from dry, flaky, rough, or chapped skin. The soothing cream helps to hydrate, nourish, and protect skin, but shouldn't be applied to any areas of broken skin.

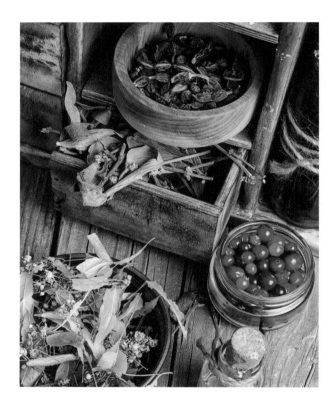

Chickweed cream

Chickweed cream is useful as it can help to soothe the skin after insect stings, sunburn, or minor burns.

Clove oil

Clove oil is handy to have in case you experience any toothache. Simply put a few drops on a cotton pad and hold it against the affected tooth or gum.

Crystallized ginger

Ginger is renowned for helping ease feelings of nausea. You can use it in many different forms— fresh ginger made into a tea, or in tablet form—but crystallized ginger is handy to keep in store and lasts a long time. If you feel nauseous, simply pop a small piece in your mouth and suck it slowly.

Echinacea

Echinacea tablets or syrup are good to have on hand ready for the first sign of a cold, cough, sore throat, or flu. It helps support your immune system and fight infections.

Eucalyptus oil

Eucalyptus is a common ingredient in vapor rubs and can help ease sinus congestion. Eucalyptus oil can be added to a bowl of hot water, so you can make your own facial steam bath. Don't apply the undiluted oil to your skin.

Garlic capsules

Garlic can help boost the immune system and ward off early signs of coughs or catarrh. You can cook with garlic and add it as an ingredient in food, but capsules can be useful too.

Peppermint capsules

Peppermint is good for digestive problems such as indigestion, wind, or nausea, and peppermint capsules are readily available. Alternatively, try peppermint tea.

Rescue Remedy®

Rescue Remedy® is a flower essence remedy that was originally developed by Dr. Edward Bach. It contains five flower essences and is designed to be used in times of emotional demand, such as when you're experiencing shock, anxiety, worry, or trauma after receiving bad news. The original product comes in the form of a diluted alcohol solution in a dropper bottle, where you put a few drops under your tongue. It's now available in various other forms, such as a spray and pastilles, which are alcohol-free.

Slippery elm bark

Slippery elm bark is a remedy that comes from the inner part of the *Ulmus rubra* tree and it's used for minor digestive complaints. Tablets and capsules are available and are convenient to keep in your home herbal medicine box.

Tea tree

Tea tree oil comes from the Australian tea tree and contains natural antiseptic and antifungal properties. Tea tree gels and creams can be used for treating fungal infections such as athlete's foot, acne, dandruff, or head lice.

Witch hazel

Witch hazel has natural anti-inflammatory properties and can be used to ease bruises, grazes, sunburn, and minor burns.

HERBAL REMEDIES FOR FIRST AID

It's useful to have herbs or homemade herbal remedies on hand alongside a traditional first-aid kit to help treat common minor ailments.

Burns

If you're going to have any houseplant in your home, make it an aloe vera plant. Keep an aloe vera plant on a windowsill in your kitchen and you'll be well equipped to deal with accidental minor burns. Simply cut a fresh leaf from the plant, squeeze out the gel inside, and apply a layer of it to the affected area of skin. It also works well as a remedy for sunburn.

Grazes

For minor grazes, first clean the wound using warm water. If it's on a hand or finger, place under a running tap; for other parts of the body, gently dab with a piece of absorbent cotton soaked in warm water. To ensure all dirt is removed from a graze, always wipe from the center to the edges. If a graze is bleeding or looks like it's going to bleed, press a clean piece of gauze over the area for a few minutes and it should stop.

There are lots of herbal creams and ointments that have antiseptic properties and are ideal for using on grazes, including ready-made creams that you can buy and keep in your home herbal medicine box, and others you can make yourself, such as tea tree, echinacea, and St. John's wort. Calendula and chamomile creams are both gentle on the skin and can help relieve the initial discomfort of a graze. If you don't have any cream on hand, you could also improvise and use a chamomile herbal tea bag, moistened in cold water and applied to the affected area.

Calendula balm

3 cups chopped calendula flowers
1 cup olive oil infused with tea tree, peppermint, and lavender
¾ cup of beeswax or vegan wax alternative

Put the chopped calendula flowers in a pan and cover with the infused olive oil. Simmer for 30–45 minutes, until the flowers have softened. Use a fine sieve or colander to strain the flowers out of the liquid, then put the liquid back into a clean pan over low heat. Add the beeswax and stir gently until all the wax has melted. Remove from the heat and pour the salve into jars or small cans (this amount should fill one large jar or several small cans). Let it set for 30 minutes, then pop it in the fridge. The balm can be used to help soothe the discomfort of skin grazes, as well as bites and stings and other minor skin concerns. It's a very good all-purpose balm to make and keep at home for skin-soothing needs.

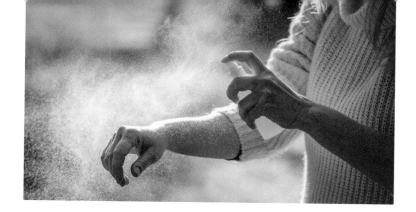

Bites and stings

Whether you're out and about, on vacation, or at home in your garden, insect bites and stings are common. Most are harmless, but even the tiniest bite from an insect can cause considerable pain and discomfort. There are various herbs available that you can use to help ease the discomfort and swelling of bites and stings.

Lemon balm can be soothing for uncomfortable bites too. Pick and chop some fresh leaves and make a poultice to apply to the bite site. For minor stings, try applying chamomile or calendula cream to your skin, as they can both help to reduce inflammation and encourage the natural healing process. They can be bought at health-food stores, but you could also try making your own calendula balm (see page 84).

If you're out in the countryside and get stung—either by nettles or an insect—then the age-old method of using a dock leaf is a good first port of call. Find a large dock leaf and press or rub it on the affected area of skin, squeezing the leaf gently to ensure all the natural juices come out.

Preventing bites and stings

If you're eating outside, entertaining, on a camping trip, or having a barbecue, you can help ward off unwanted insects by burning a citronella candle. Place it somewhere safe and remember to blow it out when you go back inside. Eucalyptus and cedarwood essential oils may also help to deter insects. If you're out walking, try sprinkling tea tree or lemon balm oils on your clothing as this may go some way to helping prevent unwanted bites.

Be aware that bites and stings can sometimes become infected—if you have any areas of redness or the symptoms are worsening, always consult a medical practitioner.

Chamomile cooler

Fill a cup halfway with fresh or dried chamomile flowers and fill to the top with cold water. Place in the fridge for half an hour to cool, then strain off the flowers. Soak a clean piece of gauze in the remaining liquid and apply it to the affected skin, holding it on the bite and resoaking in the herbal liquid as needed. Afterward, wipe away any excess with a clean cloth. The chamomile cooler can be reused throughout the day as needed and can help to reduce skin irritation and inflammation.

Thyme ice pack for mosquito bites

Add several sprigs of thyme to a bowl of water, then decant it into an ice-cube tray. Once frozen, wrap one ice cube in a clean dish towel and apply it to the site of the bite. Thyme has natural antibacterial and antifungal properties and can help ease the extreme itching that a mosquito bite can cause.

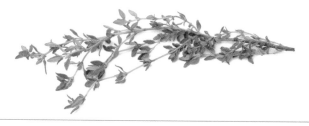

HERBAL REMEDIES FOR COMMON AILMENTS

Herbal remedies can be used to help ease the symptoms of common minor ailments, either as an alternative to other medication or used alongside in a holistic manner. In many cases you can make your own remedies using easily accessible garden herbs, although it's always useful to have the fallback of being able to purchase ready-made natural remedies too.

Colds, coughs, and sore throats

Colds, coughs, and sore throats are common ailments, especially during the colder winter months. They can come on quickly, so it's useful to be prepared with herbal remedies.

Elderberry is a traditional hedgerow remedy for coughs and colds, as it's believed to help support the immune system. If you keep a stash of dried elderberries in your herbal store cupboard, you can whip up a batch of elderberry syrup when needed. It's useful to take when you have symptoms, as well as to boost your immunity and try to ward off a cold.

Warm drinks are soothing for a sore throat and it's important to keep your fluid intake up to prevent dryness from coughing, but rather than your usual tea, why not swap it for an herbal tea instead? Marshmallow tea, made from the leaves and roots

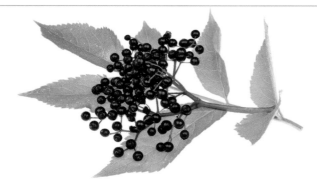

Elderberry syrup

4½ cups dried elderberries
12 cups water
½ cup honey

In advance, put the elderberries in a pan and pour the water over them, ideally leaving them to soak overnight. Heat the elderberries and soaking water and let them simmer for 30–40 minutes, then turn off the heat. When the liquid has cooled, strain out the berries using a fine sieve. Stir in as much of the honey as desired; this is to help the taste, as elderberries can be very tart. Decant the syrup into glass bottles, then store them in your fridge. Take 2 tablespoons as required, but don't take more than four times a day.

Head cold relieving steam bath

To make a steam bath, chop a bunch (approximately 1 cup) of peppermint and eucalyptus and put the herbs in a bowl. Pour 3 cups freshly boiled hot water over them. Drape a towel over your head and lean over the bowl, taking deep breaths of the fragrant steam. If you don't have fresh herbs on hand, you could use dried, or substitute the herbs with 5 drops of essential oil.

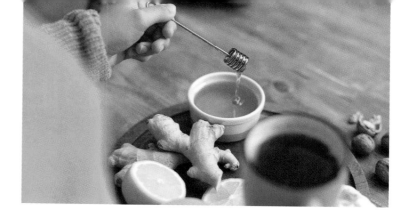

of the marshmallow plant, has anti-inflammatory properties and could help to reduce the irritation caused by coughs and sore throats. If you don't have access to a marshmallow plant, look for ready-made marshmallow tea in a health-food store.

Thyme tea is also worth trying for a cold and cough, as it's believed it can help relax the muscles in the throat. Some of the ingredients of traditional herbal remedies for colds, such as eucalyptus and peppermint, are still used in store-bought products today, and rightly so. If you're suffering from a stuffy nose and head cold, the menthol in peppermint can help your breathing become easier, and the expectorant properties of eucalyptus can loosen mucus and help clear blocked sinuses. Steam inhalations are one of the best ways of utilizing the power of menthol.

If you enjoy a hot bath before bed, you could also add eucalyptus and peppermint to water, or pop them in a muslin bag and put that into the water.

Nausea

Ginger is one of the most popular traditional remedies for nausea. Studies into the use of ginger compared to antinausea medications have found it can be just as effective, plus it has the bonus of having fewer side effects.

There are various ways in which you can use ginger to help ease nausea. If you have root ginger on hand, you can make fresh ginger tea by steeping a slice of ginger root in boiling water, before drinking when it's cool enough. Or you could simply buy ready-made ginger tea bags. Small pieces of crystallized ginger can be sucked slowly if you feel nauseous, or you could even try eating a ginger cookie.

Other useful herbs for treating nausea include lemon balm, chamomile, peppermint (particularly if it's linked to digestive problems), and dandelion.

Headaches

Willow bark extract is famous for being used in the development of the painkiller aspirin. Its anti-inflammatory and pain-relieving properties make it a practical solution for naturally treating headaches. You should be able to find natural willow bark tablets in your health-food store; sometimes it's even possible to find chewable pieces of willow bark to buy.

Coriander seeds are traditionally used in Ayurvedic medicine to relieve headaches related to sinus pain. If you like the taste of the seeds, chewing a few could help relieve your headache pain. Otherwise, make yourself an herbal infusion by adding some coriander seeds to a mug of boiling water.

Products containing menthol are often available for treating headaches, but you can access the natural properties yourself using herbs such as peppermint and eucalyptus as a tea infusion. Peppermint tea bags are widely available too, and useful if you don't have any fresh herbs. You could also try making a steam bath with peppermint, eucalyptus, or rosemary, as inhaling the aromatic steam may help to clear your head.

If any of your symptoms persist or worsen, or you develop a high fever, always consult a medical practitioner.

HERBAL REMEDIES FOR STRESS, SLEEP, AND ANXIETY

Issues regarding stress, sleep, and anxiety are common and often intertwined—you may feel anxious if you can't sleep, and lack of sleep doesn't help stress, for example—and there are various herbal remedies that can play a part in easing symptoms.

Do keep in mind that a holistic approach to health focuses on the importance of finding the underlying cause and not just purely treating the symptoms. Often causes of issues such as stress, sleep problems, and anxiety run deeper beyond the surface and it's worth working on trying to identify the causes too, especially for longer-lasting and more effective treatments. As well as herbal remedies, you could explore lifestyle changes or mind-body therapies that may be beneficial, such as taking more exercise or meditation.

Stress-calming tea

Mix together 1 teaspoon of chamomile flowers, 1 teaspoon of valerian root, ½ teaspoon of lavender flowers, 1 teaspoon of lemon balm, and 1 teaspoon of holy basil (optional). Steep the herbs in boiling water for 15 minutes, then strain and drink to help relieve feelings of stress.

Valerian tea

Put ½ teaspoon chopped dried valerian root in a cup of boiling hot water and steep for 10–15 minutes. Strain out the herb, reheat the drink, and enjoy before bed. This remedy tends to work better if you have it regularly, so try and make valerian tea a part of your daily bedtime routine.

Lavender pillow mist

Lavender sprays are widely available to purchase, but can be made just as easily at home.

2 tablespoons dried lavender flowers
30 drops of lavender essential oil
2 tablespoons witch hazel
Water

Put all the ingredients into a jug, stir well, then decant it into a brown glass spray bottle. Keep the bottle out of bright light to preserve the potency of the spray, then use on your pillow at night.

Anti-anxiety balm

5 tablespoons lavender, basil, and lemon balm infused oil
1 teaspoon beeswax or vegan alternative
4 drops of neroli essential oil
4 drops of rose otto essential oil
4 drops of sweet orange essential oil

Heat the infused oil over low heat and add the beeswax. Stir until melted. Stir in the essential oils, then pour the mixture into small jars. Leave to cool and harden. When ready, apply the balm to your temples and wrists when you feel anxious. The herbs and oils should have a calming effect.

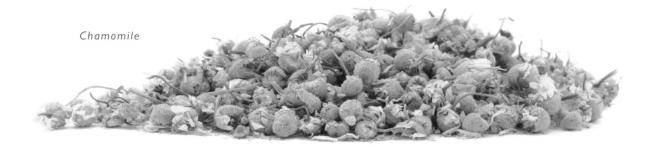

Chamomile

Stress

The calming herbs chamomile and valerian are useful to keep in stock, either grown freshly in pots or kept in your cupboard in dried form, as they're both good for tackling stress. Valerian has natural analgesic and antibacterial properties, whereas chamomile contains natural phenolic acids, quinones, and antioxidants. From an herbal perspective, they can be combined together to make healing remedies or used individually to promote a relaxed state of mind.

The herb tulsi, otherwise known as holy basil, is an Ayurvedic herb that's native to Southeast Asia. If you're able to get your hands on some, it's a very useful ingredient to have on hand to help deal with issues such as stress and anxiety. You can add the dried herb to teas or make tinctures from it.

Sleep

Valerian has been used to aid sleep for centuries. Look on the shelves of any health-food store and you'll find various valerian remedies available that could help with sleep problems. The ready-made tablets can be effective, but you can also make your own remedies using valerian root.

Lavender is renowned for its calming properties and is a popular herb to aid sleep. There are many ways to access the soothing benefits of lavender, from having a lavender bath before bed, spraying lavender on your bedding at night, or by massaging lavender balm into the soles of your feet, your forehead, or arms before going to bed. You could even get creative and make a small lavender pillow, stuffed with dried lavender, and keep it on your bed to naturally infuse your bedroom with the floral aroma.

Anxiety

The calming floral scent of lavender may also help relieve feelings of anxiety, so you could try using lavender pillow mist if you're feeling anxious. You can spray the mist on your clothes so the scent goes with you wherever you are or whatever you're doing.

Lemon balm and chamomile are both calming and can be helpful to ease mild feelings of anxiety. To make lemon balm tea, infuse 1 tablespoon of the herb in a mug of boiling water for 10–15 minutes, then strain, reheat, and drink it. Stir in 1 teaspoon of honey, if desired.

The herb passionflower, or *Passiflora*, contains naturally occurring phytochemicals and the alkaloid harmine, which can have a calming effect on the mind. Remedies include tea, tinctures, sprays, or ready-made tablets. To brew passionflower tea, infuse 1 tablespoon of the herb in a mug of boiling water and let it steep for 10–15 minutes. Strain, warm, and enjoy. As well as enjoying a single herb tea, you could pair it with complementary herbs, such as valerian or lemon balm.

Flower remedies, which tend to work on a more subtle emotional level, are also good for use with issues such as anxiety.

NOTE

If you are on any other medication for stress, sleep, anxiety, or other health conditions, always check with a medical practitioner first, as some herbs can react with medication.

MAKING HEALING HERBAL TEAS AND TISANES

One of the most accessible ways of making an easy herbal remedy is to create herbal teas or tisanes. Herbal teas have been used for centuries to act as a form of natural remedy, or simply as an alternative brew to drink, and they're still a popular drink today.

At the most basic level, simply cutting a few sprigs of fresh herbs and popping them into a mug of boiling water can create a simple herb tea. But with extra care and attention you can create drinks with more depth and flavor, that you can enjoy hot or cold, and herbal mixes that you'll return to time and time again. Tisanes or herbal teas can be made from various parts of herbs, including the flowers, leaves, bark, berries, or seeds. For example:

- Leaves are commonly chosen when using lemon balm, mint, or sage
- Seeds are used when making fennel, caraway, or cardamom teas
- Flowers are used to create chamomile, lavender, or rose teas
- Bark is used in the case of slippery elm or cinnamon teas
- Berries are used in the case of elderberry, hawthorn, or juniper teas

How to make herbal teas

The two main methods to make herbal teas are an infusion or a decoction. For an infusion, boiling water is poured over fresh or dried herbs and they're left to steep for a minimum of 10 minutes. As a rough guide, on average you'll need 1–1½ cups dried herbs and a generous 2 cups boiled water to make 2–3 mugs. If you're using fresh herbs, the quantities will differ, as there's more water in freshly picked plants, so aim for around 5–6 cups fresh herbs per 2 generous cups boiled water. After the herbs have steeped, you can strain out the plant matter, and consume it.

The method of making a decoction involves simmering the herbs in a pan for 15–20 minutes over low heat. It's more suitable for the tougher parts of herbs, such as the bark, roots, and berries. On average you'll need approximately 1 cup herbs and a generous 3 cups water, but the exact measurements differ depending on which herbs you're using.

Creating herbal infusions

One of the benefits of herbal tea infusions is that the herbal base doesn't have to be made fresh as and when you want it. Instead, you can mix up your choice of herbs in advance and store them ready for when you fancy a fresh brew. Dried herbs are best for this, and for improved depth of flavor, a mix of herbs typically works well.

A wide variety of herbs are suitable for use in infusions, including: angelica, basil, borage, burdock, chamomile, chickweed, daisy, dandelion, echinacea, elderflower, lemon balm, marigold, meadowsweet, oregano, rosemary, St. John's wort, thyme, vervain, and yarrow.

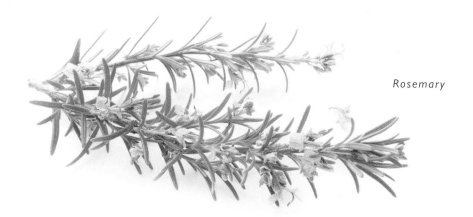

Rosemary

To find combinations you like, experiment! Aim to pick between three and five herbs that could help certain ailments such as sleep, headaches, or digestion, or alternatively pick flavors that you like and that should work well together. Mix up small quantities to start with, keeping a note of all the ingredients, and keep them in airtight jars to brew as required. To brew, spoon 1–2 teaspoons per mug. Once you find particular combinations that you love, you can make up bigger batches to keep in stock. To add sweetness to any infusions, stir in a teaspoon of honey.

Digestive herbal tea blend

1 cup dried peppermint
½ cup fennel seeds
½ cup coriander seeds

Chop the dried peppermint and mix all the ingredients together. Store in an airtight jar. Infuse for at least 10 minutes for a tea to support your digestive system.

Calming herbal blend

1 cup lemon balm leaves
1 cup chamomile flowers
½ cup dried passionflower
¼ cup dried spearmint
¼ cup dried valerian

Finely chop all the dry ingredients and mix together. Infuse for at least 10 minutes when needed for a calming brew.

Concentration blend

1 cup dried peppermint
½ cup dried rosemary
½ cup dried ginkgo biloba
¼ cup dried ginseng

Finely chop all the dry ingredients and mix together. Infuse for at least 10 minutes before drinking. This lovely combination of herbs could help boost concentration and help you focus more when you feel like you're flagging.

Refreshing summer tea

1 cup lemon balm leaves
½ cup dried eucalyptus
1 cup dried elderberries
½ cup dried lemon peel

Finely chop all the ingredients and mix together. This tea is ideal to drink warm, or poured over crushed ice with slices of fresh lemon for a refreshing summer drink.

Spicy fruit tea

3 tablespoons whole cloves
1 cinnamon stick
1 cup dried orange peel
1 cup dried orange mint
1 cup chamomile flowers
2 cups dried lemon verbena leaves

Grind the cloves and cinnamon to a fine mixture. Add to the orange peel and mint, then combine with the chamomile flowers and lemon verbena leaves. Store in an airtight jar. This spicy tea has aromas that evoke a feeling of comfort and coziness.

FLOWER ESSENCES

Flower essences, or flower remedies as they are more commonly known, are used therapeutically to harmonize the body, mind, and spirit. The essences are said to contain the life force of the flowers used to make them. Thousands of essences are available in health-food stores, and they work "vibrationally" on a mental and emotional level to relieve negative feelings, encourage the healing process, and balance the energy in the body.

What are flower essences?

Flower essences are ideal for home use, being simple to make and use. They are prepared in water and preserved with alcohol. Historically, flower water and the morning dew collected from flower petals were thought to be imbued with magical properties. That flower remedies work is indisputable for those who are regular users; but no one knows how, so there is still an element of magic associated with their use—even today, when our understanding of vibrational medicine is growing.

Flower remedies are so simple that they are often dismissed as a placebo. They do not work in any biochemical way, and because no physical part of the plant remains in the remedy, its properties and actions cannot be detected or analyzed as if it were a drug or herbal preparation. Therapists believe the remedies contain the energy, or imprint, of the plant from which it was made, and work in a way that is similar to homeopathic remedies. In this way a remedy is believed to provide the stimulus needed to kick-start your own healing mechanism.

Dr. Bach

Until recently, the name Dr. Edward Bach was almost synonymous with flower remedies. His set of thirty-eight remedies became the inspiration for the worldwide development of remedies. They are still the cornerstone of flower remedy therapy and easily available. While working in the London Homeopathic Hospital, just after the World War I, he noticed that people with similar attitudes often had similar complaints. He concluded that, independently of other factors, mood and a negative attitude predisposed people toward ill health, and that illness was a manifestation of a deeper disharmony or an indication that the personality was in conflict. Between 1928 and 1932 he identified seven main negative states and found the first twelve of the flower remedies he needed to address them.

Over the subsequent few years, Dr. Bach dedicated himself to finding natural remedies from the countryside, and by the time of his death he had made thirty-eight separate remedies.

His successors at his house in Oxfordshire, England, called Mount Vernon, continue to make his remedies today, and they are sold under the brand name of Bach Flower Remedies.

Other remedies

The Bach Flower Remedies are made from the trees and flowers Dr. Bach saw on his travels, which are native to England, with the exceptions of olive and vine. In the last twenty years, remedies from the United States and Australia have also been made.

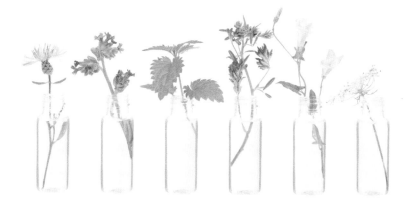

Sometimes they are called flower essences (do not confuse them with essential oils), but they are said to work in the same way as the original flower remedies.

They address the emotional self, unlocking repressions, liberating negativity, and encouraging positive well-being.

Seeing a professional

Flower remedies were created to be so simple to use that people could treat themselves. However, many practitioners of other disciplines—such as herbalism, homeopathy, and aromatherapy—use flower remedies to complement their own treatments, and a few flower essence therapists use the remedies exclusively.

Most therapists have their own ways of working. But every consultation should begin with an interview between you and the therapist. This can last from as little as 15 minutes to over an hour. During this time the therapist will explain the system to you if you do not already know how it works. He or she will ask why you have come to see a therapist and will listen while you talk about yourself and your worries. The therapist will observe your posture and appearance, and will listen to the tone of your voice and the way you say things, as these can be as revealing as what you say. While you chat, the therapist may take notes and ask questions to determine, by a process of elimination, which remedies would be best for you. He or she might ask questions about your fears, how you feel about your children or other family members, or how easily you give up when something you attempt does not work out. It is not enough for the therapist to know that you have a problem at home or at work.

At the end of the consultation the therapist will help you select the remedies. The number of remedies prescribed depends on the individual, but it is unlikely to be more than six, and will often be much fewer. Most people feel at least a little better at the end of the consultation because they have been able to talk through their problems.

The Dr. Edward Bach Foundation maintains an international register of qualified practitioners in the Bach Flower Remedies. A list of practitioners may be obtained from the Bach Centre (see Resources and Further Reading on pages 298–299).

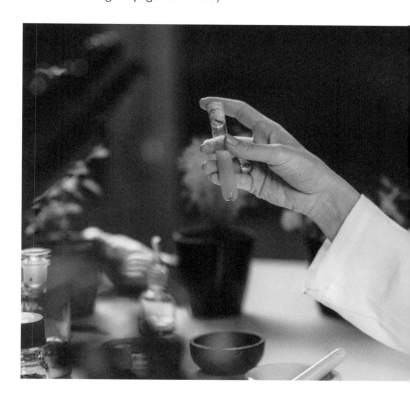

FLOWER ESSENCES FOR HEALTH AND WELL-BEING

When to use flower essences

Flower remedies are simple and effective, and they can be used to treat mental or emotional problems:

• To support in times of crisis
• To treat the emotional outlook produced by illness
• To address a particular recurring emotional or behavioral pattern
• To give strength during a brief emotional setback
• As a preventive remedy when things start to go out of balance

Remedies act swiftly for passing moods and there should be a quick improvement, although it may take months to start to change a long-standing pattern.

Choosing remedies

Successful treatment depends on accurate diagnosis. Get to know the different essences available and then aim to match the remedies to the individual character. If you find it hard to decide on a remedy, make a note of the one you think you need and then ask yourself the same questions you would ask anyone for whom you were prescribing:

• How do you feel?
• Why are you feeling like that?
• How do the symptoms affect you?
• What could have caused the problem?

Some people recommend that an appropriate affirmation is written down several times a day for a week while taking a remedy. An example of a positive affirmation for the clematis daydreamer would be: "I am awake (or becoming awake) and open to the experience of here and now."

Are they safe?

The remedies are not addictive or dangerous, nor do they interfere with any other form of treatment. They are suitable for people of all ages. Pregnant women and children can take them with confidence. Flower remedies are safe for young babies, should they need them.

Remedies and alcohol

Flower remedies and essences are preserved in alcohol. The amount of alcohol in a personal remedy made solely with water is minute, but it is enough to upset those who are alcohol-intolerant or recovering from alcoholism. Always check the status of those to whom you give a remedy. Thoughtlessness can do untold damage.

It is possible to remove the alcohol by putting the diluted drops of remedy in a boiling hot drink—the steam will evaporate the alcohol. Leave the remedy to cool before taking. Sip throughout the day.

Children and flower essences

Flower remedies are ideal for children. However, physical symptoms must be professionally treated. Consult a physician if in doubt. When treating children:

• Listen and do not trivialize children's emotional lives. Be calm and methodical.
• Notice the mood or address a previously known pattern. Give the remedy for a day or two, then reassess. Moods in children may change rapidly.
• If worried about a child (or other family member), take red chestnut, Rescue Remedy®, or any other

"I am awake (or becoming awake) and open to the experience of here and now."

remedy that seems relevant, to settle yourself before deciding on treatment.

• If the child is of breastfeeding age, give the remedy to the mother. It may also be put in the bath: for example, use impatiens to treat the hot and restless frustration of a teething baby.

• Support the parents if their child is unwell. For example, give Rescue Remedy® and walnut if the child is hospitalized.

• Treat the parents. Their emotional problems (even if suppressed) may be the root of a child's distress.

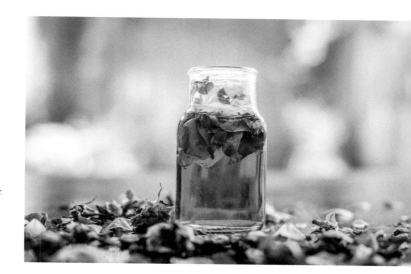

Making a personal remedy

The flower remedies or essences bought in a store are sold in stock bottles. They can be used straight from the bottle, but it is better to make a personal remedy mix. Sometimes a single flower remedy is needed, but in most cases two or more are combined.

Method

1. Decide on the remedies that are most applicable. If you think you need several, simplify to a maximum of seven covering immediate issues, and check again in a few weeks.

2. Put 2 drops of each remedy into a clean 1 fl. oz. amber glass dropper bottle. This is the standard amount, but read the label, as occasionally some of the newer essences suggest you use 4 or 7 drops.

3. If the remedies are to be used within a week, fill the bottle with clean spring water. If the remedies are to be taken for a prolonged period, add 1 teaspoon of brandy to the bottle and then fill with spring water.

4. Label the bottle with your name and the date. Give the remedy a title or a few words to remind you of the purpose. Keep remedies, like other medicines, out of the reach of children.

Dose

• The standard dose is 4 drops, on or under the tongue, four times a day.

• At times of crisis, 2 drops from the stock bottle can be put into a glass of water (or, in an emergency, any drink) and sipped as needed.

• If it is impossible to take anything by mouth, put the drops on the skin or in washing water.

MAKING YOUR OWN FLOWER ESSENCES

Basic rules

Before you begin to make your own remedies, consider these basic rules:

• Correct identification. Find the plant and site well before the day of picking. Make sure that it is legal to pick it or that you have the landowner's permission.
• Preparation. Collect the essential tools. Absolute cleanliness is vital. Wash your hands and rinse them several times. Clean utensils by boiling in spring or rain water for 20 minutes, and leave to drain and dry. Wrap them in a clean cloth to keep them ready.
• The day. For sun method remedies (see below), choose a warm, sunny day with no clouds. For boiling method remedies (see right), any bright, sunny day is good.

• On the day. Pick with respect. Pick flowers that you are drawn to. Pick from all sides of the plant, from the top and bottom branches of trees, or from a wide area with meadow plants. Work quickly so there is only a little time between picking the flowers and putting them into the water to make the remedy. If you need to carry the flowers, cover your palm with a large leaf (preferably from the plant being picked) to prevent the heat and oils from your hand contaminating the blossoms.
• Labeling. When you have finished making your remedy, label and date it clearly. Keep it in a cool, dark place, away from direct sunlight.

The sun method

This method is used for flowers other than tree blossoms. Pick when the flowers are coming into full bloom. This will depend on the climate, but the following can serve as a general guide:

• Early spring: oak, gorse, olive, vine
• Late spring: white chestnut, water violet
• Summer: rock water, mimulus, agrimony, rock rose, centaury
• Late summer: Scleranthus, wild oat, impatiens, chicory, vervain, clematis, heather
• Fall: cerato, gentian

A 3 fl. oz. bottle of mother tincture will last the average family many years. This recipe can make more, up to six bottles. Each 3 fl. oz. should contain ¼ cup of brandy and be made up as follows:

19-oz. bottle of spring or mineral water
Plain glass bowl
Natural and unbleached filter paper
3 fl. oz. amber bottle(s)
¼ cup brandy

Decide beforehand on the plants, where to pick from, and where to place the bowl (as close to the plants as possible, but away from shadows and possible contamination), then wait for a suitable sunny day. The best time for harvesting the plants is between 9:00 a.m. and midday. The flowers are dry from the dew, but not yet exhausted by the sun.

Put the water in the bowl, pick the flowers, and put them in the water as quickly as possible. Float

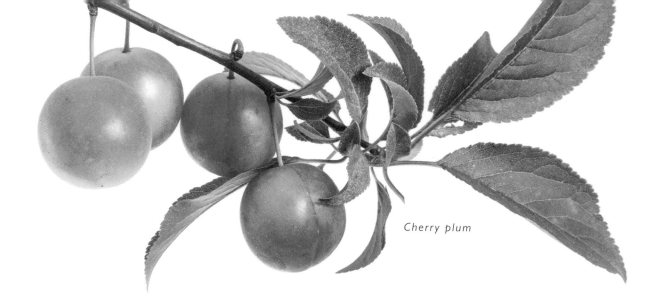

Cherry plum

the flowers on the water until the whole surface is covered. Use a twig or leaf to arrange them, not your fingers. Leave the bowl out in the open where it will receive direct sunshine for 3 hours.

Remove the flowers with a twig or leaf and filter the liquid. Pour ¼ cup of the water into a bottle with the brandy. Shake and label with the name "flower essence mother tincture" and date. This mother tincture will be used to prepare stock bottles and it will keep for many years. To prepare a stock bottle, put 2 drops of mother tincture into a 1 fl. oz. dropper bottle, and top up with brandy.

The boiling method

The boiling method is mainly used for the flowers of trees. In addition to the flowers, it is necessary to collect twigs that have a few leaves on them. Pick when the flowers are at their best:

• Early spring: cherry plum
• Mid-spring: elm, aspen
• Late spring: beech, chestnut bud, hornbeam, larch, walnut, star of Bethlehem, holly, crab apple, willow
• Early summer: red chestnut, pine, mustard
• Summer: honeysuckle, sweet chestnut, wild rose

3¼-quart saucepan with lid (use an enamel, glass, or stainless steel pan; avoid copper, aluminum, and Teflon-coated pans)
4¼ cups cold water (rain water or mineral water)
Natural and unbleached filter paper
Glass measuring jug
3 fl. oz. amber glass bottle(s) (up to six)
¼ cup brandy

If you are going to boil the remedy outside, check your camping stove and equipment.

Take everything into the field between 9:00 a.m. and 11:00 a.m. on a sunny day. Touch as little as possible. Pick twigs or flowers until the saucepan is three-quarters full. Put on the lid and take to the heat source as quickly as possible.

When the pan is on the heat, cover the flowers and twigs with the cold water and bring to a boil. Simmer for 30 minutes. Use a twig from the tree to push the flowers and twigs under the water.

Remove the pan from the heat and stand it outside to cool with the lid on. When cool, remove the twigs, then carefully filter the water into the jug.

Put ¼ cup of the flower water into an amber bottle with the brandy. Label with the name "flower essence mother tincture" and date. This is the mother tincture from which a stock bottle is made, as described under "The sun method" opposite.

COSMETICS AND SKIN CARE

Herbal remedies have been traditionally used for skin care and cosmetic purposes and are still as popular today as they were in the past. In fact, if you look at the ingredients of many store-bought skin-care and facial products, the chances are you'll see that they contain herbs and natural ingredients, although often alongside not-so-natural elements too. For the purest and most natural approach, though, you can't beat making your own skin-care products. You can make them up as you need them, or in advance, storing them in glass jars to keep them fresh until needed. As well as herbs, you'll need some basic cupboard ingredients.

Sugar scrubs

Sugar scrubs are made from a base of sugar—natural brown sugar or raw sugar are good—and can have a polishing effect that makes your skin glow after use. Sugar scrubs are particularly suitable for normal or combination skin; if you have sensitive skin, take care and do a skin patch test first to ensure it's not too harsh for you (if it doesn't suit, try an oat-based mask or scrub).

Relaxing lavender sugar scrub
1 cup sugar
½ cup coconut oil
½ cup dried lavender
1 teaspoon honey

Mix all the ingredients together in a bowl, then apply the mixture to your skin before rinsing it away. The coconut oil will help hydrate your skin, while the addition of honey will help add nourishment. The lavender will relax and calm you—this is a good scrub to use at night, before bed.

Salt scrubs

Salt scrubs are good for very dry, rough, or callused skin, such as on your knees, the soles of your feet, or on your elbows, as the salt grains tend to be harder and more abrasive in nature than sugar. If you have oily skin, the salt might help to balance the condition of your skin and could help dry it out. Avoid using salt scrubs on your face, particularly if you have sensitive skin. Always do a patch test first.

Both natural Dead Sea salt and Himalayan salt are good contenders for use in a salt scrub. Dead Sea salt contains up to sixty trace minerals, or micronutrients, and Himalayan salt has even more; together they can help the look and feel of skin, even before you add any herbs. Exfoliating your skin with salt helps to remove dead skin, improve circulation, and help your skin look brighter.

Invigorating rosemary salt scrub
1 cup Dead Sea or Himalayan salt
½ cup dried rosemary
½ cup almond or coconut oil

Mix all the ingredients together in a bowl until it forms a pastelike consistency. If you want it a bit thinner, add a drop more oil, or to thicken it, add more salt. Once made, store in a glass jar. Use the scrub in the shower or bath, where it will dissolve into your skin when it comes into contact with water. Alternatively, you can use it as a dry scrub as part of

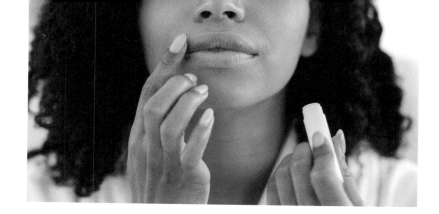

a home manicure or pedicure—scrub your hands or feet with it, then rinse with warm water.

Oat-based skin care

Skin masks made from a base of oats or cooked oatmeal are likely to be more suitable for dry or sensitive skin, as they are calming and less abrasive. Oats can help add much-needed moisture and nourishment to dry skin.

Calming oatmeal and chamomile mask
½ cup chamomile flowers
½ cup cooked oatmeal
1 teaspoon honey
1 cup warm water

Mix together the dried chamomile, cooked oatmeal, and honey. Slowly pour in the warm water, taking care to stir the ingredients as you do. You're looking to create a smooth and thick paste, so you may not need the entire cup—be guided by how the paste looks and feels. When it feels smooth and thick, apply it to your skin and gently massage it in. Leave on for approximately 5 minutes, then wash clean. The oatmeal in the mask will cleanse and moisturize your skin, while the gentle floral aroma of the chamomile could have a calming effect.

Lip balms

Lip balms are an essential skin-care product, especially during the winter months when lips can dry out even more than usual. You can make your own using beeswax or a vegan substitute wax, popping the mixture into small jars.

In advance, choose which herbs you'd like to include, as they need to be infused in an edible oil for a few days before; either pick a single herb or a combination. Good oils to use include avocado, almond, or sunflower; be aware that some oils, such as olive and coconut, have stronger aromas and could affect the flavor of your lip balm. Experiment and see what works best for you.

Soothing shea butter lip balm
½ cup beeswax
½ cup natural shea or cocoa butter
1 cup infused herb oil

Mix the ingredients together, then melt them gently in a pan over medium heat and stir. When all the ingredients have melted and combined, remove from the heat and pour into small jars. Your lip balms will need to cool for several hours before use and should be stored away from heat and direct sunlight—if they get too warm, they'll be at risk of melting.

Be creative and use these ideas to get started on making your own herbal skin-care products. A lot of the scrub bases can easily be adapted using other herbs or common home ingredients. For example, for an invigorating wake-up mask, you could try using coffee grounds with salt—the caffeine could get you going if you're feeling sluggish. Adding a drop or two of aromatherapy essential oils to the mixes not only adds extra fragrance, but the oils have their own benefits for the skin too.

HERBAL REMEDIES FOR THE HAIR

You don't need expensive salon products for your hair to look good—homemade herbal products can cleanse, moisturize, and soothe your hair and scalp too. Many herbs have traditionally been used for hair-care products due to their beneficial properties, and lots continue to be used as ingredients in branded products.

As a guide, if you have particular hair or scalp issues you're looking to improve, these are some of the herbs that could help:

• Dry hair: try comfrey, geranium, elderflower, burdock root, parsley, sage, or nettle
• Oily hair: try calendula, lemon balm, clary sage, mint, rosemary, or lavender
• Dry scalp and dandruff: try eucalyptus, lavender, peppermint, rosemary, sage, tea tree, nettle, burdock root, or thyme
• Itchy scalp: try chamomile, tea tree, or comfrey
• Fine or limp hair: try calendula, parsley, sage, nettle, or basil
• Hair growth: try ginseng, eucalyptus, basil, burdock root, or aloe vera

One of the key advantages of making your own herbal remedies for your hair is that you can experiment with different ingredients and see what suits your hair best—the results may surprise you! As with conventional hair-care products, you may find that you're best off varying the herbs you choose to use, as sometimes the benefits are less effective if you constantly use exactly the same remedies. Bear in mind that even though herbs are natural, they can still cause unexpected reactions, so it's always a good idea to do a patch test before putting anything new on your scalp. Try out your mixture on the inside of your elbow to see if the skin reacts over the next twenty-four hours. If there's no redness, itching, or other reactions, then it should be okay to use. If you have any doubts, or know you have sensitive skin or have had previous scalp issues, it might be best to avoid using homemade herbal remedies on your hair.

Herbal hair rinse

An herbal hair rinse can be used as an alternative to shampoo, or as a form of conditioner to use after shampooing your hair. Rosemary is traditionally added for those with brown hair, while chamomile is included if you have blond hair, with the idea being that these herbs will help to balance, enhance, and brighten the natural color of your hair. Rosemary is also stimulating and promotes circulation, whereas chamomile is typically relaxing and calming.

½ cup dried or 1 cup fresh rosemary or chamomile
2 cups boiling water
3 tablespoons apple cider vinegar

To make the rinse, put the herbs in a bowl and pour the boiling water into the bowl. Cover the bowl and let the herbs steep in the water until it cools. Next, use a colander or sieve to strain off the herbs. Add the apple cider vinegar to the liquid and stir in (don't be alarmed, your hair won't smell of vinegar!) The herbal rinse should be used cold on wet hair. The idea is that the cold water and the acid from the vinegar

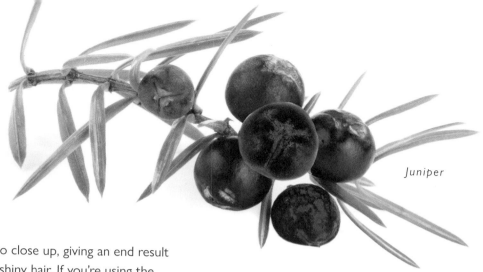

Juniper

help the hair cuticles to close up, giving an end result of clean, smooth, and shiny hair. If you're using the rinse as a conditioner after another form of shampoo, you could leave it on for super shiny hair.

Moisturizing hair mask

If your hair is in poor condition from too much coloring or styling, a weekly hair mask could help get some much-needed moisture back in. This hair mask is easy to make and includes the addition of natural yogurt to give it a creamy, luxurious feel.

1 tablespoon olive oil infused with lavender
2 tablespoons honey
2 tablespoons natural yogurt
Fresh aloe vera gel

In advance, add fresh or dried lavender to ¾ cup olive oil and let the herbs infuse for a few days. On the day you want to use the mask, pour out 1 tablespoon of infused oil, taking care to strain off the herbs. Mix in the honey and natural yogurt and stir well. Finally, cut a fresh aloe vera leaf and squeeze out the gel, stirring it into your mixture. Apply the mask onto wet hair, massaging it in, and leave on for 10 minutes. Rinse off with warm or cool water.

Herbal hair gel

Have herbal hair gel on hand whenever you need it, thanks to an aloe vera plant. Simply cut a leaf off, squeeze out the aloe gel, and apply it to your hair as needed. The gel could help you tame curly or unruly hair and style it as needed, plus it will dry with a slightly glossy finish.

Juniper hair and scalp tonic

For a rejuvenating hair and scalp tonic, infuse dried rosemary and juniper in ⅓ cup olive oil and massage the mix into your hair and scalp before you wash it.

Wrap your hair in a warm towel and leave for about 2 hours. Wash out with a mild shampoo, massaging the shampoo into the hair before you wet it to remove all the oil. Alternatively, try using rosemary and juniper essential oils.

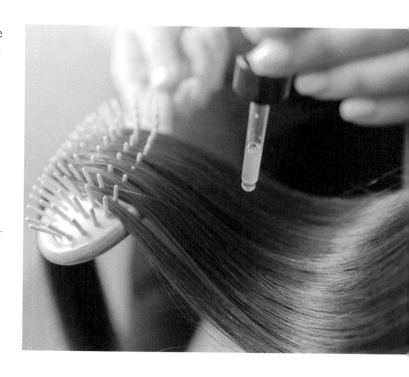

GROWING YOUR OWN MEDICINAL HERBS

Fresh herbs

Nothing beats having freshly growing herbs on hand whenever you need them for medicinal purposes. One of the benefits of using herbs for natural remedies is that many varieties are easy to grow yourself, inside or out.

If you have a garden, deck, or balcony, herbs can be grown outside in pots, planters, and window boxes, but even without outdoor space you can successfully grow herbs indoors on a sunny windowsill. If you're new to growing herbs, good options to start with include rosemary, basil, mint, sage, and cilantro.

Pots of herbs can be purchased inexpensively from grocery stores, and you can continue growing them on your windowsill in their small pots or repot them into other containers. However, for the best-quality plants, it's better to purchase plants or seeds from a reputable garden center or plant nursery. You never know exactly how store-bought herbs have been grown, and they could have been fed with pesticides and fertilizers or intensively grown in an unnatural environment.

For herbs that you'll be using for natural remedies, you need good-quality plants that haven't been subjected to additional chemicals. When you're choosing herbs, look for organically grown plants that look strong, green, and healthy with lots of new growth, yet still have room in their pot to grow more. Warning signs of unhealthy plants include yellowing leaves, wilting, and straggly stems.

Growing herbs from seed

Herbs can be grown from seeds too, but it will take a bit longer until you're able to reap the benefits and use the leaves in your natural remedies. To grow herbs from seed, start by sprinkling your chosen seeds into small plant pots and cover them with a layer of compost, then water them in. The seeds need to germinate and you can help them do so by putting a layer of plastic wrap across the top of the pot. This helps to create a warm greenhouse effect. After approximately 4–5 weeks, the green shoots of the seedlings should have appeared and have developed their first leaves. At this stage, you can take off the plastic wrap, thin out the seedlings, and replant them into their own pots.

Another option for growing herbs, especially if you're on a budget or want to boost the number of different plants you have, is to take cuttings of other people's herb plants (with permission, of course!). To take a cutting, look for side shoots on rosemary or sage plants and break or cut them off. Pop the cuttings into a pot of compost and water them well. After a few weeks, they should have rooted and you can plant out the rooted cuttings into individual pots.

Outside herbs can be grown in containers or directly in the ground, either in a dedicated herb patch or mixed in with other plants, as a form of companion planting. Just be aware that some herbs, such as mint, will spread, so unless you want a massive patch of mint in your garden, limiting their spread is worthwhile. That's why you'll often see pots being sold specifically as herb planters, with different compartments or layers where you can plant a variety of herbs, without the worry of one plant completely taking over. One useful trick for outdoor growing is to plant herbs in pots, then bury the pots in the garden; the pots will act as a form of barrier, containing the root balls and preventing unnecessary spread.

In terms of when to plant herbs, starting an herb garden in spring is a good move, as the herbs should grow well during the summer months. But some herbs, such as rosemary, lavender, sage, oregano, and thyme, are quite hardy plants, so should cope with being planted and grown throughout the year.

If you don't think you're green-fingered, don't panic! Herbs don't need loads of attention once they're planted, just regular watering and exposure to sunlight. Most herbs appreciate full sun, but some, such as mint, are happy being partially in shade.

When you're watering your herb plants, take care not to water them too much—and don't give them more water if the soil surrounding them is already damp. Keep an eye on the color of the leaves on the plants, as they can indicate whether you're over- or underwatering your herbs.

Some common signs that you're overwatering include leaves that are yellow, dark, or black in color, leaves that have mildew on them, stems and roots that are soft and break easily, and an herb that doesn't improve when you water it more. One herb that's often susceptible to overwatering is basil.

Underwatering can cause leaves to become dry and crisp, with brown edges, and feel light to the touch (overwatered leaves, in contrast, will feel soft and limp). The plant will also look like it's wilting, with the leaves hanging down, and the soil will feel dry.

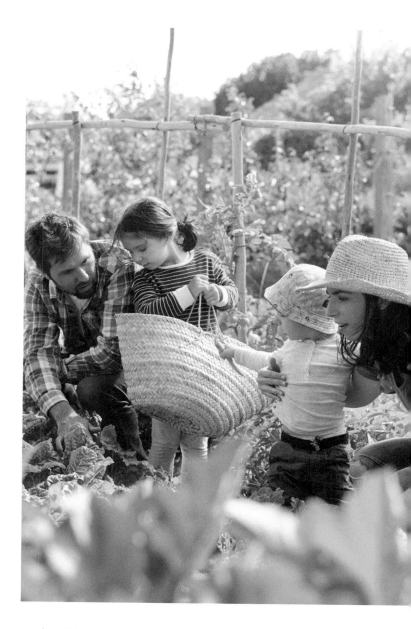

As with growing any plant, it can be a case of trial and error to get the balance right. Sometimes a plant won't thrive, and it could be due to many reasons and nothing you've done wrong. If your herbs don't grow, or keel over and die, treat it as a learning experience. Buy more seeds or more plants and start again.

Tip: Be resourceful and sustainable by saving containers to reuse for growing seeds. Empty, clean yogurt pots, for example, make ideal starter pots for herb seedlings. Washed popsicle sticks can be used for plant markers in pots and outside in the garden.

GATHERING HERBS IN THE WILD AND BUYING HERBS

The nature of herbs means that many of them grow naturally in the wild, in hedgerows, woods, or meadows, and if there are suitable areas that you can access easily, you could go into the great outdoors to source and pick them.

Gathering herbs in the wild can be a lovely ritual. There's something special about heading out to scour the hedgerows, forage for herbs, and collect the ingredients you need to take home and make special tinctures and healing remedies. It's an age-old practice that's been carried out for centuries.

In fact, there are various forms of folklore and traditions associated with picking herbs. There are tales, for example, about the best times of day, night, or month to pick herbs, with some varieties picked only during certain phases of the moon or when particular stars were visible in the sky.

These days you don't need to worry about the moon or the stars (unless you particularly want to, of course), although it's still important to be aware that some plants are seasonal. As you get to know what plants you enjoy using and the remedies you can make, you can plan in advance and pick, dry, and store your ingredients for future use. One advantage of herbs is that you often need only a small amount, so storing plants won't take up too much room.

Before going anywhere to pick herbs, it's essential to know exactly what you're looking for. Make sure you can recognize the herbs in question, know what they look like, and where they typically grow. If you're in any doubt, take a visual guide with you or save pictures of the plants on your cell phone so you can double check. You don't want to accidentally pick the wrong plants and make remedies from them, as this could be very dangerous.

Next, you'll have to check that the land they're on isn't private property and ensure that you have the right to be there. If you're unsure, err on the side of caution and find somewhere else—you don't want to be fined for trespassing on someone else's land.

If you're picking herbs from a hedgerow, choose the location carefully. Ideally, you don't want to use herbs that have grown directly next to busy roads and could have been exposed to traffic fumes and pollution. Likewise, it's best not to pick from hedges right next to public footpaths. In order to get the best out of your natural remedies, you want to find herbs that are in their purest and most natural state, so this might entail going off the beaten track.

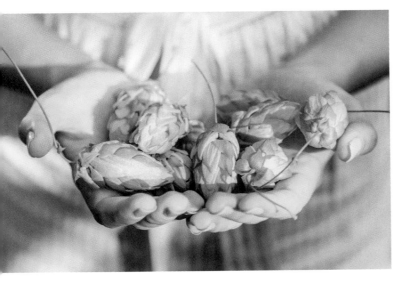

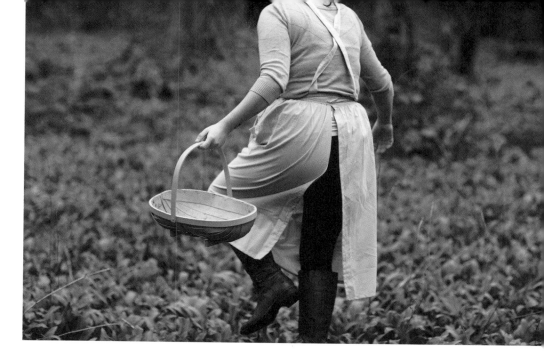

It's best to choose a dry day to go out gathering herbs, as this makes it easier to preserve the plants. As a general rule, look for herbs that are in their peak of maturity, as they're more likely to be fully potent. When you're picking flowers, aim to pick them when they're fully open or, if they're small and delicate, consider cutting the whole stem to preserve them. Try and keep flower heads whole until they've been dried, as this makes it easier to separate the parts.

Big leaves such as basil can be picked individually, whereas smaller ones may need to be picked on the stem. In the case of seeds, they're best collected when at least two-thirds of the seeds are ripe. It's a fine balance, as if they're too ripe they may have begun to disperse in the wind, fallen on the ground, or been eaten by birds, yet if they're not ripe enough you may not be able to gather enough. Likewise, if you're gathering fruits, look for specimens that are just ripe and ideal for preserving, rather than over-ripe, squishy fruits that are trickier to deal with.

Dandelion roots are traditionally gathered in the spring, but the roots of other plants may be best obtained in the fall, when their aerial parts have died down. Make sure you don't leave it too late though, as the ground can become hard as winter takes hold and roots will be more difficult to dig up.

When you're picking herbs in the wild, take care to abide by countryside rules and don't strip an area entirely of its plants. Take what you need, but always leave plenty behind, both for the natural purposes of the plant and land, and for other people to admire, enjoy, and perhaps pick for themselves.

Buying herbs

If you aren't in a position where you can go out and forage for herbs in the wild and are unable to grow your own due to lack of time, space, or gardening prowess, you can buy herbs to use for remedies.

Fresh and dried herbs are widely available to purchase from grocery stores, health-food stores, and local markets and can be used to make your own natural remedies. Some of the more unusual or hard-to-find herbs can be purchased from specialty websites online.

Look for herbs that have been grown organically, without any pesticides, as they're likely to be in their purest form. Buying pre-dried herbs can be a bonus, as you can use them immediately and you're not restricted by seasonal availability.

HARVESTING, DRYING, AND STORING HERBS

Whether you're harvesting your homegrown herbs, or going out to pick them in the wild, as a general rule herbs are best harvested on a dry day, when it's not been raining or when there hasn't been a heavy morning dew. The lack of added moisture makes it easier to pick and preserve the plant components, ensuring they have the best potency.

If you're harvesting all of the aerial parts of an herb—the leaves, flowers, stem, and seed head—then a good time to harvest is when the plant is in full flower, as this gives you the best chance of all parts being full of goodness. Snip gently using a pair of scissors. Flowers need to be handled carefully as they're highly delicate and it's easy to accidentally damage them. Make sure you're equipped with a suitable basket or container to put them in and transport them back to your kitchen. When you're harvesting leaves only, aim to harvest them before the plant flowers (with the exception of deciduous herbs, which you can harvest all year round). Herbs with small, dainty leaves, such as lemon balm, are best left on the stems. In the case of plants with larger leaves, such as basil, these can be picked individually.

Aim to harvest berries and fruit before they get too ripe, otherwise they'll be trickier to pick as the fruit will be too soft. Seeds need to be harvested when they're already ripe. Inevitably, not all seeds will be ready at exactly the same time, so look for plants that have about 75 percent of ripe seeds on their heads before picking.

The roots of plants are normally picked during the fall months, when the aerial parts have peaked. If you leave it until winter, the chances are the ground will have become too hard to dig them up. The only herb that's best to pick earlier in the year is the humble dandelion—its roots are best picked in the spring, as that's when they're the most potent.

Drying methods

In order to preserve the potency of herbs and keep them at the best levels, they need to be kept away from bright sunlight and dried as quickly as possible after harvesting.

Tie herbs in small bunches so that air can circulate around them, then hang them up on a drying rack for a few days. Ideal places include in a garden shed, garage, or utility room, or even an airing cupboard if you have space; the temperature should be in the region of 70–90°F (21–32°C). If the room you're using isn't naturally warm, add a small heater to bring up the temperature and improve drying.

Aim to keep flowers whole until they're fully dried, as they are easier to manage. Wash flower heads carefully to ensure all insects are removed, drain in a sieve or colander, then place the flower heads on trays and leave in a warm, dry place for a few days. When they are fully dried, you can separate the petals as needed. In the case of herbs such as lavender, the stems are best tied together and hung to be dried—loosely place a paper bag over the flowers so they can fall into it as they dry.

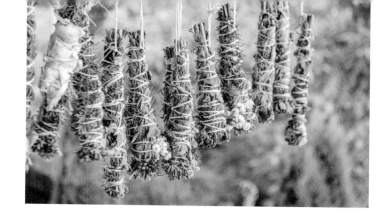

On average, herbs should take around 4–6 days to sufficiently dry. You can tell if they're ready by gently touching the leaves—if they're brittle and naturally start crumbling, they're ready.

Seed heads should be kept whole during the drying process too, but it's a good idea to put a paper bag over them and hang them up, so the seeds can drop into the bag as they dry.

Berries can be lightly washed, patted dry, and laid out on trays to be dried. Space them out so they're not touching one another and check them regularly for signs of mold; discard any berries that become moldy. Turn the berries every few days to ensure that all of the fruit dries out properly.

If you've harvested roots for medicinal purposes they'll naturally be covered in soil, so will need a good clean. Soak them in a bowl of cold water first to take off the majority of the soil, then remove them from the bowl, put them in a colander, and give them another wash with cold water. Pat them dry, then chop the roots into smaller pieces, as roots can become tough and harder to cut once fully dried. Depending on the roots, you may need to use garden clippers to chop through them. Once chopped, lay the roots onto a wooden board or tray, spacing them out where possible, and place them in a warm, dry place. Roots take about 4–7 days to completely dry out and need to be turned every few days.

How to store herbs

Once all your herbs are fully dried, it's time to store them. Leaves can be gently crumbled into glass jars or bottles and sealed with airtight lids. Darker colored bottles, such as amber or brown glass, may help preserve the contents for longer. Remember to clearly label the herbs with their name and the date. Most herbs keep well, but may begin to lose potency after 12–24 months. Always make sure herbs are fully dried before you store them, as any moisture could cause unwanted mold or make them go off.

Flowers and dried berries can be stored in airtight jars and bottles too, and seeds and flowers can be kept dried in paper bags or moved to jars as needed. Roots need to be stored in airtight containers, taking care that no moisture is able to get into them.

The joy of harvesting and drying your own herbs is that they tend to last longer than store-bought

herbs, which often take weeks or months from being harvested to reaching the shelves. So, you may well notice that your herbs taste and perform better than commercially dried herbs, making the process even more rewarding.

Freezing herbs

Herbs such as basil, dill, and parsley—particularly if you plan to use them for culinary purposes—can be washed, chopped, and frozen while still fresh. Try freezing them in ice-cube trays or small bags, so you can get them out of the freezer and add them to dishes as you cook.

HOW TO MAKE HOT- AND COLD-PRESSED OILS

As a home herbalist, you're likely to use herbal oils regularly when creating herbal remedies and home solutions. Ready-made oils are widely available to purchase, but there may be times when you want to experiment with creating your own.

Cold-pressed oils

Cold-pressed oils are traditionally made without the use of heat, which keeps them pure, natural, and raw. If you're using cold-pressed oils for culinary purposes, such as the base for dressings to drizzle over salads, then the flavor can be perceived as being better in a cold-pressed oil, plus it can be healthier as it's not been subject to high levels of heat. Common types of cold-pressed oils include sunflower, coconut, olive, avocado, pumpkin, nut, and flaxseed.

Cold-pressed oils are made by using seeds, nuts, or fruits, which are ground up until they form a paste. Traditionally this was done by hand, using a mortar and pestle, but it can be laborious work and small presses, juicers, or food processors can make the process easier. Sometimes the seeds are pressed completely raw, while on other occasions nuts may be roasted first at very low temperatures, then pressed.

This results in an oil that has a low acidic level that doesn't need refining, and it can be used immediately. The oil is also considered more nutritious than hot-pressed oil and it loses less of its natural, active ingredients.

Cold-pressed coconut oil
6 fresh coconuts
3 cups water

First, use a sharp tool to make a hole in the coconut shells, so you can pour out the coconut water. Once

they are drained, crack open the shells and scoop out the coconut flesh. Chop the coconut flesh and blend it using a food processor. Add the water and blend again until it forms into a cream. Put the coconut cream into a muslin bag and squeeze out all the water.

Next, decant the coconut into a bowl, cover, and put it somewhere warm (such as an airing cupboard) for up to 48 hours. You need to wait for the coconut cream to ferment, so that the curd will separate

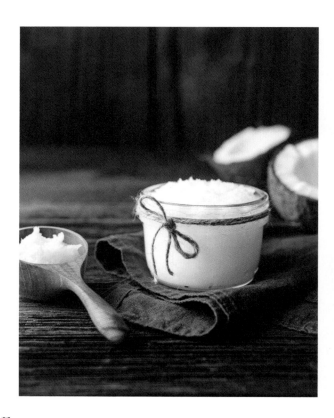

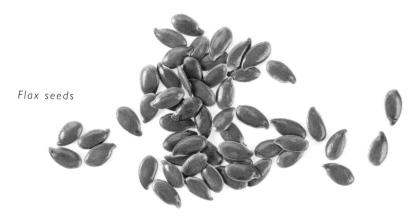

Flax seeds

from the oil. When it is ready, the oil will be on top and the coconut curd will be in the middle. At the bottom of the bowl you'll find some water, which can be discarded. Carefully spoon out the oil from the top, taking care not to spoon out any of the curd. Use a fine sieve to filter the oil once more, then pour it into an airtight jar.

The exact amount of oil you'll be able to make will vary according to the size of the coconuts, but on average you can expect to produce at least 1 cup of oil from six standard coconuts. Your cold-pressed coconut oil should be sealed in an airtight jar and could last for up to three months.

Hot-pressed oils

In contrast to cold-pressed oils, hot-pressed oils are made using heat. In a commercial setting, the seeds, nuts, or fruits are roasted and pressed using very high temperatures. Where oils are made commercially, chemicals are often added to the seeds before they're pressed, causing the eventual product to be acidic and refined. The high temperatures used in the process means that the oil loses it nutritional value, especially compared to cold-pressed oil.

In a home environment, it's largely impractical to make hot-pressed oils and most people tend to focus on the healthier cold-pressed oils instead. It's also worth noting that it can take a lot of seeds, nuts, or fruits to make only a small amount of oil, so it may work out as a more expensive process than choosing to purchase a good-quality oil from a grocery or health-food store.

Ways to use hot- and cold-pressed oils

Hot- and cold-pressed oils can be used for a wide variety of purposes. They can form the base of herbal infusions, be used for herbal skin and hair-care products (cold-pressed is favored for this), or to make herbal dressings for food or various herbal remedies.

Herbal vinegars and oils

Almost all culinary herbs can be used to flavor vinegars and oils. This has been done for centuries, particularly in Mediterranean countries. Some herbs are better suited to flavor vinegars, including basil, bay, chervil, chives, dill, fennel, garlic, juniper, lavender, lovage, marjoram, mint, oregano, rosemary, sage, savory, tarragon, and thyme. For steeping in oil, the best herbs are basil, bay, chervil, dill, fennel, garlic, juniper, lavender, lovage, marjoram, mint, parsley, rosemary, sage, savory, and thyme.

Herbal vinegars
Use good white wine vinegar. Pound a handful of your favorite herb and bruise it well with the pestle and mortar. Add 2½ cups vinegar to a handful of herbs in a wide-necked jar, then seal. Leave for a week, then strain. Repeat the process if you require a stronger flavor. After the second week, strain off all the leaves and stems and bottle the vinegar. Finally, add a few fresh sprigs of the herb for identification and a decorative effect.

Herbal oils
Follow the method above, but substitute the white wine vinegar with a good-quality cold-pressed oil such as coconut, olive, or sunflower.

USING HERBS IN YOUR HOME

As you progress with your herbal journey and build up a repertoire of remedies, you'll discover more and more ways in which you can use herbs in your daily life. These wonderful plants are super versatile, meaning that you can cook with them, create healing remedies, use them as ingredients for natural skin-care products, for decorative purposes, or to make into herbal gifts.

If you enjoy having pretty vases of fresh or dried flowers in your home, herbs can be added to the arrangements, providing extra texture, contrasting colors, or aromatic scents. Try including herbs such as rosemary, sage, chives, lavender, or dill flowers into your arrangements, or cut bunches of fresh herbs to display in small glass jars or jam pots. Herbs can be used to create herbal wreaths to hang in your home or on the outside of your front door as a form of scented decoration. You may also find that herbs are used as the base scent for many home diffusers.

Home scents

Aromatic dried herbs, such as rosemary or lavender, can be used to create mini bags to put inside drawers, wardrobes, or on coat hangers to naturally scent and freshen fabrics. Herbs can be used to make your own natural room sprays, using a base of witch hazel (2 tablespoons), water, and your choice of dried herbs: mix together and add to a spray bottle. Different aromas can be chosen according to the mood you want to evoke. Scents such as rosemary, sage, or oregano are clean scents for purifying the air, whereas lemon and mint can be uplifting, and lavender is relaxing. Experiment with using single fresh or dried herbs in room sprays, or a combination of different herbs and see what works best for you.

Culinary uses

From a culinary point of view, there are many ways to use herbs at home. They can be added to:

- Jellies, jams, and syrups
- Teas, wines, cocktails, and cordials
- Sweet and savory baked goods
- Oils and vinegars
- Butters and spreads
- Salt and sugar
- Pickles and chutneys
- Soups, stews, and stir-fries
- Sorbets and ice creams

Plus they can be used as trimmings and garnishes, to add the final touches to meals before serving.

Fresh chopped herbs can be frozen in ice-cube trays and added to drinks—the addition of herbs can transform a simple glass of water and make getting your daily H_2O more pleasurable.

Herb butter
1 tablespoon fresh chervil
1 tablespoon fresh chives
1 tablespoon fresh tarragon
1 tablespoon chopped shallots
1 teaspoon lemon juice
2 cups butter

Steam the chervil, chives, and tarragon lightly for a few minutes. Drop the shallots into boiling water

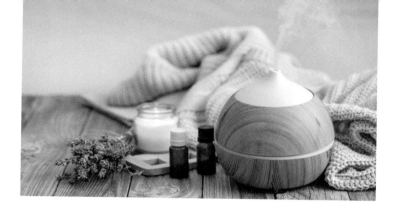

briefly, then drain and blend with the mixed herbs. Blend the herbs, lemon juice, and shallots with the butter. This herb butter is excellent with vegetables, baked potatoes, or roast meats.

Lemon verbena jelly

2 cups fresh lemon verbena leaves
¼ cup cider vinegar
4½ cups superfine sugar
⅓ cup liquid pectin

Shred the lemon verbena leaves. Pour 2½ cups boiling water over the leaves, cover, and leave to stand for 15 minutes. Strain the mixture and pour into a saucepan. Add the cider vinegar and sugar and bring to a boil. Stir well. Add the pectin and boil thoroughly for about 1 minute, stirring all the while. Pour into sterilized jars and seal.

Lavender honey

1½ cups honey
1 cup lavender leaves

Pour the honey over the lavender leaves and heat gently in a double boiler, simmering for 30 minutes. Strain into sterilized jars and seal. Keep for at least a month before using. This honey is great for coughs and sore throats, as well as delicious with herbal teas.

Borage summer wine

Fresh borage leaves and flowers
Cucumber-flavored water
White wine
Sugar, to taste
Lemon slices

Steep the borage leaves in a small quantity of boiling water. Leave to cool, then strain off the leaves. Add the cucumber-flavored water to white wine, sweeten with sugar to taste, and add a couple of slices of lemon. Serve with blue borage flowers as decoration.

Rose petal wine

20 cups scented rose petals
12¾ cups superfine sugar
Juice of 1 lemon
¼-oz. sachet wine yeast and nutrient

Mix together the rose petals, sugar, and lemon juice. Add 19 cups boiling water. Steep until the water is lukewarm. Then add the wine yeast and nutrient. Leave the mixture in a warm place for one week to ferment. Stir once a day. Strain into a fermentation jar and fit an airlock. Once a firm deposit has formed, strain into a sterilized jar. When fermentation has stopped and the wine is clear, strain into sterilized bottles. Lay by for six months before drinking.

Mint punch

10 cups fresh mint leaves
1¼ cups superfine sugar (or more to taste)
2 cups grape juice
Lemon juice, to taste
4¼ cups ginger ale
Mint leaves and glacé cherries to garnish

Grind the washed mint leaves in a bowl until soft. Dissolve the sugar in boiling water, add to the mint leaves and steep for 10 minutes. Strain off the mint leaves, and add the grape juice with lemon juice to taste. Check the sweetness and add more sugar if needed. Add the ginger ale. Refrigerate until cold. In summer, serve with ice together with fresh mint leaves and glacé cherries as a garnish.

PART TWO

Aromatherapy and Essential Oils

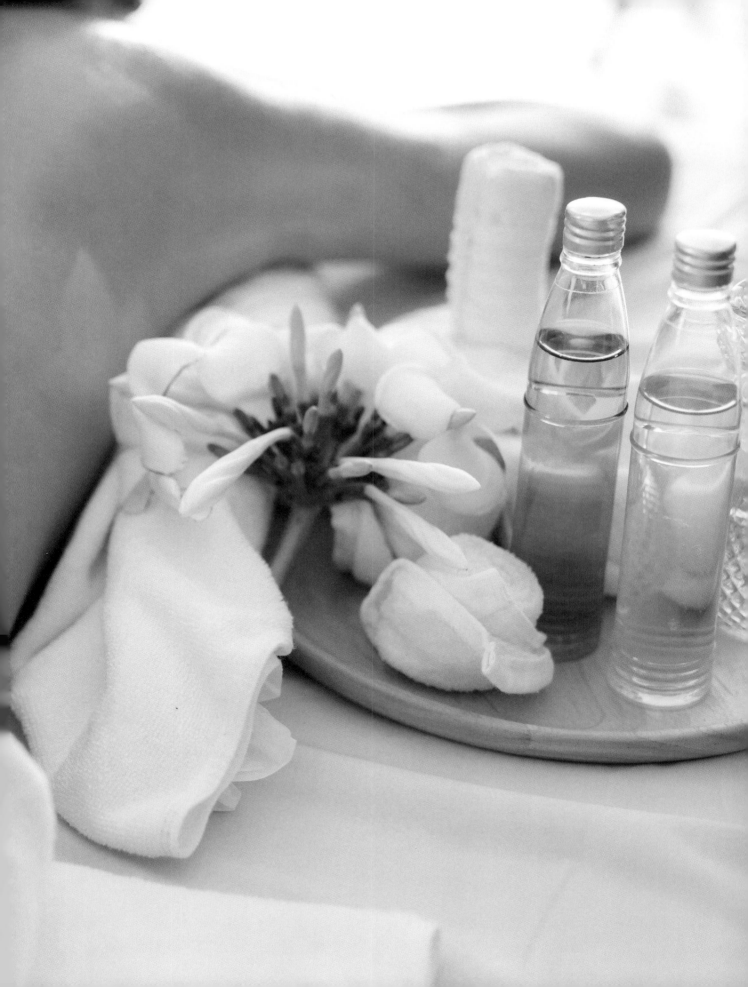

AN INTRODUCTION TO AROMATHERAPY

Aromatic oils have been used for centuries in cultures around the world to treat minor ailments, promote health, and improve well-being. The ancient Egyptians used aromatic oils when they were embalming the deceased, the Bible makes multiple mentions of using oils for anointing purposes, and the tenth-century Persians were involved in the distillation of essential oils.

It was the French chemist Reneé-Maurice Gattefossé who is largely known for bringing aromatherapy techniques into the twentieth century. When he burned his hand, he used lavender essential oil on the burn and found it effective, leading him to carry out research into the therapeutic benefits of plant oils. His published research was later expanded on in the 1960s by Dr. Jean Valnet and Marguerite Maury, and some French doctors began to use essential oils alongside other medical techniques. Aromatherapy is widely used today as a form of complementary therapy.

What is aromatherapy?

Aromatherapy is based on the idea that the medicinal properties of plants and flowers can have a beneficial effect on health and well-being. Essential oils are extracted from the flowers, leaves, roots, and stalks of plants through a distillation process and can be used in various ways.

The sense of smell is an important element of aromatherapy. The aromas released by the oils stimulate the olfactory centers in the brain that are linked with the hypothalamus, the part of the brain that's concerned with mood. Research has shown that different scents can evoke different moods, feelings, and emotions, such as being uplifting, relaxing, energizing, or promoting sleep. The absorption of oils through the skin is a key factor too. Most essential oils can't be used directly on the skin, but they can be massaged in when a few drops are included in a base of carrier oil and they are absorbed into the body through the pores on your skin.

There are many ways in which you can use aromatherapy to treat minor ailments and for self-care purposes. The oils work well popped into an oil burner or diffuser, where they can gradually scent the air, or made into a steam bath to help treat common symptoms such as colds and blocked noses. For self-care purposes, you can use the oils to create hair- and skin-care products, including lotions, face masks, and pampering products, all tailored to your individual needs, or add them to a bath to help ease aching muscles.

As a complementary therapy, it works effectively alongside other treatments, although you may wish to consult your medical practitioner first if you're taking any prescribed medication, as some oils may cause reactions.

What happens at an aromatherapy treatment?

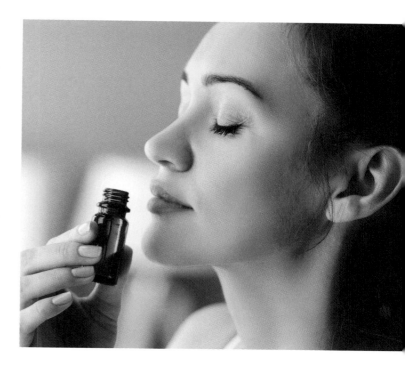

Visiting a professionally trained aromatherapist is worthwhile if you have specific health concerns or ailments that you'd like to be treated. Although you can use basic aromatherapy on your own at home, it's hard to massage some areas of your body that may benefit from it, and especially to the degree that a professional offers.

Aromatherapy can be useful for a range of health concerns, including:

• Headaches
• Backache
• Colds and sinus issues
• Menstrual issues
• Insomnia
• Fatigue
• Menopause
• Inflammation
• Muscle and joint pain

First off, it's important to find a properly trained and qualified professional (check out the Resources on page 298 to find relevant organizations). When you go for your first appointment, your aromatherapist will do a thorough consultation with you, asking questions about your health and lifestyle. It's the chance to explain any concerns you have and find out how treatments could help you.

In some cases, you may wish to have only a one-off pampering session, while in others it may be beneficial to have regular sessions as part of a treatment regime to help a particular ailment. Whatever you decide, make sure you're comfortable with your chosen practitioner and ensure that any aromatherapy treatments will work hand-in-hand with any other medical treatment you may be having (if in doubt, consult your medical practitioner before embarking on aromatherapy treatments).

The cost of treatments varies considerably, depending on the experience of your therapist and where they're located. You can expect to pay more for the first appointment, as it's normally longer due to the consultation process. Some therapists may offer discounts for bulk bookings of multiple sessions, rather than one-offs.

An aromatherapy appointment will be tailored to your individual needs. It's likely to include massage techniques using essential oil blends, but may also involve other forms of treatments, such as the use of compresses, inhalations, salves, and soaks. There may be some treatment ideas that you can take away and do yourself at home.

Inhaling the aromas and having aromatherapy massage can be a highly relaxing experience, so it's not unusual to leave a session feeling like you're floating in the air. If you need a rest or a nap after a session, that's perfectly normal too.

USING AROMATHERAPY AND ESSENTIAL OILS

There's something magical about aromatherapy and the way that different blends of oils can transform the way you feel physically, emotionally, and mentally. As you explore the vast array of different aromatic oils available, you'll gradually discover new scents—some you'll like, others you may not take to—and learn new ways in which you can use them in your life.

One of the benefits of aromatherapy is that there are a variety of ways in which you can utilize the natural healing power of the oils. For example, aromatherapy can involve the use of:

• Diffusers—plug-in electrical gadgets or candle burners in which you can put a few drops of single or multiple aromatherapy oils. Good to use for general scent purposes in your home or to set the mood for holistic practices such as meditation or yoga.
• Massage oils—blends of oils that can be massaged into your skin to help aching muscles, sore joints, or to ease stress.
• Facial baths—mini steam baths that you can create to inhale essential oils. Good for skin-care needs or for blocked sinuses.
• Hot and cold compresses—pieces of cloth with drops of essential oils on them that can be applied to some minor ailments.
• Bath products—essential oils are ideal for making bath salts, bath bombs, or other scented bath products.
• Spritzer sprays—a mix of oils can be added to water and put in spray bottles to help scent your home.
• Body creams and lotions—drops of essential oils can be used to make natural skin-care products such as creams, lotions, and salves.

CAUTION

Always consult a professional first if you're pregnant, breastfeeding, or on any prescription medications, as some essential oils may cause unwanted side effects or reactions. When you're using oils with a carrier oil for the first time, always do a small patch test first to ensure it's suitable for your skin.

Undiluted application

In general, essential oils should not be applied to the skin undiluted as they are highly concentrated. Some oils can cause irritation or a burning or tingling sensation when they are applied in an undiluted form. However, there are exceptions to this rule. (See Aromatherapy for first aid, pages 152–155; Using essential oils in your home, pages 174–175.)

Carrier oils

If you are planning to use aromatherapy oils for massage purposes, you need to mix them with a carrier or base oil first. Essential oils are pure and concentrated, so are too harsh to put directly onto the skin. The best carrier oils are those that are cold-pressed (see pages 108–109 for how you could make your own), pure, organic, and additive-free.

While most carrier oils are unscented, some do have a distinctive scent to them. Sometimes this can affect the smell when you add the essential oils, so you may want to experiment with a few different oils to see what works best for your sense of smell. Other considerations for using carrier oils are how the oil is absorbed into your skin, as this can differ from oil to oil and depending on your skin type. If you have existing skin issues or sensitive skin, then do a patch test first, as some carrier oils may not be suitable for you to use. Some of the popular carrier oil choices for aromatherapy include:

• Sweet almond oil—made from sweet almonds, this oil tends to have a strong nutty scent. It's good for skin-care purposes and can help moisturize dry skin.
• Jojoba oil—made from jojoba plant seeds, this oil has a light nutty aroma. It can reduce the production of oil in the skin and doesn't tend to clog pores, so it's good for massage and skin-care products.
• Coconut oil—unrefined oil is made from the flesh of ripe coconuts. It's a good source of fatty acids.

• Sunflower oil—made from pressed sunflower seeds, this oil tends to have a very light and unoffensive scent. It's good to use for massage purposes.
• Olive oil—made from olives, with a slightly fruity aroma. It's a good source of fatty acids and can help dry skin.
• Apricot kernel oil—made from apricot seeds, it's a good source of vitamin E and fatty acids. It has a slightly sweet and nutty scent.
• Avocado oil—made from avocado fruits, this oil can have a nutty scent to it. The oil contains oleic acid, which can help dry and damaged skin.

The cost of carrier oils varies, with some more expensive than others. Sunflower oil can be a good basic oil for a beginner to start with and tends to be at the lower end of the price scale. If you have access to a store selling good-quality aromatherapy carrier oils, it's always worth going to smell the products before buying to ensure you like the scent of the carriers.

Preparing a compress

Prepare a hot compress by dipping a clean facecloth or piece of absorbent cotton in a small bowl containing about 2 cups steaming water to which has been added 5 or 6 drops of an essential oil such as lavender. Squeeze out any excess water, and then apply to the affected area. Apply a bandage if required and repeat as necessary. Make a cold compress by dipping a clean facecloth or cotton pad in a bowl of cold water to which has been added 5 or 6 drops of a cooling oil such as peppermint, squeezing out any excess water. Alternatively, wrap the dipped and squeezed cloth around an ice cube before applying to the affected area. Refresh the compress regularly and apply until the swelling or pain subsides.

A TO Z OF ESSENTIAL OILS

ANGELICA ROOT *Angelica archangelica*
Family: Umbelliferae

DESCRIPTION: A large, hairy plant with rhizome-like roots, ferny leaves, and umbels of white flowers. The whole plant has a strong, aromatic scent.

ACTIONS: Antispasmodic, carminative, depurative, diaphoretic, digestive, diuretic, emmenagogue, expectorant, febrifuge, nervine, stimulant, stomachic, tonic, bactericidal, fungicidal.

EXTRACTION: The essential oil is produced by steam distillation from the roots.

CHARACTERISTICS: The root oil is colorless, or pale yellow, turning yellowish-brown with age. It has a rich, herbaceous, earthy body note. The seed oil is a colorless liquid, with a fresher, spicy top note. Blends well with patchouli, clary sage, vetivert, and citrus oils.

AROMATHERAPY USE: Skin care: Dull and congested skin, irritated conditions, psoriasis. Circulation, muscles, and joints: Accumulation of toxins, arthritis, gout, rheumatism, water retention. Respiratory system: Bronchitis, colds, coughs. Digestive system: Anemia, flatulence, indigestion. Nervous system: Fatigue, migraine, nervous tension, stress-related disorders.

PERFUME: Scent: Balsamic, musky, herbaceous, bittersweet, powerful, earthy, spicy, long-lasting. Acts as a fixative. Key qualities: Restorative, tonic, revitalizing, purifying, comforting, stimulating (in small quantities), sedating (in large quantities), warming, grounding, aphrodisiac. Odor intensity: High.

CAUTION: Not to be used during pregnancy or by young children or people with diabetes. The root oil is phototoxic. Use with care, in low dilutions only (1 percent).

BASIL, SWEET/FRENCH *Ocimum basilicum*
Family: Lamiaceae

DESCRIPTION: A tender annual herb up to 2.5 inches high, with dark green, ovate leaves, grayish-green beneath. It bears whorls of two-lipped, greenish or pinky-white flowers. The whole plant has a powerful aromatic scent.

ACTIONS: Antiseptic, antispasmodic, carminative, digestive, emmenagogue, expectorant, febrifuge, galactagogue, nervine, prophylactic, stimulant of adrenal cortex, stomachic, tonic, insecticide.

EXTRACTION: The oil is extracted by steam distillation from the flowering herb.

CHARACTERISTICS: Sweet basil oil is a colorless or pale-yellow liquid, with a light, fresh, sweet-spicy scent, and balsamic undertones. It blends well with bergamot, clary sage, lime, citronella, geranium, hyssop, and other green notes.

AROMATHERAPY USE: Skin care: Insect bites, insect repellent. Circulation, muscles, and joints: Gout, muscular aches and pains, rheumatism. Respiratory system: Bronchitis, colds, coughs, earache, sinusitis. Digestive system: Dyspepsia, flatulence, nausea. Reproductive system: Cramps, scanty periods. Immune system: Colds, fever, flu, infectious disease. Nervous system: Anxiety, depression, fatigue, insomnia, migraine, nervous tension.

PERFUME: Scent: Fresh, slightly spicy, clove-like. Key qualities: Restorative, tonic, antidepressant, refreshing, uplifting, fortifying, purifying, clearing, warming, cephalic, stupefying (in excess). Odor intensity: High.

CAUTION: Possible sensitization. Use in moderation. Avoid prolonged use. Do not use during pregnancy.

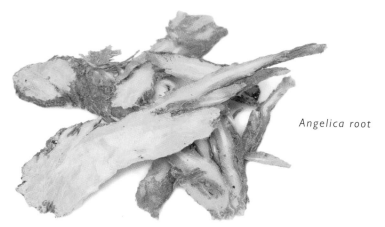

Angelica root

BERGAMOT *Citrus bergamia*
Family: Rutaceae

DESCRIPTION: A small tree, about 15 feet high, with smooth oval leaves, bearing small, round fruit that ripens from green to yellow.

ACTIONS: Analgesic, anthelmintic, antiseptic, antispasmodic, antitoxic, carminative, digestive, diuretic, deodorant, febrifuge, laxative, parasiticide, rubefacient, stimulant, stomachic, tonic, vermifuge, vulnerary, insecticide.

EXTRACTION: Bergamot oil is extracted from the peel of the nearly ripe fruit by cold expression. Bergapten-free oil is produced by a process known as fractionation.

CHARACTERISTICS: A light greenish-yellow liquid, with a fresh, sweet-fruity scent and slightly spicy-balsamic undertone. It blends well with lavender, neroli, jasmine, cypress, geranium, clary sage, chamomile, juniper, coriander, and other citrus oils.

AROMATHERAPY USE: Skin care: Acne, boils, cold sores, eczema, insect bites, oily complexion, psoriasis, scabies, spots, varicose ulcers, wounds.

PERFUME: Scent: Fresh, citrus, sweet, light, warm, slightly spicy-floral, green. Key qualities: Reviving, refreshing, calming, soothing, uplifting, sedative, regulating, balancing, antidepressant. Odor intensity: Low.

CAUTION: Phototoxic. Extreme care must be taken when using the oil in dermal applications, or a rectified, bergapten-free oil should be substituted.

CARAWAY *Carum carvi*
Family: Umbelliferae

DESCRIPTION: A biennial herb up to 2.5 feet high with a much-branched stem, finely cut leaves, and umbels of white flowers, with a thick and tapering root. The small seeds are curved with five distinct pale ridges.

ACTIONS: Antihistaminic, antimicrobial, antiseptic, aperitif, astringent, carminative, diuretic, emmenagogue, expectorant, galactagogue, larvicidal, stimulant, spasmolytic, stomachic, tonic, vermifuge.

EXTRACTION: The essential oil is extracted by steam distillation from the dried ripe seed or fruit (approximately 2–8 percent yield).

CHARACTERISTICS: Crude caraway oil is a pale yellowish-brown liquid with a harsh, spicy odor. The redistilled oil is colorless to pale yellow, with a strong, warm, sweet-spicy odor, like rye bread. It blends well with jasmine, cinnamon, cassia, and other spices; however, it is very overpowering.

AROMATHERAPY USE: Respiratory system: Bronchitis, coughs, laryngitis. Digestive system: Dyspepsia, colic, flatulence, gastric spasm, nervous indigestion, poor appetite. See also sweet fennel (page 126). Immune system: Colds.

PERFUME: Scent: Strong, warm, sweet-spicy. Key qualities: Warming, stress-relieving, stimulating, antiseptic, expectorant. Odor intensity: High.

CAUTION: May cause dermal irritation in concentration.

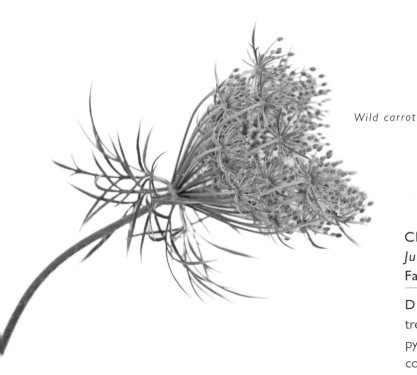
Wild carrot

CARROT SEED *Daucus carota*
Family: Umbelliferae

DESCRIPTION: Annual or biennial herb, with a small, inedible, tough whitish root. It has a much-branched stem, up to 5 feet high, with hairy leaves and umbels of white, lacy flowers.

ACTIONS: Anthelmintic, antiseptic, carminative, depurative, diuretic, emmenagogue, hepatic, stimulant, tonic, vasodilatory, smooth muscle relaxant.

EXTRACTION: The oil is extracted by steam distillation from the dried seeds.

CHARACTERISTICS: A yellow or amber liquid, with a warm, dry, woody-earthy odor. It blends well with cedarwood, geranium, citrus, and with the spice oils.

AROMATHERAPY USE: Skin care: Dermatitis, eczema, oily skin, psoriasis, rashes, wrinkles, mature complexions—revitalizing and toning. Circulation, muscles, and joints: Anemia, accumulation of toxins, arthritis, gout, edema, rheumatism. Digestive system: Colic, indigestion, liver congestion. Reproductive and endocrine system: Amenorrhea, dysmenorrhea, glandular problems, PMS.

PERFUME: Scent: Woody-earthy, herbaceous, slightly spicy, strong, warm. Key qualities (mind): Clearing, comforting, reviving. Odor intensity: Medium–high.

CEDARWOOD, VIRGINIAN
Juniperus virginiana
Family: Cupressaceae

DESCRIPTION: A slow-growing evergreen coniferous tree, up to 108 feet high, with a narrow, dense, and pyramidal crown, a reddish heartwood, and brown cones.

ACTIONS: Abortifacient, antiseborrheic, antiseptic (pulmonary, genitourinary), antispasmodic, astringent, balsamic, diuretic, emmenagogue, expectorant, insecticide, sedative (to the nervous system), stimulant (to the circulation).

EXTRACTION: The oil is extracted by steam distillation from lumber waste, sawdust, and shavings.

CHARACTERISTICS: A pale yellow or orange, oily liquid, with a mild, sweet-balsamic, pencilwood scent. It blends well with sandalwood, rose, juniper, cypress, vetiver, patchouli, and benzoin.

AROMATHERAPY USE: Skin care: Acne, dandruff, eczema, greasy hair, oily skin, psoriasis (can cause acute local irritation in some individuals). Circulation, muscles, and joints: Arthritis, rheumatism. Respiratory system: Bronchitis, catarrh, congestion, coughs, sinusitis. Genitourinary system: Cystitis, leukorrhea. Nervous system: Nervous tension, stress-related disorders. Other: insect repellent.

PERFUME: Scent: Sweet-balsamic, pencilwood, tenacious, tobacco, clean, sporty. Key qualities (mind): Restorative, uplifting, warming. Odor intensity: Medium–low.

CAUTION: Use this oil in dilution only, with care, and in moderation. The oil is a powerful abortifacient— avoid during pregnancy.

CELERY SEED *Apium graveolens*
Family: Umbelliferae

DESCRIPTION: A familiar biennial plant, 2–3 feet high, with a grooved, fleshy, erect stalk, shiny pinnate leaves, and umbels of white flowers.

ACTIONS: Antioxidant, antirheumatic, antiseptic (urinary), antispasmodic, aperitif, depurative, digestive, diuretic, carminative, cholagogue, emmenagogue, galactagogue, hepatic, nervine, sedative (to nervous system), stimulant (uterine), stomachic, tonic (digestive).

EXTRACTION: The oil is extracted by steam distillation from the whole or crushed seeds.

CHARACTERISTICS: A pale yellow or orange, spicy-warm, sweet, long-lasting odor. It blends well with lavender, pine, tea tree, coriander, and other spices.

AROMATHERAPY USE: Circulation, muscles, and joints: Arthritis, buildup of toxins in the blood, gout, rheumatism. Digestive system: Dyspepsia, flatulence, indigestion, liver congestion, jaundice. Reproductive and endocrine systems: Amenorrhea, glandular problems, increases milk flow. Urinary system: Cystitis. Nervous system: Neuralgia, sciatica.

PERFUME: Scent: Spicy-warm, sweet, long-lasting. Key qualities (mind): Warming, refreshing, reviving. Odor intensity: Medium.

CAUTION: Avoid using during pregnancy. Possible sensitization.

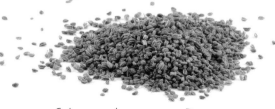

Celery seed

CHAMOMILE, GERMAN/BLUE *Chamomilla matricaria/matricaria recutita*
Family: Asteraceae

DESCRIPTION: An aromatic annual herb, up to 2 feet tall, with a hairless, erect, branching stem. It has delicate feathery leaves and white flowers.

ACTIONS: Analgesic, anti-allergenic, anti-inflammatory, antiphlogistic, antispasmodic, bactericide, calminative, cicatrizant, cholagogue, digestive, febrifuge, fungicidal, hepatic, nerve sedative, stimulant of leukocyte production, stomachic, sudorific, vermifuge, vulnerary.

EXTRACTION: The oil is extracted by steam distillation from the flower heads.

CHARACTERISTICS: An inky-blue, viscous liquid, with a strong, sweetish, warm herbaceous odor. It blends well with geranium, lavender, patchouli, rose, benzoin, neroli, bergamot, marjoram, lemon, ylang ylang, jasmine, and clary sage.

AROMATHERAPY USE: Skin care: Acne, allergies, boils, burns, cuts, chilblains, dermatitis, earache, eczema, hair care, inflammation, insect bites, rashes, sensitive skin, teething pain, toothache, wounds. Circulation, muscles, and joints: Arthritis, inflamed joints, muscular pain, neuralgia, rheumatism, sprains. Digestive system: Dyspepsia, colic, indigestion, nausea. Reproductive system: Dysmenorrhea, menopausal problems, menorrhagia. Nervous system: Headache, insomnia, nervous tension, migraine, stress-related complaints.

PERFUME: Scent: Warm, herbaceous, sweet, slightly bitter, green. Key qualities: Relaxing, soothing, calming, balancing, tonic (nerve). Odor intensity: Very high.

CAUTION: Generally nontoxic, nonirritant, but can cause dermatitis in some individuals.

The oil is produced by steam distillation from the flower heads.

CHAMOMILE, ROMAN *Chamaemelum nobilis/anthemis nobilis*
Family: Asteraceae

DESCRIPTION: A stocky, perennial herb, up to 10 inches high, with a much-branched, hairy stem, half creeping. It has feathery, pinnate leaves, and white flowers.

ACTIONS: Analgesic, antianemic, antineuralgic, antiphlogistic, antiseptic, antispasmodic, bactericide, carminative, cholagogue, cicatrizant, digestive, emmenogogue, febrifuge, hepatic, hypnotic, nerve sedative, stomachic, sudorific, tonic, vermifuge, vulnerary.

EXTRACTION: The oil is produced by steam distillation from the flower heads.

CHARACTERISTICS: A pale blue liquid (turning yellow over time), with a warm, sweet, fruity, herbaceous scent. It blends well with bergamot, clary sage, jasmine, neroli, rose, geranium, and lavender.

AROMATHERAPY USE: Skin care: Acne, boils, burns, cuts, chilblains, dermatitis, earache, eczema, inflammation, insect bites, rashes, sensitive skin, wounds. Circulation, muscles, and joints: Arthritis, inflamed joints, muscular pain, neuralgia, sprains, rheumatism. Digestive system: Dyspepsia, colic, indigestion, nausea. Reproductive system: Dysmenorrhea, menopausal problems, menorrhagia. Nervous system: Headache, insomnia, nervous tension, migraine, and stress-related complaints.

PERFUME: Scent: Slightly fruity, sweet, fresh, warm, herbaceous, rich, grassy, fragrant, apple-like. Key qualities: Restorative, calming, sedative, relaxing, soothing, warming, balancing, comforting, mild, slightly soporific or hypnotic in large doses.

Odor intensity: High.

CAUTION: Generally nonirritant, but can cause dermatitis in some individuals.

CINNAMON LEAF *Cinnamomum zeylanicum*
Family: Lauraceae

DESCRIPTION: A tropical evergreen tree, up to 50 feet high, with stiff, sharp spines, smooth ovate leaves, and small white flowers and bluish-white berries.

ACTIONS: Anthelmintic, antidiarrheal, antidote, antimicrobial, antiseptic, antispasmodic, antiputrescent, astringent, digestive, emmenagogue, hemostatic, parasiticide, refrigerant, spasmolytic, stimulant, stomachic, vermifuge.

EXTRACTION: Essential oil is extracted by water or steam distillation from the leaves and twigs.

CHARACTERISTICS: Leaves and twigs yield a yellow to brownish oil, with a warm-spicy, somewhat harsh odor. It blends well with frankincense, ylang ylang, orange, mandarin, and benzoin.

AROMATHERAPY USE: Skin care: Lice, scabies, tooth and gum care, warts, wasp stings. Circulation, muscles, and joints: Poor circulation, rheumatism. Digestive system: Colitis, diarrhea, dyspepsia, intestinal infection, sluggish digestion, spasm. Reproductive system: Childbirth (stimulates contractions), frigidity, leukorrhea, metrorrhagia). Immune system: Chills, colds, flu, infectious diseases. Nervous system: Debility, nervous exhaustion, stress-related conditions.

PERFUME: Scent: Sweet-spicy, peppery, hot, dry, tenacious, slightly woody, herbaceous, diffusive, powerful, warm. Key qualities (mind): Warming,

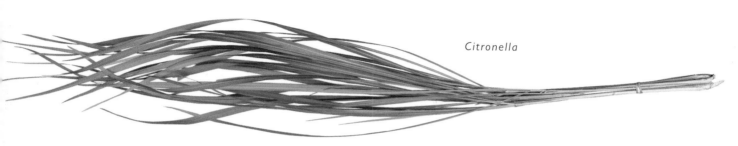

Citronella

reviving, tonic, strengthening, aphrodisiac, restorative, uplifting. Odor intensity: High.

CAUTION: The leaf oil is relatively nontoxic, though possibly a skin irritant. Its major component, eugenol, causes irritation to the mucous membrane. Use in moderation. Do not use bark oil on the skin.

CITRONELLA *Cymbopogon nardus*
Family: Poaceae

DESCRIPTION: A tall, cultivated, aromatic, perennial grass, derived from the wild managrass found in Sri Lanka.

ACTIONS: Antiseptic, antispasmodic, bactericidal, deodorant, diuretic, emmenagogue, febrifuge, fungicidal, insecticide, stomachic, tonic, vermifuge.

EXTRACTION: Oil is extracted by steam distillation of the fresh, part-dried, or dried grass. Java citronella yields twice as much oil as the Sri Lanka type.

CHARACTERISTICS: A yellowish-brown, mobile liquid, with a fresh, powerful, lemony scent. The Java oil is colorless to pale yellow, with a fresh, woody-sweet fragrance; it is considered of superior quality in perfumery work. It blends well with geranium, lemon, bergamot, orange, cedarwood, and pine.

AROMATHERAPY USE: Skin care: Excessive perspiration, oily skin. Immune system: Colds, flu, minor infections. Nervous system: Fatigue, headaches, migraine, neuralgia. Other: Insect repellent. Mixed with Virginia cedarwood oil, it is a popular remedy against mosquitoes.

PERFUME: Scent: Fresh, lemony, slightly herbaceous, green, powerful. Key qualities (mind): Refreshing, active, penetrating. Odor intensity: High.

CLARY SAGE *Salvia sclaria*
Family: Lamiaceae

DESCRIPTION: Stout biennial or perennial herb, up to 3 feet high, with large, hairy leaves, green with a hint of purple, and small blue flowers.

ACTIONS: Anticonvulsive, antidepressant, antiphlogistic, antiseptic, aphrodisiac, astringent, bactericidal, carminative, cicatrizant, deodorant, digestive, emmenagogue, hypotensive, nervine, sedative, stomachic, uterine tonic.

EXTRACTION: The oil is extracted by steam distillation from the flowering tops and leaves.

CHARACTERISTICS: A colorless or pale yellowish-green liquid, with a sweet, nutty, herbaceous scent. It blends well with juniper, lavender, coriander, cardamom, geranium, sandalwood, cedarwood, pine, jasmine, frankincense, bergamot, and all the citrus oils.

AROMATHERAPY USE: Skin care: Acne, boils, dandruff, hair loss, inflamed conditions, oily skin and hair, ulcers, wrinkles. Circulation, muscles, and joints: High blood pressure, muscular aches and pains. Respiratory system: Asthma, throat infections, whooping cough. Digestive system: Colic, cramps, dyspepsia, flatulence. Reproductive system: Amenorrhea, labor pain, dysmenorrhea, leukorrhea. Nervous system: Depression, frigidity, impotence, migraine, nervous tension, stress-related disorders.

PERFUME: Scent: Musky-amber, mellow, rich, warm, herbaceous, sweet; imperative in eau de cologne. Key qualities: Relaxing, rejuvenating, balancing, inspiring, revitalizing, aphrodisiac, intoxicating, euphoric, warming. Odor intensity: Medium–high.

CAUTION: Avoid during pregnancy and while drinking alcohol.

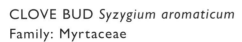

Cloves are stimulating, revitalizing, warming, and comforting.

CLOVE BUD *Syzygium aromaticum*
Family: Myrtaceae

DESCRIPTION: A slender evergreen tree with a smooth, gray trunk, up to 40 feet high. It has large, bright green leaves, standing in pairs on short stalks. At the start of the rainy season, long buds appear, with a rosy-pink corolla at the tip; as the corolla fades, the calyx slowly turns deep red.

ACTIONS: Anthelmintic, antibiotic, antiemetic, antirheumatic, antineuralgic, antioxidant, antiseptic, antiviral, carminative, expectorant, larvicidal, spasmolytic, stimulant, stomachic, vermifuge.

EXTRACTION: The oil is obtained by water distillation from the flower buds.

CHARACTERISTICS: Clove bud oil is a pale yellow liquid, with a sweet-spicy odor that has a fruity, fresh top note. Used in perfumery, it blends well with rose, lavender, clary sage, bergamot, bay, and ylang ylang.

AROMATHERAPY USE: Skin care: Acne, athlete's foot, bruises, burns, cuts, toothache, ulcers, wounds. Circulation, muscles, and joints: Arthritis, rheumatism, sprains. Respiratory system: Asthma, bronchitis. Digestive system: Colic, dyspepsia, nausea. Immune system: Colds, flu, minor infections. Other: Insect repellent (mosquitoes).

PERFUME: Scent: Hot, fruity, floral, fresh, fragrant, peppery, sweet-spicy, diffusive, powerful, clean, medicinal. Key qualities: Tonic, stimulating, revitalizing, aphrodisiac, warming, comforting, purifying, active. Odor intensity: High.

CAUTION: Clove bud oil can cause skin and mucous membrane irritation, and may cause dermatitis in some individuals. Use this oil in moderation only, and in low dilution (less than 1 percent).

CUMIN *Cuminum cyminum*
Family: Umbelliferae

DESCRIPTION: A small, delicate, annual herb about 20 inches high, with a slender stem, dark green feathery leaves and small pink or white flowers followed by small oblong seeds.

ACTIONS: Antioxidant, antiseptic, antispasmodic, antitoxic, aphrodisiac, bactericidal, carminative, depurative, digestive, diuretic, emmenagogue, larvicidal, nervine, stimulant, tonic.

EXTRACTION: The essential oil is extracted by steam distillation from the ripe seeds.

CHARACTERISTICS: A pale yellow or greenish liquid with a warm, soft, spicy-musky scent. It blends well with lavender, lavandin, rosemary, galbanum, rosewood, and cardamom.

AROMATHERAPY USE: Circulation, muscles, and joints: Accumulation of fluids or toxins, poor circulation. Digestive system: Colic, dyspepsia, flatulence, indigestion, spasm. Nervous system: Debility, headaches, migraine, nervous exhaustion. Other: Used in veterinary medicine in digestive preparations. As a fragrance component in cosmetics and perfumes, and a flavor ingredient in many foods and drinks, especially meat products and condiments.

PERFUME: Scent: Warm, soft, spicy-musky. Key qualities: Antiseptic, tonic, relaxing, soothing, cleansing. Odor intensity: Medium.

CAUTION: The oil is phototoxic, so do not expose treated skin to direct sunlight. Avoid during pregnancy.

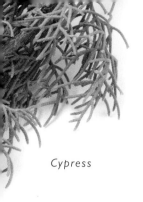

Cypress

CYPRESS *Cupressus sempervirens*
Family: Cupressaceae

DESCRIPTION: A tall evergreen tree, with slender branches and a statuesque, conical shape. It bears small flowers and round, brownish-gray cones or nuts.

ACTIONS: Antirheumatic, antiseptic, antispasmodic, antisudorific, astringent, deodorant, diuretic, hepatic, styptic, tonic, vasoconstrictive.

EXTRACTION: The oil is extracted by steam distillation from the needles and twigs. An oil from the cones is available occasionally.

CHARACTERISTICS: A pale yellow to greenish-olive mobile liquid, with a smoky, sweet-balsamic, tenacious odor. It blends well with cedarwood, pine, lavender, mandarin, clary sage, lemon, cardamom, juniper, benzoin, bergamot, orange, marjoram, and sandalwood.

AROMATHERAPY USE: Skin care: Oily and over-hydrated skin, perspiration, wounds, bruises. Circulation, muscles, and joints: Hemorrhoids, varicose veins, cellulitis, muscular cramps, edema, poor circulation, rheumatism. Respiratory system: Asthma, bronchitis, spasmodic coughing. Reproductive system: Dysmenorrhea, menopausal problems, menorrhagia. Nervous system: Nervous tension, stress-related conditions. Other: Treats pyorrhea (inflamed/bleeding gums); insect repellent.

PERFUME: Scent: Smoky, sweet, balsamic, tenacious, woody, dry, slightly nutty, austere, spicy. Key qualities: Refreshing, purifying, relaxing, warming, reviving, restorative, comforting, protective, soothing. Odor intensity: Medium–low.

EUCALYPTUS BLUE GUM *Eucalyptus globulus*
Family: Myrtaceae

DESCRIPTION: An evergreen tree, up to 50 feet high. Long narrow, yellowish leaves, white flowers, and a smooth, gray bark covered in a white dust.

ACTIONS: Analgesic, antineuralgic, antiseptic, antiviral, cicatrizant, decongestant, deodorant, depurative, diuretic, expectorant, febrifuge, hypoglycemic, parasiticide, prophylactic, rubefacient, stimulant, vermifuge, vulnerary, insecticide.

EXTRACTION: The oil is extracted by steam distillation from the leaves and young twigs.

CHARACTERISTICS: A colorless mobile liquid that yellows on aging, with a camphoraceous odor and woody-sweet undertone. Blends well with thyme, rosemary, lavender, and marjoram.

AROMATHERAPY USE: Skin care: Burns, blisters, cuts, herpes, insect bites, lice, skin infections, wounds. Circulation, muscles, and joints: Muscular aches and pains, poor circulation, rheumatoid arthritis, sprains. Respiratory system: Asthma, bronchitis, catarrh, coughs, sinusitis, throat infections. Immune system: Chicken pox, colds, epidemics, flu, measles. Genitourinary system: Cystitis, leukorrhea. Nervous system: Debility, headaches, neuralgia. Other: Insect repellent.

PERFUME: Scent: Woody-camphoraceous, penetrating, fresh, slightly sweet. Key qualities: Stimulating, refreshing, clearing, purifying, balsamic, regulating. Odor intensity: High.

CAUTION: Apply in dilution only: in concentration, the oil can irritate the skin. Do not use on young children. The oil is toxic if taken internally.

FENNEL, SWEET *Foeniculum vulgare*
Family: Umbelliferae

DESCRIPTION: Biennial or perennial herb, up to 6.5 feet high, with feathery leaves and golden yellow flowers. There are two varieties of fennel: bitter and sweet. Bitter fennel is not recommended for aromatherapy use.

ACTIONS: Aperitif, anti-inflammatory, antimicrobial, antiseptic, antispasmodic, carminative, depurative, diuretic, emmenagogue, expectorant, galactagogue, laxative, stimulant (to circulation), splenetic, stomachic, tonic, vermifuge.

EXTRACTION: The oil is extracted by steam distillation from the crushed seeds.

CHARACTERISTICS: Sweet fennel is a colorless to pale yellow liquid, with a very sweet, anise-like, slightly earthy, peppery scent. It blends well with rose geranium, lavender, rose, and sandalwood.

AROMATHERAPY USE: Skin care: Bruises; dull, oily, mature complexions. Circulation, muscles, and joints: Cellulitis, obesity, edema, rheumatism. Respiratory system: Asthma, bronchitis. Digestive system: Colic, constipation, dyspepsia, flatulence, hiccups, nausea. Reproductive system: Amenorrhea, insufficient milk in nursing mothers, menopausal problems. Other: Treats pyorrhea.

PERFUME: Scent: Sweet, anise-like, earthy, peppery. The name derives from the Latin *foenum*, meaning hay, descriptive of the plant's musty fragrance. Key qualities: Stimulating, balancing, restorative, revitalizing, purifying, cleansing. Odor intensity: High.

CAUTION: This oil should not be used by people who suffer from epilepsy, children under six, or pregnant women.

FRANGIPANI *Plumeria rubra*
Family: Apocynaceae

DESCRIPTION: *Plumeria rubra* is a small tree up to 16 feet tall with a "candelabrum" shape, having a single trunk and branches that spread to form an open canopy. The deciduous pointed leaves, dark green on top and a lighter shade underneath, cluster at the tips of branches. The grayish-green, scaly bark produces a milky, sticky sap that is poisonous, much like oleander. The frangipani flowers, which appear in clusters, each with five waxy petals, are most fragrant at night in order to lure moths to pollinate them.

ACTIONS: Anti-inflammatory, antioxidant, antimicrobial, antifungal, antitumoral, antiviral, aphrodisiac, astringent, nervine.

EXTRACTION: Frangipani absolute is obtained by alcoholic or solvent extraction from the concrete prepared from *P. rubra* (*acutifolia*).

CHARACTERISTICS: The absolute has a heavy, sweet, floral-green aroma, with a soft-spicy background and hints of apricot. It blends with sandalwood, rose, patchouli, tuberose, clove bud, jasmine, neroli, bergamot, ginger, ylang ylang, and most citrus oils.

AROMATHERAPY USE: Skin care: Inflamed and sensitive skin, mature skin, wrinkles, and general skin

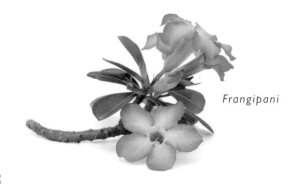

Frangipani

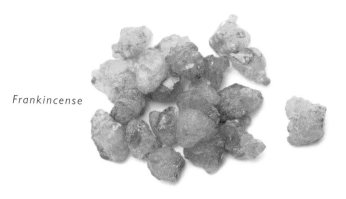

Frankincense

care. Nervous system: Anxiety, depression, fear, insomnia, nervous debility and tension, mood swings, stress.

PERFUME: Scent: Strong, rich, heavy, sweet, floral, spicy, apricot. Key qualities: Romantic, relaxing, aphrodisiac, astringent, purifying. Odor intensity: High.

CAUTION: Avoid using in pregnancy and for children. May cause skin irritation in concentration.

FRANKINCENSE/OLIBANUM
Boswellia carteri
Family: Burseraceae

DESCRIPTION: A small tree or shrub, with pinnate leaves, and white or pale pink flowers. It yields a natural oleo-gum-resin.

ACTIONS: Anti-inflammatory, antiseptic, astringent, carminative, cicatrizant, cytophylactic, digestive, diuretic, emmenagogue, expectorant, sedative, tonic, uterine, vulnerary.

EXTRACTION: The oil is extracted by steam distillation from selected oleo-gum-resin (around 3–10 percent oil to 60–70 percent resin).

CHARACTERISTICS: A pale yellow or greenish mobile liquid, with a fresh terpeney top note, and a warm, rich, sweet-balsamic undertone. It blends well with sandalwood, pine, vetivert, geranium, lavender, neroli, orange, bergamot, and other citrus oils, camphor, basil, pepper, cinnamon, and other spice oils.

AROMATHERAPY USE: Skin care: Blemishes, dry and mature complexions, scars, wounds, wrinkles. Respiratory system: Asthma, bronchitis, catarrh, colds, coughs, flu, laryngitis. Genitourinary system: Cystitis, dysmenorrhea, leukorrhea, metrorrhagia.

Nervous system: Anxiety, nervous tension, stress-related conditions. Frankincense has the ability to slow down and deepen the breath—very conducive to prayer and meditation.

PERFUME: Scent: Balsamic, long-lasting, woody, slightly camphoraceous, resinous, rich, sweet, incense-like, dry. This oil is a fixative and preservative. Key qualities: Clearing, purifying, restorative, warming, sedative, uplifting, tonic, cephalic, revitalizing. Odor intensity: High.

GARDENIA *Gardenia jasminoides*
Family: Rubiaceae

DESCRIPTION: Native to China, gardenia is a large evergreen shrub with deep, glossy green leaves and large, fragrant white flowers in summer and fall.

ACTIONS: Antibacterial, antifungal, antiviral.

EXTRACTION: Oil is extracted from the delicate flower petals using the enfleurage method.

CHARACTERISTICS: A yellowish amber oil. It blends well with other floral fragrances such as jasmine, ylang ylang, and lavender, as well as citrus oils such as bergamot, lemon, and orange.

AROMATHERAPY USE: Skin care: Dermatitis, mature complexions—toning and revitalizing. Circulation, muscles, and joints: Inflammation. Nervous system: Anxiety, depression.

PERFUME: Scent: Floral, sweet, fresh, green, earthy. Key qualities: Antidepressant, calming, soothing, exotic. Odor intensity: Medium.

CAUTION: Can cause skin rashes and irritation, especially in sensitive skin. Always dilute with a carrier oil, such as jojoba. Should be avoided during pregnancy and breastfeeding.

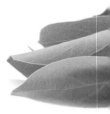

GERANIUM, ROSE *Pelargonium graveolens*
Family: Geraniaceae

DESCRIPTION: A perennial hairy shrub, up to 3 feet high, with lobed leaves, serrated at the edges, and small pink flowers. The whole plant is aromatic.

ACTIONS: Antihemorrhagic, anti-inflammatory, antiseptic, astringent, cicatrizant, deodorant, diuretic, fungicidal, hemostatic, stimulant (to adrenal cortex and lymphatic system), styptic, tonic, vermifuge, vulnerary.

EXTRACTION: The oil is extracted by steam distillation from the leaves, stalks, and flowers.

CHARACTERISTICS: Greenish-olive liquid with a green, rosy-sweet, minty scent. (The Bourbon oil is generally preferred in perfumery work.) It blends well with lavender, patchouli, clove, rose, sandalwood, jasmine, juniper, neroli, bergamot, and other citrus oils.

AROMATHERAPY USE: Skin care: Acne, bruises, broken capillaries, burns, congested skin, cuts, dermatitis, eczema, hemorrhoids, lice, oily complexion, mature skin, ringworm, ulcers, wounds. Circulatory system: Cellulitis, engorgement of breasts, edema, poor circulation. Respiratory system: Sore throat, tonsillitis. Reproductive and endocrine system: Adrenocortical glands and menopausal problems, PMS. Nervous system: Nervous tension, neuralgia, stress-related conditions. Other: Insect repellent (especially mosquitoes).

CAUTION: Generally nonsensitizing, but may cause contact dermatitis in hypersensitive individuals (especially the Bourbon type).

GINGER *Zingiber officinale*
Family: Zingiberaceae

DESCRIPTION: An erect perennial herb, up to 3 feet high, with a thick, spreading, tuberous rhizomatous root, which is very pungent. The green, reed-like stalk, with narrow, spear-shaped leaves and white or yellow flowers, grows up from the root.

ACTIONS: Analgesic, antioxidant, antiseptic, antispasmodic, aperitif, aphrodisiac, bactericidal, carminative, cephalic, expectorant, febrifuge, laxative, rubifacient, stimulant, stomachic, tonic.

EXTRACTION: The oil is extracted by steam distillation from the unpeeled, dried ground root.

CHARACTERISTICS: A pale yellow, amber, or greenish liquid with a warm, slightly green, fresh, woody-spicy scent. It blends well with sandalwood, vetivert, patchouli, frankincense, rosewood, rose, cedarwood, coriander, lime, neroli, orange, and lemon.

AROMATHERAPY USE: Circulation, muscles, and joints: Arthritis, fatigue, muscular aches and pains, poor circulation, rheumatism, sprains, strains. Respiratory system: Catarrh, congestion, coughs, sinusitis, sore throat. Digestive system: Diarrhea, colic, cramp, flatulence, indigestion, loss of appetite, nausea, travel sickness. Immune system: Chills, colds, flu, fever, infectious disease. Nervous system: Debility, nervous exhaustion.

PERFUME: Scent: Fresh, woody-spicy, rich, slightly green, peppery, fiery, penetrating, diffusive, exotic. Key qualities: Tonic, aphrodisiac, stimulating, warming, cephalic, comforting. Odor intensity: High.

CAUTION: Nonirritant (except in high concentration), but may cause some sensitization—use in low dilutions only. Slightly phototoxic.

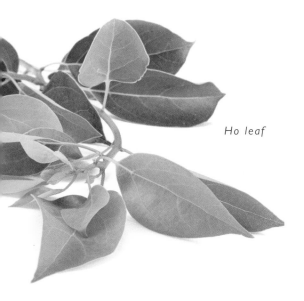

Ho leaf

GRAPEFRUIT *Citrus x paradisi*
Family: Rutaceae

DESCRIPTION: A cultivated tree, often over 33 feet high, with glossy leaves and familiar large, yellow fruits.

ACTIONS: Antiseptic, antitoxic, astringent, bactericidal, diuretic, depurative, stimulant (to lymphatic and digestive systems), tonic.

EXTRACTION: The oil is extracted by cold expression from the fresh peel.

CHARACTERISTICS: A yellow or greenish mobile liquid, with a fresh, sweet, citrus aroma. It blends well with lemon, palmarosa, bergamot, neroli, rosemary, cypress, lavender, geranium, cardamom, and other spice oils.

AROMATHERAPY USE: Skin care: Acne, congested and oily skin, promotes hair growth, tones the skin and tissues. Circulation, muscles, and joints: Cellulitis, exercise preparation, muscle fatigue, obesity, stiffness, water retention. Immune system: Chills, colds, flu. Nervous system: Depression, headaches, nervous exhaustion, performance stress.

PERFUME: Scent: Citrus, fruity, bitter, powerful, lemony, fresh. Key qualities (mind): Cleansing, stimulating, refreshing, uplifting. Odor intensity: Medium.

CAUTION: Slightly phototoxic. This oil has a short shelf life—it oxidizes quickly.

HO WOOD *Cinnamomum camphora linalool*
Family: Lauraceae

DESCRIPTION: A tall, tropical evergreen tree, quite dense with small white flowers and black berries, which grows up to 100 feet in height. This is the same tree that produces camphor, which comes from the wood of the tree.

ACTIONS: Analgesic, antifungal, anti-infectious, anti-inflammatory, antioxidant, antiseptic, antispasmodic, bactericidal, immune support, sedative, tonic. It is also believed to be a mild aphrodisiac.

EXTRACTION: The oil is extracted by steam distillation from the leaves (ho leaf oil) and wood (ho wood oil).

CHARACTERISTICS: Ho wood oil is a pale-yellow liquid with a soft, warm, floral, spicy-woody scent with a slightly camphor-like undertone. The leaf oil has a sweet-fresh, green-floral, and woody scent. It blends well with basil, bergamot, cedarwood, chamomile, lavender, lime, geranium, juniper, neroli, petitgrain, myrtle, sandalwood, ylang ylang, and spice oils.

AROMATHERAPY USE: Skin care: Acne, cuts, dermatitis, stretch marks, scars, wounds, and general skin care; dry, oily, mature, and sensitive skin. Circulation, muscles, and joints: Aches and pains caused by inflammation. Respiratory system: Chills, coughs and colds, flu. Immune system: Low libido, boosts vitality. Nervous system: Anxiety, depression, insomnia, nervous tension, stress. Other: An effective insect repellent.

PERFUME: Scent: Soft, warm, floral, spicy, woody. Key qualities: Calming, relaxing. Odor intensity: Medium.

CAUTION: Possible sensitization in some individuals.

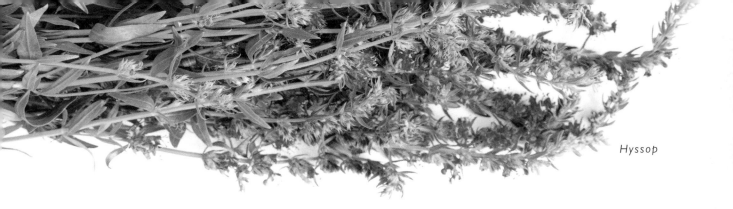

HYSSOP *Hyssopus officinalis*
Family: Lamiaceae

DESCRIPTION: An attractive perennial, almost evergreen, sub-shrub, up to 2 feet high, with a woody stem, small, lance-shaped leaves, and purplish-blue flowers.

ACTIONS: Astringent, antiseptic, antispasmodic, antiviral, bactericide, carminative, cephalic, cicatrizant, digestive, diuretic, emmenagogue, expectorant, febrifuge, hypertensive, nervine, sedative, sudorific, tonic (to heart and circulation), vermifuge, vulnerary.

EXTRACTION: The oil is extracted by steam distillation from the leaves and flowering tops.

CHARACTERISTICS: A colorless to pale yellowish-green liquid, with a sweet, camphoraceous top note and warm, spicy-herbaceous undertone. It blends well with lavender, rosemary, myrtle, bay, sage, clary sage, geranium, and the citrus oils.

AROMATHERAPY USE: Skin care: Bruises, cuts, dermatitis, eczema, inflammation, wounds (nonirritant, nonsensitizing). Circulatory system: Low or high blood pressure, rheumatism. Respiratory system: Asthma, bronchitis, catarrh, cough, flu, sore throat, tonsillitis, whooping cough. Digestive system: Colic, indigestion. Reproductive system: Amenorrhea, leukorrhea. Nervous system: Anxiety, fatigue, nervous tension, stress-related conditions.

PERFUME: Scent: Sweet, warm, herbaceous, slightly camphoraceous. Key qualities: Tonic, cephalic, nervine, warming, calming, purifying, cleansing, aphrodisiac, mental stimulant, balancing. Odor intensity: High.

CAUTION: Use oil in moderation. Avoid during pregnancy and by people suffering from epilepsy. Do not use on children.

JASMINE *Jasminum officinale*
Family: Oleaceae

DESCRIPTION: An evergreen shrub or vine up to 33 feet high, with delicate, bright green leaves and star-shaped, very fragrant white flowers.

ACTIONS: Analgesic (mild), anti-inflammatory, antiseptic, antispasmodic, carminative, cicatrizant, expectorant, galactagogue, parturient, sedative, tonic (uterine).

EXTRACTION: A concrete is produced from the flowers by solvent extraction. The absolute is obtained from the concrete by separation with alcohol. A second essential oil is produced by steam distillation of the absolute.

CHARACTERISTICS: The absolute is a dark orange-brown, viscous liquid, with an intensely rich, warm, floral scent and a tea-like undertone. It blends well with rose, sandalwood, clary sage, and all citrus oils.

AROMATHERAPY USE: Skin care: Dry, greasy, irritated, sensitive skin. Circulation, muscles, and joints: Muscular spasm, sprains. Respiratory system: Catarrh, coughs, hoarseness, laryngitis. Reproductive system: Dysmenorrhea, frigidity, labor pains, uterine disorders. Nervous system: Depression, nervous exhaustion, stress-related conditions.

PERFUME: Scent: Rich, warm, floral, sweet, tea-like, exquisite, exotic, long-lasting. Key qualities: Intoxicating, uplifting, antidepressant, euphoric, aphrodisiac, tonic, balancing, warming. Odor intensity: High.

CAUTION: An allergic reaction has been known to occur in some individuals.

Juniper berry oil is has a sweet, fresh, woody-balsamic odor.

JUNIPER *Juniperus communis*
Family: Cupressaceae

DESCRIPTION: An evergreen shrub or tree, up to 20 feet high, with bluish-green, narrow, stiff needles. It has small flowers and little round black berries.

ACTIONS: Antirheumatic, antiseptic, antispasmodic, antitoxic, aphrodisiac, astringent, carminative, cicatrizant, depurative, diuretic, emmenagogue, nervine, parasiticide, rubefacient, sedative, stomachic, sudorific, tonic, vulnerary.

EXTRACTION: The oil is extracted by steam distillation from the berries, the needles, or the wood.

CHARACTERISTICS: Juniper berry oil is a water-white or pale yellow mobile liquid, with a sweet, fresh, woody-balsamic odor. It blends well with vetivert, sandalwood, cedarwood, galbanum, elemi, cypress, clary sage, pine, lavender, rosemary, benzoin, geranium, and citrus oils.

AROMATHERAPY USE: Skin care: Acne, dermatitis, eczema, hair loss, hemorrhoids, wounds, tonic for oily complexions (nonsensitizing, but may be slightly irritating). Circulation, muscles, and joints: Accumulation of toxins, arteriosclerosis, cellulite, gout, obesity, rheumatism. Immune system: Colds, flu, infections. Genitourinary system: Amenorrhea, cystitis, dysmenorrhea, leukorrhea. Nervous system: Anxiety, nervous tension, stress-related conditions.

PERFUME: Scent: Sweet, fresh, woody, balsamic, turpentine-like, peppery, smoky. Key qualities: Aphrodisiac, purifying, clearing, depurative, tonic (nerve), reviving, protective, restorative. Odor intensity: Medium.

CAUTION: This oil stimulates the uterine muscle (an abortifacient) and must not be used during pregnancy. It should not be used by those with kidney disease, as it is nephrotoxic. It is not suitable for young children. Use in moderation.

LABDANUM *Cistus ladaniferus*
Family: Cistaceae

DESCRIPTION: A small, sticky shrub up to 10 feet high, with lance-shaped leaves that are white and furry on the underside, and fragrant white flowers. Labdanum gum, a dark brown solid mass, is a natural oleoresin, which is obtained by boiling the plant material in water.

ACTIONS: Antimicrobial, antiseptic, antitussive, astringent, emmenagogue, expectorant, tonic, balsamic.

EXTRACTION: The oil is extracted by steam distillation from the crude gum, the absolute, or from the leaves and twigs of the plant directly.

CHARACTERISTICS: A dark yellow or amber viscous liquid with a warm, sweet, dry-herbaceous, musky scent. It blends well with oakmoss, clary sage, pine, juniper, calamus, opopanax, lavender, lavandin, bergamot, cypress, vetivert, sandalwood, patchouli, olibanum, and chamomile maroc.

AROMATHERAPY USE: Skin care: Mature skin, wrinkles. Respiratory system: Coughs, bronchitis, rhinitis. Immune system: Colds.

PERFUME: Scent: Amber, warm, sweet, herbaceous, musky. Key qualities: Calming, soothing, uplifting, rejuvenating. Odor intensity: High.

CAUTION: Avoid during pregnancy.

Laurel leaves were used to crown Olympians and emperors.

LAUREL *Laurus nobilis*
Family: Lauraceae

DESCRIPTION: An evergreen tree up to 65 feet high, with dark green, glossy leaves and black berries; often cultivated as an ornamental shrub.

ACTIONS: Antirheumatic, antiseptic, bactericidal, diaphoretic, digestive, diuretic, emmenagogue, fungicidal, hypotensive, sedative, stomachic.

EXTRACTION: The oil is extracted by steam distillation from the dried leaf and branchlets. (An oil from the berries is produced in small quantities.)

CHARACTERISTICS: A greenish-yellow liquid with a powerful, spicy-medicinal odor. It blends well with pine, cypress, juniper, clary sage, rosemary, olibanum, labdanum, lavender, citrus, and spice oils.

AROMATHERAPY USE: Digestive system: Dyspepsia, flatulence, loss of appetite. Genitourinary system: Scanty periods. Immune system: Colds, flu, tonsillitis, and viral infections.

PERFUME: Scent: Spicy, medicinal, sweet, floral. Key qualities: Uplifting, confidence-inspiring, energizing, analgesic, antiseptic. Odor intensity: Medium.

CAUTION: Can cause dermatitis in some individuals. Use in moderation due to possible narcotic properties. Should not be used during pregnancy.

LAVENDER, TRUE *Lavandula angustifolia/ L. officinalis*
Family: Labiatae

DESCRIPTION: An evergreen, woody shrub, up to 3 feet tall, with gray-green, narrow, linear leaves and blue flower spikes.

ACTIONS: Analgesic, anticonvulsive, antimicrobial, antirheumatic, antiseptic, antispasmodic, antitoxic, carminative, cholagogue, choleretic, cytophylactic, deodorant, diuretic, emmenagogue, hypotensor, insecticide, nervine, parasiticide, rubefacient, sedative, stimulant, sudorific, tonic, vermifuge, vulnerary.

EXTRACTION: The oil is extracted by steam distillation from the fresh flowering tops.

CHARACTERISTICS: The oil is colorless to pale yellow, with a sweet, floral-herbaceous scent and balsamic-woody undertone. Blends well with most oils, especially citrus, florals, cedarwood, clove, clary sage, pine, geranium, vetivert, and patchouli.

AROMATHERAPY USE: Skin care: Abscess, acne, allergies, athlete's foot, boils, bruises, burns, dermatitis, eczema, inflammation, insect bites and stings, lice, psoriasis, ringworm, scabies, spots, sunburn, wounds. Circulation, muscles, and joints: Lumbago, rheumatism, sprains. Respiratory system: Asthma, bronchitis, catarrh, flu, halitosis, throat infections, whooping cough. Digestive system: Colic, dyspepsia, flatulence, nausea. Genitourinary system: Cystitis, dysmenorrhea, leukorrhea. Nervous system: Depression, headache, hypertension, insomnia, migraine, nervous tension, stress.

PERFUME: Scent: Light, floral, classic, soft, mellow. Key qualities: Soothing, sedative, antidepressant, calming, relaxing, balancing, restorative, cephalic, appeasing, cleansing, purifying. Odor intensity: Medium.

LEMON *Citrus limon*
Family: Rutaceae

DESCRIPTION: A small evergreen tree, up to 20 feet high, with serrated oval leaves, stiff thorns, and fragrant flowers. The fruit ripens from green to yellow.

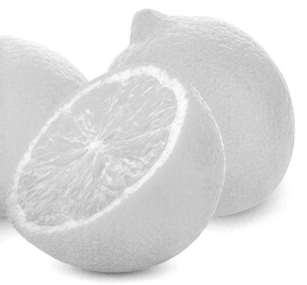

Lemon

ACTIONS: Antianemic, antimicrobial, antirheumatic, antisclerotic, antiseptic, antispasmodic, antitoxic, astringent, bactericide, carminative, cicatrizant, depurative, diaphoretic, diuretic, febrifuge, hemostatic, hypotensive, insecticide, rubefacient, tonic, vermifuge.

EXTRACTION: The oil is extracted by cold expression from the outer part of the fresh peel.

CHARACTERISTICS: A pale greenish-yellow liquid, with a light, fresh, citrus scent. It blends well with lavender, neroli, ylang ylang, rose, sandalwood, olibanum, chamomile, benzoin, fennel, geranium, eucalyptus, juniper, elemi, and other citrus oils.

AROMATHERAPY USE: Skin care: Acne, anemia, brittle nails, boils, chilblains, corns, cuts, greasy skin, herpes, insect bites, mouth ulcers, spots, throat infections, warts. Circulation, muscles, and joints: Arthritis, cellulitis, high blood pressure, nosebleeds, obesity (congestion), poor circulation, varicose veins, rheumatism. Respiratory system: Asthma, bronchitis, catarrh. Digestive system: Dyspepsia. Immune system: Colds, flu, fever, infections.

PERFUME: Scent: Fresh, clean, lemony, light, penetrating, fruity, diffusive. Key qualities: Refreshing, mental stimulant, cephalic, purifying, reviving, strengthening, soothing. Odor intensity: Medium.

CAUTION: This oil is phototoxic—do not use on skin before exposing to direct sunlight or sunbeds. May cause irritation or sensitization. Use in moderation.

LEMONGRASS, WEST INDIAN
Cymbopogon citratus
Family: Graminaceae

DESCRIPTION: A fast-growing, tall, aromatic, perennial grass, up to 5 feet high, producing a network of roots and rootlets that rapidly exhaust the soil.

ACTIONS: Analgesic, antidepressant, antimicrobial, antioxidant, antipyretic, antiseptic, astringent, bactericidal, carminative, deodorant, febrifuge, fungicidal, galactagogue, insecticide, nervine, sedative (nervous system), tonic.

EXTRACTION: The oil is extracted by steam distillation from the fresh and partially dried leaves (grass).

CHARACTERISTICS: A yellow, amber, or reddish-brown liquid, with a fresh, grassy-citrus scent and an earthy undertone. Blends well with geranium, bergamot, and the other citrus oils.

AROMATHERAPY USE: Skin care: Acne, athlete's foot, excessive perspiration, open pores, pediculosis, scabies, tissue toner. Circulation, muscles, and joints: Muscular pain, poor circulation and muscle tone, slack tissue. Digestive system: Colitis, indigestion, gastroenteritis. Immune system: Fevers, infectious diseases. Nervous system: Headaches, nervous exhaustion, stress-related conditions. Other: Insect repellent (fleas, lice, ticks).

PERFUME: Scent: Citrus, clean, green, hay-like, slightly bitter, lemony, pungent. Key qualities (mind): Refreshing, active, stimulating, soothing. Odor intensity: High.

CAUTION: Possible dermal irritation and/or sensitization in some individuals—use with care.

MANDARIN *Citrus reticulata*
Family: Rutaceae

DESCRIPTION: A small evergreen tree, up to 20 feet high, with glossy leaves, fragrant flowers, and bearing fleshy fruit. The fruit is larger than other tangerines, and is rounder, with a more yellowish skin.

ACTIONS: Antiseptic, antispasmodic, carminative, digestive, diuretic (mild), laxative (mild), sedative, stimulant (to digestive and lymphatic systems), tonic.

EXTRACTION: The oil is extracted by cold expression from the outer peel.

CHARACTERISTICS: Mandarin oil is a yellowish-orange mobile liquid with a blue-violet hint. It has a sweet, almost floral, citrus scent. It blends well with other citrus oils, especially neroli, and spice oils such as nutmeg, cinnamon, and clove.

AROMATHERAPY USE: Skin care: Acne, congested and oily skin, scars, spots, stretch marks, toner. Circulatory system: Fluid retention, obesity. Digestive system: Digestive problems, dyspepsia, hiccups, intestinal problems. Nervous system: Insomnia, nervous tension, restlessness.

PERFUME: Scent: Fresh, warm, sweet, fruity, soft, mild. Key qualities (mind): Warming, comforting, soothing, uplifting. Odor intensity: Low.

CAUTION: Slightly phototoxic.

MARJORAM, SWEET *Origanum marjorana/ Marjorana hortensis*
Family: Lamiaceae

DESCRIPTION: A tender, bushy perennial plant, up to 2 feet high, with a hairy stem, dark green oval leaves, and small grayish-white flowers growing in clusters.

ACTIONS: Analgesic, anaphrodisiac, antioxidant, antiseptic, antispasmodic, antiviral, bactericidal, carminative, cephalic, cordial, diaphoretic, digestive, diuretic, emmenagogue, expectorant, fungicidal, hypotensor, laxative, nervine, sedative, tonic, vasodilatator, vulnerary.

EXTRACTION: The oil is extracted by steam distillation from the dried flowering herb.

CHARACTERISTICS: A pale yellow or amber-colored mobile liquid with a warm, woody, spicy, camphoraceous odor. Blends well with lavender, rosemary, bergamot, chamomile, cypress, tea tree, and eucalyptus.

AROMATHERAPY USE: Skin care: Chilblains, bruises, tics. Circulation, muscles, and joints: Arthritis, lumbago, muscular aches and stiffness, rheumatism, sprains, strains. Respiratory system: Asthma, bronchitis, colds, coughs. Digestive system: Colic, constipation, dyspepsia, flatulence. Reproductive system: Amenorrhea, dysmenorrhea, leukorrhea,

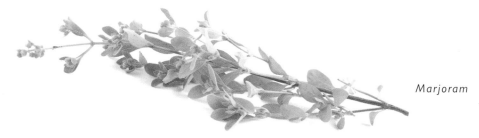

Marjoram

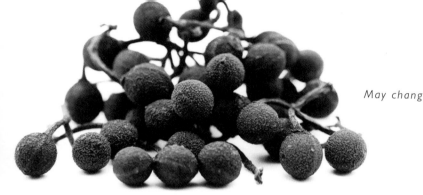
May chang

PMS. Nervous system: Headache, hypertension, insomnia, migraine, nervous tension, stress-related conditions.

PERFUME: Scent: Warm, woody, spicy, nutty, camphoraceous, herbaceous, penetrating. Key qualities: Anaphrodisiac, stupefying in large doses, cephalic, sedative, nervine, restorative, warming, comforting. Odor intensity: Medium.

CAUTION: This oil should not be used during pregnancy.

MAY CHANG *Litsea cubeba*
Family: Lauraceae

DESCRIPTION: A small tropical tree with fragrant, lemongrass-scented leaves and flowers. The small fruits are shaped like peppers, from which the name "cubeba" derives.

ACTIONS: Antiseptic, deodorant, digestive, disinfectant, insecticidal, stimulant, stomachic.

EXTRACTION: The oil is extracted by steam distillation from the fruits.

CHARACTERISTICS: A pale yellow mobile liquid with an intense, lemony, fresh-fruity odor (sweeter than lemongrass but less tenacious).

AROMATHERAPY USE: Skin care: Acne, dermatitis, excessive perspiration, greasy skin, insect repellent, spots. Digestive system: Flatulence, indigestion. Immune system: Epidemics, sanitation.

PERFUME: Scent: Lemony, fresh-fruity, spicy. Key qualities: Refreshing, stimulating, uplifting, tonic, cleansing, antiseptic, antiviral, astringent. Odor intensity: Medium.

CAUTION: Possible sensitization in some individuals.

MELISSA/LEMON BALM *Melissa officinalis*
Family: Labiatae

DESCRIPTION: A sweet-scented herb about 2 feet high, soft and bushy, with bright green, serrated leaves, square stems, and tiny white or pink flowers.

ACTIONS: Antidepressant, antihistaminic, antispasmodic, bactericidal, carminative, cordial, diaphoretic, emmenagogue, febrifuge, hypertensive, nervine, sedative, stomachic, sudorific, tonic, uterine, vermifuge, insect repellent.

EXTRACTION: The oil is extracted by steam distillation from the leaves and flowering tops.

CHARACTERISTICS: A pale yellow liquid with a light, fresh, lemony fragrance. It blends well with lavender and geranium oil and with all floral and citrus oils.

AROMATHERAPY USE: Skin care: Allergies, insect bites. Respiratory system: Asthma, bronchitis, chronic coughs. Digestive system: Colic, indigestion, nausea. Reproductive system: Menstrual problems. Nervous system: Anxiety, depression, hypertension, insomnia, migraine, nervous tension, shock, vertigo. Other: Insect repellent.

PERFUME: Scent: Lemony, light, fresh, green, herbaceous, honey-sweet. Key qualities: Soothing, calming, uplifting, regulating, sedative, appeasing, comforting, heart tonic, strengthening, revitalizing, protecting, antidepressant. Odor intensity: High.

CAUTION: Skin irritant. Use in low dilutions (up to 1 percent). Narcotic in large doses, causing headaches. Available information suggests possible sensitization and skin irritation.

MIMOSA *Acacia dealbata*
Family: Mimosaceae

DESCRIPTION: An attractive small tree up to 40 feet high, having a grayish-brown bark with irregular longitudinal ridges, delicate foliage, and clusters of ball-shaped, fragrant yellow flowers.

ACTIONS: Antiseptic, astringent.

EXTRACTION: A concrete and absolute by solvent extraction from the flowers and twig ends.

CHARACTERISTICS: The concrete is a hard, wax-like yellow mass. The absolute is an amber-colored viscous liquid with a slightly green, woody-floral scent. It blends well with lavandin, lavender, ylang ylang, violet, styrax, citronella, Peru balsam, cassie, floral, and spice oils.

AROMATHERAPY USE: Skin care: Oily, sensitive, general skin care. Nervous system: Anxiety, nervous tension, oversensitivity, stress.

PERFUME: Scent: Sweet, floral, woody, honey-like, leathery. Key qualities: Calming, warming, soothing, relaxing, uplifting, balancing. Odor intensity: Medium.

Mimosa

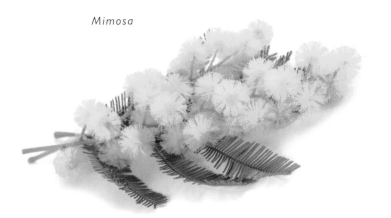

MYRRH *Commiphora myrrh*
Family: Burseraceae

DESCRIPTION: Shrubs or small trees up to 33 feet high, with knotted branches, aromatic leaves, and small white flowers The trunk yields oleoresin (myrrh).

ACTIONS: Anti-inflammatory, antimicrobial, antiphlogistic, antiseptic, astringent, balsamic, carminative, cicatrizant, expectorant, fungicidal, sedative, stimulant, stomachic, tonic, uterine, vulnerary.

EXTRACTION: Resinoid (and resin absolute) are obtained by solvent extraction from the crude myrrh. The oil is extracted by steam distillation.

CHARACTERISTICS: The essential oil is a pale yellow to amber, oily liquid with a warm, slightly spicy, medicinal odor. It blends well with frankincense, sandalwood, benzoin, cypress, juniper, mandarin, geranium, patchouli, thyme, mints, lavender, and pine.

AROMATHERAPY USE: Skin care: Athlete's foot, chapped and cracked skin, eczema, ringworm, wounds, wrinkles, mature complexions (nonirritant, nonsensitizing). Circulation, muscles, and joints: Arthritis. Respiratory system: Asthma, bronchitis, catarrh, colds, coughs, sore throat, voice loss. Digestive system: Diarrhea, dyspepsia, flatulence, hemorrhoids, loss of appetite. Genitourinary system: Amenorrhea, leukorrhea, pruritus, thrush. Other: Treats gum infections, mouth ulcers.

PERFUME: Scent: Bitter-spicy, rich, balsamic, resinous, long-lasting. Key qualities: Purifying, uplifting,

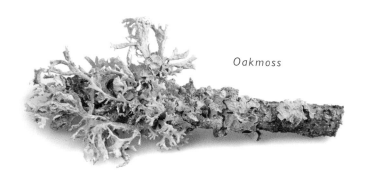

Oakmoss

revitalizing, sedative (to nervous system), restorative, soothing. Odor intensity: High.

CAUTION: This oil should not be used during pregnancy. Do not use in high concentrations.

NEROLI *Citrus aurantium* var. *amara*
Family: Rutaceae

DESCRIPTION: An evergreen tree, up to 33 feet high, with dark green, glossy, oval leaves, paler beneath, and with long, but not very sharp, spines. It has a smooth, grayish trunk and branches, and very fragrant white flowers. The fruits are smaller and darker than those of the sweet orange.

ACTIONS: Antiseptic, antispasmodic, bactericidal, carminative, cicatrizant, cordial, deodorant, digestive, mildly fungicidal, stimulant (nervous), tonic.

EXTRACTION: Essential oil is extracted by steam distillation from the freshly picked flowers.

CHARACTERISTICS: The oil is a pale yellow mobile liquid, with a light, sweet-floral fragrance and terpeney top note. Blends well with virtually all oils, especially jasmine, lavender, rose, lemon, and other citrus oils.

AROMATHERAPY USE: Skin care: Scars, stretch marks, thread veins, mature and sensitive skin, wrinkles, tones the complexion. Circulatory system: Palpitations, poor circulation. Digestive system: Diarrhea (chronic), colic, flatulence, spasm, nervous dyspepsia. Nervous system: Anxiety, depression, nervous tension, PMS, shock, stress-related conditions, and especially problems of emotional origin.

PERFUME: Scent: Floral, soft, delicate, pervasive, sweet, warm, rich. Key qualities: Aphrodisiac, hypnotic, sedative, soothing, tonic, restorative, uplifting, antidepressant. Odor intensity: Medium–high.

OAKMOSS *Evernia prunastri*
Family: Usneaceae

DESCRIPTION: A light green lichen found growing primarily on oak trees, and sometimes on other species.

ACTIONS: Antiseptic, demulcent, expectorant, fixative.

EXTRACTION: A range of products is produced: a concrete and an absolute by solvent extraction from the lichen that has often been soaked in lukewarm water prior to extraction; an absolute oil by vacuum distillation of the concrete; resins and resinoids by alcohol extraction of the raw material. Most important of these products is the absolute.

CHARACTERISTICS: The absolute is a dark green or brown, very viscous liquid with an extremely tenacious, earthy-mossy odor and a leather-like undertone. The absolute oil is a pale yellow or olive viscous liquid with a dry-earthy, bark-like odor, quite true to nature. The concrete, resin, and resinoids are a very dark-colored semisolid or solid mass with a heavy, rich-earthy, extremely tenacious odor. They have a high fixative value and blend with virtually all other oils: they are extensively used in perfumery to lend body and rich natural undertones to all perfume types.

AROMATHERAPY USE: As a fixative.

PERFUME: Scent: Green, woody, slightly fruity, earthy. Key qualities: Soothing, restorative, antiseptic, antiaging, refreshing, reinvigorating. Odor intensity: High.

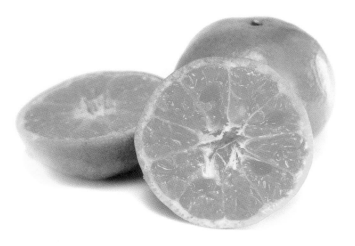

ORANGE, SWEET *Citrus sinensis/Citrus aurantium* var. *dulcis*
Family: Rutaceae

DESCRIPTION: An evergreen tree, smaller than the bitter variety, less hardy, and with fewer (or no) spines. The fruit has a sweet pulp and nonbitter membranes.

ACTIONS: Antidepressant, anti-inflammatory, antiseptic, bactericidal, carminative, choleretic, digestive, fungicidal, hypotensor, sedative (to the nervous system), stimulant, stomachic, tonic.

EXTRACTION: By cold expression (by hand or machine) or steam distillation of the fresh, ripe, or almost ripe outer peel.

CHARACTERISTICS: The oil is a yellowish-orange or dark orange mobile liquid, with a sweet, fresh-fruity scent. It blends well with lavender, neroli, lemon, clary sage, myrrh, and spice oils such as nutmeg, cinnamon, and cloves.

AROMATHERAPY USE: Skin care: Dull and oily complexions (nonirritant, generally nonsensitizing, but can cause dermatitis in some individuals). Circulatory system: Obesity, palpitations, water retention. Respiratory system: Bronchitis, chills, colds, flu. Digestive system: Constipation, dyspepsia, spasm. Nervous system: Nervous tension, stress-related conditions. Other: Used to treat mouth ulcers.

PERFUME: Scent: Sweet, warm, sensual, radiant, fresh, citrus, fruity, tangy. Key qualities: Tonic (to the nervous system), refreshing, warming, uplifting, soothing, sedative, comforting. Odor intensity: Medium–low.

CAUTION: Distilled orange oil should not be used on the skin before exposure to sunlight or use of a sunbed.

PALMAROSA *Cymbopogon martinii* var. *martinii*
Family: Poaceae

DESCRIPTION: A wild herbaceous plant, with long, slender stems and terminal flowering tops; the grassy leaves are very fragrant.

ACTIONS: Antiseptic, bactericidal, cicatrizant, digestive, febrifuge, hydrating, stimulant (to the digestive and circulatory systems), tonic.

EXTRACTION: The oil is extracted by steam or water distillation of the fresh or dried grass.

CHARACTERISTICS: A pale yellow or olive liquid, with a sweet, floral, rosy, geranium-like scent. It blends well with ylang ylang, rose geranium, bois de rose, sandalwood, cypress, cedarwood, and floral oils.

AROMATHERAPY USE: Skin care: Acne, dermatitis and minor skin infections, scars, sores, wrinkles; valuable for all types of treatment for the face, hands, feet, neck, and lips (moisturizes the skin, stimulates cellular regeneration, regulates sebum production). Digestive system: Digestive atonia, intestinal infections. Nervous system: Nervous exhaustion, stress-related conditions.

PERFUME: Scent: Rosy, sweet, fresh, warm, slightly green, floral. Key qualities (mind): Refreshing, balancing, comforting. Odor intensity: Medium–high.

The berries turn from red to black as they mature—black pepper is the dried, unripe fruit.

PATCHOULI *Pogostemon patchouli*
Family: Laminaceae

DESCRIPTION: A perennial bushy herb, up to 3 feet high, with large, fragrant, furry leaves and white flowers tinged with purple.

ACTIONS: Antidepressant, anti-inflammatory, antiemetic, antimicrobial, antiphlogistic, antiseptic, antitoxic, antiviral, astringent, bactericidal, carminative, cicatrizant, deodorant, digestive, diuretic, febrifuge, fungicidal, nervine, prophylactic, stimulant, stomachic, tonic.

EXTRACTION: The oil is extracted by steam distillation of the dried leaves.

CHARACTERISTICS: An amber or dark orange viscous liquid with a sweet, rich, herbaceous, earthy odor that improves with age. It blends well with vetivert, sandalwood, cedarwood, geranium, clove, lavender, rose, neroli, bergamot, myrrh, frankincense, and clary sage.

AROMATHERAPY USE: Skin care: Acne, athlete's foot, cracked and chapped skin, dandruff, dermatitis, eczema (weeping), fungal infections, hair care, impetigo, sores, oily hair and skin, open pores, wounds, wrinkles. Nervous system: Frigidity, nervous exhaustion, stress-related complaints. Other: Insect repellent (moths).

PERFUME: Scent: Earthy, musky, spicy, woody, diffusive, warm, medicinal, powerful. Key qualities: Stimulant in small amounts, sedative in large doses, aphrodisiac, nerve tonic, appeasing, calming, uplifting. Odor intensity: Very high.

CAUTION: Its overuse can cause loss of appetite, insomnia, and nervous attacks.

PEPPER, BLACK *Piper nigrum*
Family: Piperaceae

DESCRIPTION: A perennial woody vine, up to 16.5 feet high, with heart-shaped leaves and small, white flowers. The berries turn from red to black as they mature—black pepper is the dried, unripe fruit.

ACTIONS: Analgesic, antimicrobial, antiseptic, antitoxic, aperitif, bactericidal, carminative, diaphoretic, digestive, diuretic, febrifuge, laxative, rubefacient, stimulant, stomachic, tonic.

EXTRACTION: The oil is extracted by steam distillation from the black peppercorns, which have been dried and crushed.

CHARACTERISTICS: A water-white to pale olive mobile liquid, with a fresh, dry-woody, warm, spicy scent. It blends well with frankincense, sandalwood, lavender, rosemary, marjoram, spices, and florals when used in minute quantities.

AROMATHERAPY USE: Skin care: Chilblains. Circulation, muscles, and joints: Anemia, arthritis, muscular aches and pains, neuralgia, poor circulation, poor muscle tone, rheumatic pain, sprains, stiffness. Respiratory system: Catarrh, chills. Immune system: Colds, flu, infections, viruses. Digestive system: Colic, constipation, diarrhea, flatulence, heartburn, loss of appetite, nausea.

PERFUME: Scent: Spicy, camphoraceous, fresh, woody, active, masculine, sensual, warm. Key qualities: Aphrodisiac, stimulant (mental), tonic (nerve), restorative, strengthening, comforting, analgesic, antiseptic. Odor intensity: High.

CAUTION: This oil is toxic and an irritant in concentration—use in low dilutions only (up to 1 percent).

Petitgrain is a classic ingredient in eau de cologne.

PEPPERMINT *Mentha x piperita*
Family: Lamiaceae

DESCRIPTION: A perennial herb, up to 3 feet high. White peppermint has green stems and leaves; black peppermint has dark green, serrated leaves, purplish stems, and reddish-violet flowers.

ACTIONS: Analgesic, anti-inflammatory, antimicrobial, antiphlogistic, antipruritic, antiseptic, antispasmodic, antiviral, astringent, diaphoretic, carminative, cephalic, cordial, emmenagogue, expectorant, febrifuge, hepatic, nervine, stomachic, sudorific, vasoconstrictor, vermifuge.

EXTRACTION: The oil is extracted by steam distillation from the flowering herb.

CHARACTERISTICS: A pale yellow or greenish liquid with a highly penetrating, grassy-minty, camphoraceous odor. It blends well with benzoin, rosemary, lavender, marjoram, lemon, eucalyptus, and bergamot.

AROMATHERAPY USE: Skin care: Acne, dermatitis, ringworm, scabies, toothache. Circulation, muscles, and joints: Neuralgia, muscular pain, palpitations. Respiratory system: Asthma, bronchitis, sinusitis, spasmodic cough. Digestive system: Colic, cramps, dyspepsia, flatulence, nausea. Immune system: Colds, flu, fevers. Nervous system: Fainting, headache, mental fatigue, migraine, nervous stress, vertigo. Other: Treats halitosis, insect repellent.

PERFUME: Scent: Fresh, bright, minty, penetrating, clean. Key qualities: Refreshing, restorative, nerve tonic, cephalic, aphrodisiac, stimulant (mental). Odor intensity: High.

CAUTION: Do not use oil with homeopathic remedies. Use in low dilutions on the skin.

PETITGRAIN, ORANGE *Citrus aurantium var. amara*
Family: Rutaceae

DESCRIPTION: The oil of orange petitgrain is produced from the leaves and twigs of the same tree that produces both bitter orange oil and neroli oil.

ACTIONS: Antiseptic, antispasmodic, deodorant, digestive, nervine, stimulant (to both digestive and nervous systems), stomachic, tonic.

EXTRACTION: The oil is extracted by steam distillation from the leaves and twigs.

CHARACTERISTICS: A pale yellow to amber liquid, with a fresh-floral citrus scent and a woody, herbaceous undertone. It blends well with rosemary, lavender, geranium, bergamot, orange, neroli, clary sage, jasmine, benzoin, palmarosa, and clove, and is a classic ingredient in eau de cologne and toilet waters.

AROMATHERAPY USE: Skin care: Acne, excessive perspiration, greasy skin and hair, toning. Digestive system: Dyspepsia, flatulence. Nervous system: Convalescence, insomnia, nervous exhaustion, stress-related conditions.

PERFUME: Scent: Citrus and floral. Key qualities: Calming and refreshing. Odor intensity: Medium.

PINE, LONGLEAF *Pinus palustris*
Family: Pinaceae

DESCRIPTION: A tall evergreen tree with long needles and a straight trunk, grown extensively for its timber. It exudes a natural oleoresin from the trunk, which provides the largest source for the production of turpentine in the United States.

ACTIONS: Analgesic (mild), antirheumatic, antiseptic, bactericidal, expectorant, insecticidal, stimulant.

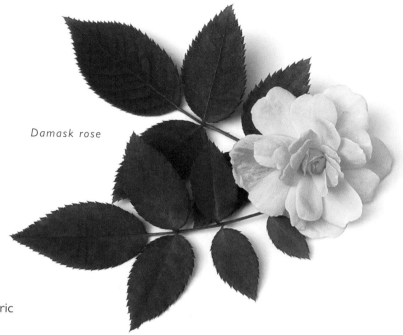

Damask rose

EXTRACTION: The crude oil is obtained by steam distillation from the sawdust and wood chips from the heartwood and roots of the tree (wastage from the timber mills), and then submitted to fractional distillation under atmospheric pressure to produce pine essential oil.

CHARACTERISTICS: A water-white or pale yellow liquid with a sweet-balsamic, pinewood scent. It blends well with rosemary, pine needle, cedarwood, citronella, rosewood, ho leaf, and oakmoss.

AROMATHERAPY USE: Circulation, muscles, and joints: Arthritis, debility, lumbago, muscular aches and pains, poor circulation, rheumatism, stiffness. Respiratory system: Asthma, bronchitis, catarrh, sinusitis. Other: Used extensively in medicine, particularly in veterinary antiseptic sprays, disinfectants, detergents, and insecticides (as a solvent carrier).

PERFUME: Scent: Balsamic, camphoraceous, woody, sweet, resinous, fresh, evergreen. Key qualities: Stimulating, strengthening, energizing, stress-relieving, uplifting, cleansing, antiseptic, anti-inflammatory. Odor intensity: Medium.

CAUTION: Nonirritant except in concentration.

ROSE, DAMASK *Rosa damascena*
Family: Rosaceae

DESCRIPTION: Small prickly shrub between 3–6 feet high, with pink, very fragrant blooms with thirty-six petals, and whitish hairy leaves. It requires a very specific soil and climate.

ACTIONS: Antidepressent, antiphlogistic, antiseptic, antispasmodic, antitubercular agent, antiviral, aphrodisiac, astringent, bactericidal, choleretic,

cicatrizant, depurative, emmenagogue, hemostatic, hepatic, laxative, regulator of appetite, sedative, stomachic, tonic.

EXTRACTION: The essential oil is obtained by water or steam distillation from the fresh petals.

CHARACTERISTICS: A pale yellow or olive yellow liquid with a very rich, deep, sweet-floral, slightly spicy scent. It blends well with most oils, and is useful for "rounding off" blends. The Bulgarian type is considered superior in perfumery work, but in therapeutic practice it is more a matter of differing properties between the various types of rose.

AROMATHERAPY USE: Skin care: Broken capillaries, conjunctivitis (rose water), dry skin, eczema, herpes, mature and sensitive complexions, wrinkles. Circulation, muscles, and joints: Palpitations, poor circulation. Respiratory system: Asthma, coughs, hay fever. Digestive system: Cholecystitis, liver congestion, nausea. Genitourinary system: Irregular menstruation, leucorrhoea, menorrhagia, uterine disorders. Nervous system: Depression, impotence, headache, nervous tension, and stress-related complaints.

PERFUME: Scent: Deep, rosy, floral, sweet, fresh. Key qualities: Soothing, harmonizing, relaxing, de-stressing, hydrating, uplifting, stimulating, astringent, antiseptic, healing, aphrodisiac. Odor intensity: High.

Rosemary is widely regarded as an herb of remembrance.

ROSEMARY *Rosmarinus officinalis*
Family: Lamiaceae

DESCRIPTION: An aromatic, shrubby evergreen bush, up to 6 feet high, with silvery-green leaves and pale blue flowers.

ACTIONS: Analgesic, antimicrobial, antioxidant, antiseptic, antispasmodic, astringent, carminative, choleretic, cicatrizant, cordial, diaphoretic, digestive, diuretic, emmenagogue, fungicidal, hepatic, hypertensor, restorative, rubefacient, stimulant, stomachic, sudorific, tonic.

EXTRACTION: The oil is extracted by steam distillation from the fresh flowering tops or (more commonly in Spain) from the whole plant.

CHARACTERISTICS: A colorless or pale yellow mobile liquid with a strong, minty-herbaceous, woody-balsamic scent. It blends well with frankincense, lavender, citronella, basil, thyme, pine, peppermint, elemi, cedarwood, petitgrain, and spice oils.

AROMATHERAPY USE: Skin care: Acne, dermatitis, eczema, lice, scabies, hair, and scalp. Circulation, muscles, and joints: Arteriosclerosis, fluid retention, gout, muscular pain, neuralgia, palpitations, poor circulation, varicose veins, rheumatism. Respiratory system: Asthma, bronchitis, whooping cough. Digestive system: Colitis, dyspepsia, flatulence, hepatic disorders, jaundice. Reproductive system: Dysmenorrhea, leukorrhea. Immune system: Colds, flu, infections. Nervous system: Headaches, hypotension, nervous exhaustion, stress-related disorders.

PERFUME: Scent: Penetrating, fresh, camphoraceous, woody-balsamic, strong. Key qualities: Stimulant (nervous and mental), analgesic, tonic (to the nervous system), strengthening, restorative, purifying, protective, reviving, refreshing. Odor intensity: Medium–high.

CAUTION: This oil should not be used by people suffering from epilepsy, or during pregnancy.

ROSEWOOD *Aniba rosaeodora*
Family: Lauraceae

DESCRIPTION: Medium-size tropical evergreen tree, with a reddish bark and heartwood, bearing yellow flowers; used extensively for timber.

ACTIONS: Mildly analgesic, anticonvulsant, antidepressant, antimicrobial, antiseptic, aphrodisiac, bactericidal, cellular stimulant, cephalic, deodorant, immune system stimulant, tissue regenerator, tonic.

EXTRACTION: The oil is extracted by steam distillation from the wood chippings.

CHARACTERISTICS: Colorless to pale yellow liquid, with a very sweet, woody-floral fragrance that has a spicy hint. Blends well with most oils, especially citrus, woods, and florals; it helps give body, and rounds off sharp edges.

AROMATHERAPY USE: Skin care: Acne, dermatitis, scars, wounds, wrinkles, and good for general skin care of all skin types. Immune system: Colds, coughs, fever, infections, immune system stimulant. Nervous system: Frigidity, headaches, nausea, nervous tension, stress-related conditions.

PERFUME: Scent: Rosy, woody, dry, floral, slightly green, fresh, mild. Key qualities (mind): Warming, comforting, pleasing. Odor intensity: Low.

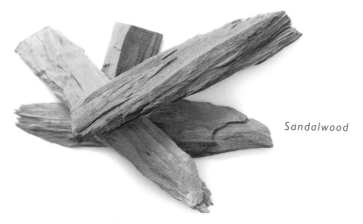

Sandalwood

SANDALWOOD *Santalum album*
Family: Santalaceae

DESCRIPTION: A small, parasitic evergreen tree, up to 30 feet high, with brown-gray trunk and many smooth, slender branches. It has small, pinkish-purple flowers.

ACTIONS: Antidepressant, antiphlogistic, antiseptic, antispasmodic, aphrodisiac, astringent, bactericidal, carminative, cicatrizant, diuretic, expectorant, fungicidal, insecticide, sedative, tonic.

EXTRACTION: The oil is extracted by water or steam distillation from the powdered and dried roots and heartwood.

CHARACTERISTICS: A pale yellow, greenish or brownish viscous liquid, with a deep, soft, sweet-woody, balsamic scent. It blends well with rose, clove, lavender, black pepper, bergamot, rosewood, geranium, benzoin, vetivert, patchouli, myrrh, and jasmine.

AROMATHERAPY USE: Skin care: Acne; dry, cracked, and chapped skin, aftershave (for barber's rash), greasy skin, moisturizer. Respiratory system: Bronchitis, catarrh, coughs (dry, persistent), laryngitis, sore throat. Digestive system: Diarrhea, nausea. Genitourinary system: Cystitis. Nervous system: Depression, insomnia, nervous tension, stress-related complaints.

PERFUME: Scent: Dry-woody, amber, balsamic, musky, sensual, masculine, tenacious, warm. Key qualities: Aphrodisiac, soothing, relaxing, uplifting, purifying, warming, grounding, opening, elevating, sedative (to the nervous system). Odor intensity: Low–medium.

SPEARMINT *Mentha spicata*
Family: Lamiaceae

DESCRIPTION: A hardy-branched perennial herb, with bright green, lance-shaped, sharply toothed leaves, quickly spreading underground runners and pink- or lilac-colored flowers in slender cylindrical spikes.

ACTIONS: Anesthetic (local), antiseptic, antispasmodic, astringent, carminative, cephalic, cholagogue, decongestant, digestive, diuretic, expectorant, febrifuge, hepatic, nervine, stimulant, stomachic, tonic.

EXTRACTION: Essential oil by steam distillation from the flowering tops.

CHARACTERISTICS: A pale yellow or olive mobile liquid, with a warm, spicy-herbaceous, minty odor. It blends well with lavender, lavandin, jasmine, eucalyptus, basil, and rosemary, and is often used in combination with peppermint.

AROMATHERAPY USE: Skin care: Acne, dermatitis, congested skin. Respiratory system: Asthma, bronchitis, catarrhal conditions, sinusitis. Digestive system: Colic, dyspepsia, flatulence, hepatobiliary disorders, nausea, vomiting. Immune system: Colds, fevers, flu. Nervous system: Fatigue, headache, migraine, nervous strain, neurasthenia, stress.

PERFUME: Scent: Crisp, minty, fresh, soft, sweet. Key qualities: Refreshing, cleansing, uplifting, energizing, cooling. Odor intensity: Low.

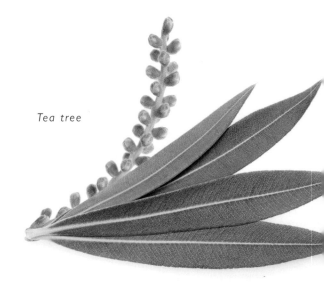

Tea tree

TEA TREE *Melaleuca alternifolia*
Family: Myrtaceae

DESCRIPTION: A small tree or shrub (the smallest of the melaleuca family), with needle-like leaves, similar to those of cypress, and heads of stalkless yellow or purplish-colored flowers.

ACTIONS: Anti-infectious, anti-inflammatory, antiseptic, antiviral, bactericidal, balsamic, cicatrizant, diaphoretic, expectorant, fungicidal, immunostimulant, parasiticide, vulnerary.

EXTRACTION: The oil is extracted by steam or water distillation from the leaves and twigs.

EXTRACTION: A pale yellowish-green or water-white mobile liquid, with a warm, fresh, spicy-camphoraceous odor. It blends well with lavender, clary sage, rosemary, pine, ylang ylang, geranium, marjoram, and spice oils, especially clove and nutmeg.

AROMATHERAPY USE: Skin care: Abscess, acne, athlete's foot, blisters, burns, bruises, chicken pox rash, cold sores, dandruff, herpes, insect bites, oily skin, rashes (nappy rash), spots, verrucae, warts, wounds (infected). Respiratory system: Asthma, bronchitis, catarrh, coughs, sinusitis, tuberculosis, whooping cough. Reproductive system: Thrush (vaginal), vaginitis. Immune system: Colds, fever, flu, infectious illnesses. Urinary system: Cystitis, pruritus.

PERFUME: Scent: Medicinal, fresh, powerful, camphoraceous, pungent, slightly spicy. Key qualities: Penetrating, medicinal, stimulating, refreshing. Odor intensity: High.

CAUTION: There are indications of possible sensitization in some individuals.

TUBEROSE *Polianthes tuberosa*
Family: Agavaceae

DESCRIPTION: A tender, tall, slim perennial up to 20 inches high, with long, slender leaves, a tuberous root, and large, very fragrant, lily-like white flowers.

ACTIONS: Narcotic.

EXTRACTION: A concrete and absolute by solvent extraction from the fresh flowers, picked before the petals open. (An essential oil is also obtained by distillation of the concrete.)

CHARACTERISTICS: The absolute is a dark orange or brown soft paste, with a heavy, sweet-floral, sometimes spicy, tenacious fragrance. It blends well with gardenia, violet, opopanax, rose, jasmine, carnation, orris, Peru balsam, neroli, and ylang ylang.

AROMATHERAPY USE: Perfume.

PERFUME: Scent: Floral, rich, intense. Key qualities: Aphrodisiac, relaxation, de-stressing, sedative, warming, moisturizing. Odor intensity: High.

TURMERIC *Curcuma longa*
Family: Zingiberaceae

DESCRIPTION: A perennial tropical herb up to 3 feet high, with a thick rhizome root, deep orange inside, lanceolate root leaves tapering at each end, and dull yellow flowers.

ACTIONS: Analgesic, anti-arthritic, anti-inflammatory, antioxidant, bactericidal, cholagogue, digestive, diuretic, hypotensive, insecticidal, laxative, rubefacient, stimulant.

EXTRACTION: Essential oil by steam distillation from the "cured" rhizome—boiled, cleaned, and sun-dried. (An oleoresin, absolute, and concrete are also produced by solvent extraction.)

CHARACTERISTICS: A yellowish-orange liquid with a faint blue fluorescence and a fresh spicy-woody odor. It blends well with cananga, labdanum, elecampane, ginger, orris, cassie, clary sage, and mimosa.

AROMATHERAPY USE: Circulation, muscles, and joints: Arthritis, muscular aches and pains, rheumatism. Digestive system: Sluggish digestion, liver congestion.

PERFUME: Scent: Fresh, spicy, woody, warm. Key qualities: Anti-inflammatory, soothing, protective, detoxifying, antioxidant, immune-boosting, soothing. Odor intensity: Medium.

CAUTION: The ketone "tumerone" is moderately toxic and an irritant in high concentration. Possible sensitization problems. Use with moderation and care.

VALERIAN *Valeriana officinalis*
Family: Valerianaceae

DESCRIPTION: A perennial herb, up to 5 feet high, with a hollow, erect stem, deeply dissected dark leaves, and many purplish-white flowers. It has short, thick, grayish roots, showing above ground; these have a strong odor.

ACTIONS: Anodyne (mild), antidandruff, antidiuretic, antispasmodic, bactericidal, carminative, depressant of the central nervous system, hypnotic, hypotensive, regulator, sedative, stomachic.

EXTRACTION: The oil is extracted by steam distillation from the roots.

CHARACTERISTICS: An olive to brown liquid, darkening with age, with a warm-woody, balsamic, musky odor; fresh oils have a green top note. It blends well with patchouli, pine, lavender, cedarwood, mandarin, petitgrain, and rosemary.

AROMATHERAPY USE: Nervous system: Insomnia, nervous indigestion, migraine, restlessness, tension states.

PERFUME: Scent: Warm, woody, balsamic, musky, earthy, green. Key qualities (mind): Sedative (mental and nervous), depressant of the central nervous system, mildly hypnotic, regulator, calming, soothing, grounding. Odor intensity: Very high.

CAUTION: In large amounts, valerian can cause headaches, mental agitation, and delusions. Use in moderation, and do not use over long periods of time (more than a month) without a break. Can cause possible sensitization.

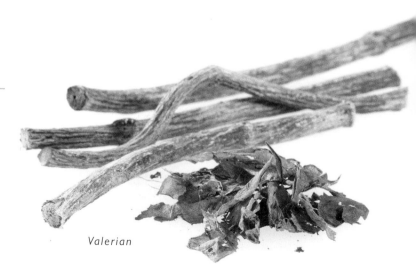

Valerian

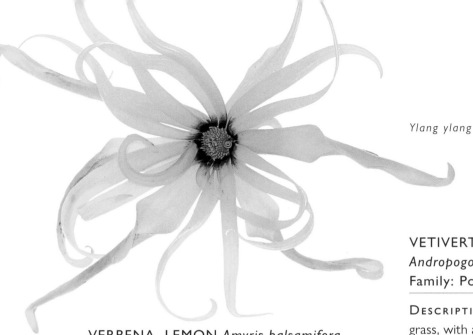
Ylang ylang

VERBENA, LEMON *Amyris balsamifera*
Family: Rutaceae

DESCRIPTION: A handsome deciduous perennial shrub up to 16 feet high, with a woody stem, very fragrant, delicate, pale green, lanceolate leaves arranged in threes, and small, pale purple flowers. Often grown as an ornamental bush in gardens.

ACTIONS: Antiseptic, antispasmodic, carminative, detoxifying, digestive, febrifuge, hepatobiliary stimulant, sedative (nervous), stomachic.

EXTRACTION: Essential oil by steam distillation from the freshly harvested herb.

CHARACTERISTICS: A pale olive or yellow liquid with a sweet, fresh, lemony, fruity-floral fragrance. It blends well with neroli, palmarosa, olibanum, Tolu balsam, elemi, lemon, and other citrus oils.

AROMATHERAPY USE: Digestive system: Cramps, indigestion, liver congestion. Nervous system: Anxiety, insomnia, nervous tension and stress-related conditions.

PERFUME: Scent: Sweet, fresh, lemony, fruity-floral. Key qualities: Antiseptic, cleansing, uplifting, refreshing, reviving, energizing. Odor intensity: Medium.

CAUTION: Possible sensitization; phototoxicity due to high citral levels. However, true verbena oil is virtually nonexistent. Most so-called verbena oil is either from the Spanish verbena (an inferior oil) or a mix of lemongrass, lemon, citronella, etc.

VETIVERT *Vetiveria zizanioides/ Andropogon muricatus*
Family: Poaceae

DESCRIPTION: A tall, tufted, perennial, scented grass, with a straight stem, long, narrow leaves, and an abundant, complex lacework of underground white rootlets.

ACTIONS: Antiseptic, antispasmodic, depurative, rubefacient, sedative (to the nervous system), stimulant (circulatory, and to blood itself), tonic, vermifuge.

EXTRACTION: The oil is extracted by steam distillation from the roots and rootlets—which have been washed, chopped, dried, and soaked.

CHARACTERISTICS: A dark brown, olive, or amber viscous oil, with a deep, smoky, earthy-woody odor, and a sweet, persistent undertone. The color and scent can vary according to the source. It blends well with sandalwood, rose, jasmine, patchouli, lavender, clary sage, and ylang ylang.

AROMATHERAPY USE: Skin care: Acne, cuts, oily skin, wounds. Circulation, muscles, and joints: Arthritis, muscular aches and pains, rheumatism, sprains, stiffness. Nervous system: Debility, depression, insomnia, nervous tension—known as the oil of tranquility.

PERFUME: Scent: Smoky, rich, earthy, dry-woody, sweet, green, diffusive, masculine, sporty, warm. Key qualities: Sedative (nervous and mental), soothing, calming, tonic (nervous), grounding, uplifting, protective. Odor intensity: High.

YLANG YLANG *Cananga odorata*
Family: Annonaceae

DESCRIPTION: A tall tropical tree up to 68 feet high, with large, tender, fragrant flowers that can be pink, mauve, or yellow.

ACTIONS: Aphrodisiac, antidepressant, anti-infectious, antiseborrheic, antiseptic, euphoric, hypotensive, nervine, regulator, sedative (nervous), stimulant (to the circulatory system), tonic.

EXTRACTION: The oil is extracted by water or steam distillation from freshly picked flowers. Yellow flowers yield the best oil.

CHARACTERISTICS: A colorless to pale yellow liquid with a light, fresh-balsamic, slightly spicy scent. A good oil has a creamy, rich top note. A very intriguing perfume oil in its own right, it also blends well with sandalwood, jasmine, bois de rose, vetivert, bergamot, rose, and floral bases. It is also an excellent fixative.

AROMATHERAPY USE: Skin care: Acne, hair growth, hair rinse, insect bites, irritated and oily skin, general skin care. Circulation: High blood pressure, hyperpnoea (abnormally fast breathing), tachycardia, palpitations. Nervous system: Depression, frigidity, impotence, insomnia, nervous tension, and stress-related disorders.

PERFUME: Scent: Exotic, sweet, balsamic, floral, slightly spicy, sensual, heady, rich, voluptuous. Key qualities: Powerfully sedative, soothing, calming, regulating, euphoria-inducing, and narcotic when used in large quantities, aphrodisiac. Odor intensity: High.

CAUTION: A few cases of sensitization have been reported. Use in moderation, since the oil's heady scent can cause headaches or nausea.

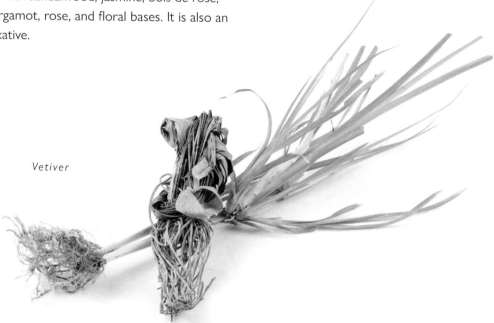

Vetiver

HEALING AND HEALTH AROMATHERAPY MASSAGE

Massage is one of the most fundamental forms of therapy, and has been utilized by many diverse cultures for thousands of years. The need to be touched is itself an essential and primitive human instinct, for without physical contact, the overall health of the individual suffers. Recent research has shown that a lack of tactile contact is associated with immune depression, and positive touch with immune stimulation.

Over the course of time, many different massage techniques have been developed, each having its own individual therapeutic approach. The art of shiatsu massage, for example, works primarily with specific pressure points along the lines of the meridians or channels of energy in the body, to influence the overall balance of energy within the body, much like acupuncture. In contrast, the Western style of Swedish massage concentrates more on releasing areas of tension trapped within the muscles, joints, and connective tissues of the body. Even performing the same stroke in different ways can produce different effects. A single movement performed vigorously can stimulate the body, while a similar movement performed slowly can promote relaxation.

Massage not only improves circulation and relaxes muscles, but also has psychological benefits, making the recipient feel comforted and cared for, and produces a unique sense of well-being. However, when the general benefits of massage are combined with the effects of specific essential oils being rubbed into the skin, the healing dynamics already at work can take on a completely new dimension.

The actual techniques of aromatherapy massage are adapted mainly from the Swedish massage style, combined with a more individualistic approach to body work, adopted from the intuitive massage style initiated in the early 1960s. The theory behind the preparation of the essential oils themselves is based largely on the ideas of the French dermatologist Marguerite Maury. Her concept of the individual prescription is still utilized by most professional aromatherapists working today, and they always prepare an individually chosen blend of essential oils for each client and for each massage session, depending on the needs of the client on each separate occasion.

There are three distinct but overlapping aspects of an aromatherapy massage treatment, and this form of therapy can therefore be seen as being beneficial in three quite distinct but interrelated ways:

• The massage itself and its effects on the body
• The interaction between therapist and recipient
• The effect of the essential oils

Each aspect supports the others in such a way as to provide a multidimensional therapeutic action. During a treatment, the essential oils themselves also interact with the body in two ways:

• Through inhalation (primarily psychological effects)
• Through absorption into the bloodstream via the skin (primarily physiological effects)

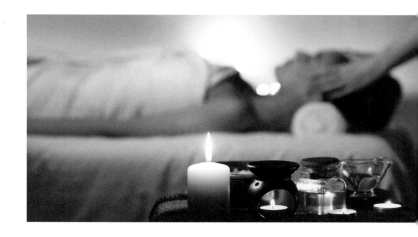

Touch and smell: a healing synergy

The synergy of essential oils and massage has been shown to be a very effective combination in the treatment of stress-related disorders, due to the powerful interaction of touch and smell. During the course of a massage, a certain amount of the essential oils will be absorbed through the skin and into the bloodstream to affect the nervous system, as well as other parts of the body directly, by toning, sedating, or stimulating. When this is backed up by a comforting and supportive relationship between patient and therapist, it can provide a vital key to breaking the stress cycle of anxiety, insomnia, and nervous fatigue that underlies so many common physical complaints.

There is increasing evidence to show that stress affects not just the mind, but also the nervous, immune, and endocrine systems, and that it constitutes a factor in physical as well as mental health.

It is not surprising that stress-related problems are an area in which aromatherapy massage enjoys a great deal of success, because it simultaneously operates on both a physical and psychological level. An aromatic massage, for example, is especially valuable for those who suffer from a number of different responses to stress at the same time. Stress-related illness often presents a wide range of contradictory symptoms. Aromatherapy, rather than dealing separately with individual symptoms such as high blood pressure, indigestion, and back pain, deals with the stress itself. In the words of Dr. Ann Coxon:

"Obviously, the approach of holistic treatment is to help enable people to manage their primary life situation, and the ability of aromatherapy to get at the knot, at the stress reaction itself within the body without using yet more pharmacological treatment is terribly important."

Evidence of the widespread sense of "disease" experienced today in the West is shown in the high consumption of tranquilizers and stimulants, although it is well known that addiction, toxicosis, and other side effects can be caused by these products if taken regularly. Any treatment that can help to revitalize and de-stress the organism, without producing detrimental side effects, is therefore of great value. Essential oils, used in the appropriate doses, are safe and harmless, and it is widely agreed that, while they can be highly effective, they "do not cause troubles like those produced by the ordinary psychological drugs."

CAUTION

Although aromatherapy massage is effective for both the prevention and treatment of stress-related disorders, it is also very important for the individual to be helped to assess factors such as lifestyle, work patterns, and emotional relationships, and to try to make necessary changes to combat the causes behind the stress reaction directly.

THERAPEUTIC MASSAGE AND BODY OILS

Therapeutic aromatic massage is the main method used by professional aromatherapists, but it can also be practiced at home—either on oneself, or on a friend or partner. Body oils are best applied after a warm bath, when the pores of the skin are still open, to encourage rapid absorption.

For the purpose of massage or general application to the skin, a few drops of essential oil are always mixed with a larger measure of base or carrier oil, usually a light vegetable oil such as sweet almond oil or grapeseed oil. When preparing a body oil or massage oil, the dilution should be in the region of 5 to 30 drops of essential oil in a bottle of ⅓ cup of base oil, depending upon the type of essential oil used and its specific purpose. For general massage purposes, a dilution of 2.5 percent (see below) is suitable for adult use.

Special dilutions	
For ⅓ cup of base oil:	
Blend percentage	Essential oil in drops
0.5 percent	5
1 percent	10
1.5 percent	15
2 percent	20
2.5 percent	25
3 percent	30

Standard dilution (2.5 percent)	
Base oil amount	Essential oil drops
1 teaspoon	2–3
1 tablespoon	6–7
2 tablespoons	12–13
⅓ cup	25
⅔ cup	50

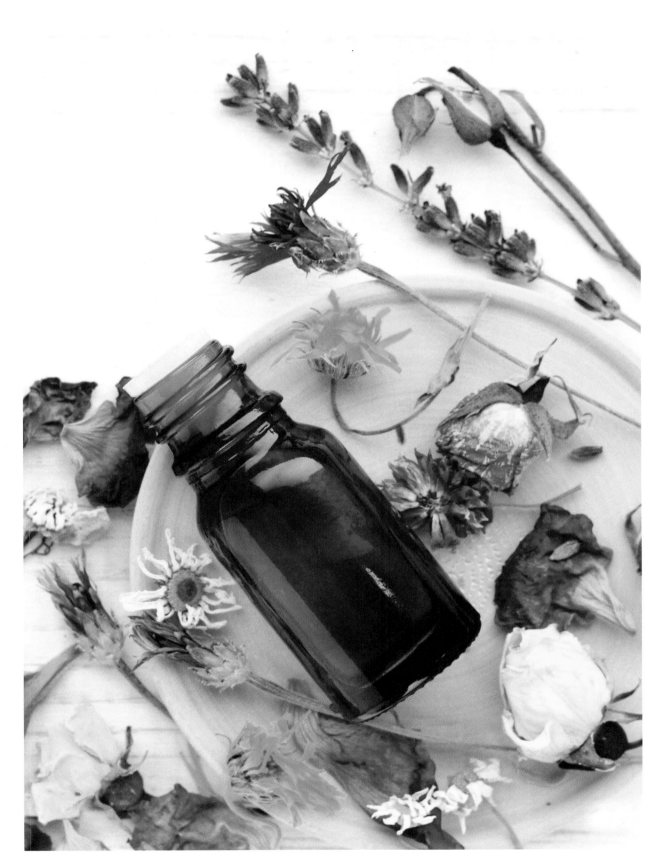

AROMATHERAPY FOR FIRST AID

Bruises

Initial pain and swelling are followed by blue, purple, or blackish discoloration of the skin, fading to yellow or brown. This indicates that the underlying tissue is damaged as a result of a knock or pressure. The skin becomes especially prone to bruising when the diet is lacking in vitamin C. Obese and anemic people are most susceptible to bruising. Frequent bruising of the skin may also indicate a kidney complaint.

CLINICAL NOTES: Case study notes show tea tree to be an effective bruise remedy: "Suppurating bruise checked in 24 hours using solution diluted 1:40 as a compress. Condition cured in one week by continuing this treatment."

Methods of use:

• For minor bruises, an application of undiluted lavender or tea tree oil reduces inflammation and speeds up the healing process.

• If the swelling is severe, apply an ice compress to ease inflammation. Then gently apply witch hazel lotion to which has been added a few drops of chamomile (Roman or German) or lavender oil. Apply this treatment 2–3 times a day until the condition clears.

• Arnica ointment is one of the most effective bruise remedies.

AROMATHERAPY OILS: Lavender, tea tree, chamomile (Roman and German), fennel, hyssop, geranium, cypress, yarrow.

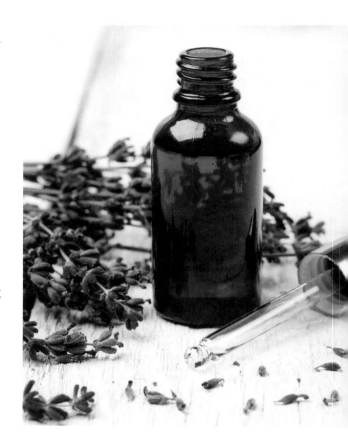

CAUTION

Severe bruising can cause considerable internal bleeding—if worried, seek medical help. Arnica must not be applied to broken skin.

Burns

Burns are classified into three degrees of severity: superficial (redness and swelling); intermediate (swelling and blistering); and deep (numbness and charring). They can be caused by dry heat or moist heat (scalds), and are among the most common household injuries. Burns can also be caused by contact with chemicals, radiation, or electricity.

CLINICAL NOTES: Minor burns respond extremely well to treatment with essential oils, which reduces pain, prevents blistering or infection, and promotes healing without scarring. Both lavender and tea tree oil are increasingly being employed for treating burns in hospitals.

Natural bisabolol, found in German chamomile, has been shown to be "more effective than synthetic racemic bisabolol in healing burns" (*Potter's New Cyclopaedia of Botanical Drugs and Preparations*).

Methods of use:

• Immediately hold the affected area under the cold tap for 10 minutes, then apply undiluted lavender or tea tree oil to the burn. Reapply at least three times a day until the skin has healed.

• For larger areas, especially if there is inflammation, apply an ice compress. Then gently apply a lotion made from 8 to 10 drops each of lavender and German chamomile oil in a 1½ fl. oz. bottle of distilled water, lavender water, or rose water, shaken well. Shake the bottle before each application.

• Cover with a sterile gauze treated with a few drops of lavender, tea tree, or German chamomile. Replace the dressing every few hours. Do not use adhesive plasters.

• Calendula cream or oil helps the skin to heal in the latter stages and prevents scarring.

AROMATHERAPY OILS: Lavender, tea tree, German chamomile, eucalyptus blue gum, geranium, yarrow.

CAUTION

Severe burns, especially if accompanied by shock, require immediate medical attention. Avoid fatty oils or ointments when treating burns during the initial stages, as they can cause the skin to "fry."

Cuts/wounds

Small cuts, grazes, and scratches are some of the most common injuries. Where glass, rust, splinters, or dirt are concerned, special care should be taken to avoid secondary infection.

CLINICAL NOTES: Tea tree and lavender are excellent first-aid remedies for all skin abrasions and wounds, due to their excellent antiseptic and wound-healing properties. They do not sting the exposed raw skin, even applied undiluted, while encouraging a rich flow of blood to the damaged area. They also prevent scarring.

Clinical research has shown tea tree to be especially effective for septic conditions, pus-filled infections, and dirty wounds: ". . . it dissolved pus and left the surfaces of infected wounds clean, so that its germicidal action became more effective without any apparent damage to the tissues . . . most effective germicides destroy tissue as well as bacteria."

Methods of use:

• Cleanse with water, to which a few drops of any of the below essential oils have been added, removing any dirt or fragments.

• Apply a few drops of undiluted lavender or tea tree oil. Cover with a plaster if required—but let the skin breathe whenever possible. Reapply several times a day until the skin has healed.

• For splinters, clean the area gently, then apply undiluted lavender or tea tree oil. Cover with a warm clay poultice and leave for 2 hours.

• Remove the splinter with tweezers, then apply a few drops of lavender or tea tree oil and cover with a plaster.

• For swelling, apply a cold compress of witch hazel lotion to which has been added a few drops of chamomile or lavender oil. Apply 2–3 times a day.

• Cover larger injuries with a sterile gauze semi-saturated with lavender or tea tree oil. If the wound is weepy or slow to heal, include a few drops of myrrh or yarrow. Myrrh can also be applied undiluted to weepy wounds.

• Calendula cream or oil helps the skin to heal in the latter stages, and prevents scarring.

AROMATHERAPY OILS: Tea tree, lavender, chamomile (both Roman and German), yarrow, myrrh, patchouli, benzoin, palmarosa, eucalyptus blue gum, clove.

CAUTION

Seek immediate medical help in cases of severe bleeding or very deep wounds, which may require stitching. Do not apply fatty oils or ointments to broken skin during the initial stages of healing, as these can delay the formation of scar tissue.

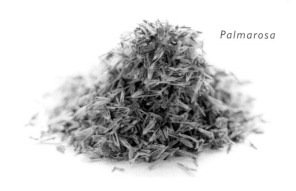

Palmarosa

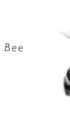

Bee

Stings/bites

Stings and bites vary from minor to severe, and there may be swelling or a gash. Poisoning or an allergic reaction can cause further inflammation and pain, fever, or headaches. Among the more common bites and stings are those of jellyfish, dogs, bees, wasps, ticks, bedbugs, fleas, horseflies, gnats, sandflies, hornets, and mosquitoes. It is important to try to identify the exact cause, since the different types require individual antidotes.

CLINICAL NOTES: Tea tree oil is traditionally used in Australia for bites and stings, including those of mosquitoes, sandflies, fleas, horseflies, wasps, and bees, and some types of spider and jellyfish. In France, lavender oil has been traditionally used. Lavender has also successfully treated adder bites.

Methods of use:

• Bee stings: Remove the sting with tweezers (avoid squeezing the venom sac). Apply an ice-cold compress saturated in a solution containing 1 teaspoon baking soda and 1 tablespoon chamomile or lavender water (or distilled water mixed with a few drops of chamomile or lavender oil). Reapply frequently until the swelling subsides.

• Ant bites and hornet stings: Treat with a compress as described for bee stings (above).

• Jellyfish/sea urchin stings: Remove any spikes or tentacles carefully, then apply undiluted tea tree or lavender oil. Repeat at intervals.

• Mosquito and other insect bites: Apply undiluted lavender or tea tree oil (or a blend of the two). Repeat every hour, or as required. If there is inflammation, apply an ice-cold compress with a few drops of chamomile, lavender, or melissa oil. To soothe irritation and avoid infection, add 8 to 10 drops of the above oils to bath water daily.

• Ticks and leeches: Apply undiluted tea tree oil to the live tick or leech and surrounding skin and leave. After 20 minutes, remove by hand those ticks or leeches that have not already fallen off. Apply the undiluted oil to the bite three times a day for a week to soothe irritation and prevent infection.

• Spider bites: Mix 2 to 3 drops each of tea tree and lavender oil in 1 teaspoon alcohol or cider vinegar and apply three times a day.

• Wasp stings: Apply a cold compress saturated with cider vinegar and 2 drops of lavender or tea tree oil. Reapply fresh compresses frequently until the swelling subsides.

AROMATHERAPY OILS: Lavender, tea tree, chamomile (Roman and German), melissa, basil, bergamot.

CAUTION

Bee stings can cause an allergic reaction, with severe swelling—seek medical help immediately if this happens. Snake bites can be extremely dangerous, especially in tropical countries. Get help immediately. Bites from rabies-infected animals or poisonous snakes, and severe insect stings inside the mouth or throat, require immediate medical attention.

TREATING SPRAINS, STRAINS, AND MUSCULAR PAIN

Sprains/strains

Sprains cause pain and tenderness around the joint, made worse by movement, with swelling and bruising. A strain is characterized by a sudden sharp pain at the site of the injury. There can be swelling, stiffness, and cramping. A sprain occurs at a joint where the ligaments and surrounding tissues are wrenched or torn. A strain occurs when a muscle or group of muscles is overstretched by a violent or sudden movement. It is most commonly caused by lifting heavy weights or by performing strenuous exercise.

CLINICAL NOTES: The traditional remedy for application to slow-healing sprains, *Oleum spicae*, was made by combining spike lavender oil and turpentine (pine oil).

CAUTION
Severe sprains or strains are difficult to distinguish from fractures: in all doubtful cases, seek medical help immediately.

Methods of use:

• Apply a cold compress (with ice) to which a few drops of chamomile oil have been added. Repeat as often as possible to reduce the swelling. Do not massage. Wrap in a bandage moistened with witch hazel lotion and rest as much as possible.

• As the swelling subsides, gently apply the following cream or oil: 4 drops each of pine, lavender, and rosemary oil in 2 tablespoons calendula cream or oil. Alternatively, use a liniment moistened with a few drops of any of the recommended oils (or a blend).

• Apply arnica ointment to the skin locally for bruising—unless the skin is broken.

• To encourage healing, soak in a warm bath containing 8 to 10 drops of one of the recommended oils and 3 tablespoons sea salt.

AROMATHERAPY OILS: Spike lavender, lavender, chamomile, pine, rosemary, eucalyptus blue gum, thyme, marjoram.

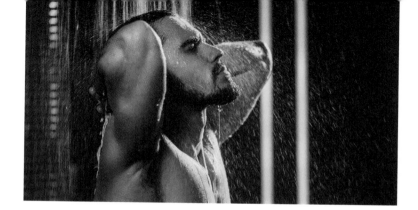

Muscular pain

Muscular aches and pains can affect any part of the body. Many people carry tension in their necks and shoulders, which causes the muscles to become tight and painful. Muscular pain can be caused by overexertion, poor posture, cold or damp, injury, stress, and tension. It can also be related to other complaints, such as rheumatism, arthritis, lumbago (lower back pain), or a slipped disk.

CLINICAL NOTES: It is well known among athletes that the combination of essential oils and massage is very effective for muscular aches and pains, as well as a valuable preventive treatment: "Rosemary is . . . a very good oil to use for tired, stiff, and over-worked muscles. I have used it very successfully for massage [before and] after training or competing."

Methods of use:

• Muscular aches and pains respond well to local massage—make a massage oil by adding about 7 to 10 drops each of lavender, marjoram, and rosemary oils to ⅓ cup of carrier oil, and rub into the affected area. Best after a warm shower or bath.

• Soaking in a hot bathtub is an easy and effective way of relaxing the muscles and bringing instant pain relief. Adding 8 to 10 drops of any of the recommended oils to the water will increase the benefits further.

• As a preventive treatment, and to tone the muscles before strenuous exercise, make a massage oil by mixing 10 drops each of rosemary and pine oils with 5 drops each of grapefruit and black pepper oils in ⅓ cup of a vegetable carrier oil. Rub gently into the whole body, concentrating on the muscles that will have to work the most.

AROMATHERAPY OILS: Marjoram, rosemary, black pepper, chamomile, lavender, ginger, pine, juniper, bergamot, grapefruit.

REMEDIES FOR COLDS AND COUGHS

The symptoms of a cold include sore throat, coughing, feverishness, aching limbs, sneezing, fatigue, and catarrh. Secondary infections such as bronchitis, sinusitis, or ear infections may arise. There are at least thirty different strains of the virus that can cause the common cold—or in medical terms, coryza. It is a highly contagious infection affecting the upper respiratory tract, and is picked up by breathing infected air. Exposure to cold, damp conditions, and to stuffy or smoky atmospheres, stress, and being generally run down are all contributing factors.

Methods of use:

• For colds with a cough or chills, make up a warming, concentrated chest rub by mixing 4 to 5 drops each of ginger, thyme, and lavender or hyssop in 2 tablespoons of carrier oil, and apply to the chest and upper back. Repeat at least twice a day.

• Use tea tree, thyme, or eucalyptus oil in vaporizers throughout the duration of the illness, but especially at the onset of the cold—this may prevent it from developing at all. Add a few drops of one of these oils to a handkerchief for inhalation throughout the day. Use drops of soothing oils such as myrtle or lavender on the pillow at night.

• Add 5 to 6 drops (in total) of tea tree, eucalyptus, or Spanish sage or thyme oil to a bowl of steaming water, cover the head with a towel, and breathe deeply for 5–10 minutes,

keeping the eyes closed. (Very hot steam is in itself a hostile environment for viruses.) Repeat at least twice a day.

• Take a daily hot bath, adding 8 to 10 drops of tea tree, rosemary, or thyme to the water—this combats congestion and fights infection. Lavender, marjoram, or bergamot oil can also be used in baths to soothe aching limbs and encourage restful sleep.

• For a sore throat, add 4 to 5 drops of tea tree or Spanish sage or clary sage or thyme to a glass of warm water, mix, and gargle at least three times daily.

AROMATHERAPY OILS: Tea tree, eucalyptus blue gum, myrtle, rosemary, marjoram, lavender, cajeput, lemon, pine, thyme, peppermint, bergamot, black pepper, ginger, cinnamon leaf, clove, Spanish sage, hyssop.

Use drops of soothing oils such as myrtle or lavender on the pillow at night.

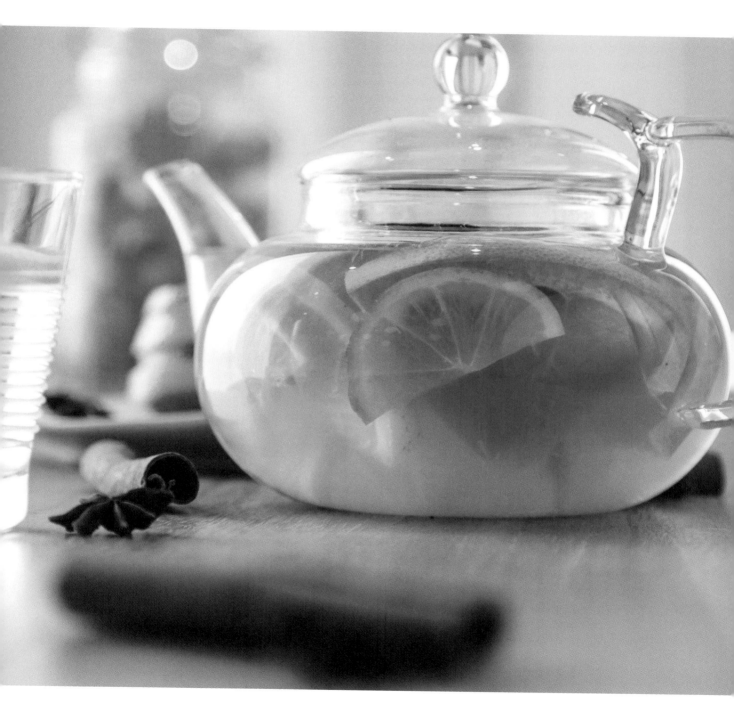

ESSENTIAL OILS FOR SELF-CARE AND WELLNESS

Aromatherapy is a wonderful approach to use when practicing self-care and looking after your physical, mental, and emotional wellness. With a variety of methods available and a vast choice of essential oils to help relax, invigorate, and stimulate your body and mind, there's something for all your self-care needs.

Self-care involves focusing on yourself and your individual needs, taking some time out from the demands of your family, life, or work, and making time for you. It can be a chance to do something you enjoy for a change, go running, catch up on craft projects, or read a good book. While you're relaxing you could have some of your favorite essential oils in an oil burner or add them to a spray bottle so you can infuse a room with an aromatic blend.

Self-care isn't all about pampering yourself, but a little bit of spa-style pampering is always pleasant. Essential oils can be used to create your own skin-care and pampering products to help you relax and unwind, such as bath salts, bath bombs, skin-care lotions, or face masks. Or you could try out simple massage techniques on your hands, feet, face, or arms.

Essential oils for meditation and relaxation

Meditation and relaxation techniques are an ideal form of self-care, helping you on physical, emotional, and mental levels, and essential oils are perfect to use too. The different properties in essential oils can help set the mood for more relaxing pursuits, or clear the air in a space to make it feel more sacred for meditation. There are oils you could use to help clear your mind and help you feel more focused, or to evoke feelings of peace and calm.

Here are some examples of essential oils that may be beneficial to use when meditating or relaxing:
• The sweet and woody scent of sandalwood helps to calm and focus the mind for meditation, helping to focus your attention on the task at hand and promote inner peace.

• The floral citrus scent of bergamot essential oil is an uplifting oil to scent a space when you're meditating. The scent can help lift a low mood and evoke feelings of self-worth and self-acceptance.
• The scent of lavender helps create a calm atmosphere and aids relaxation. It can be put into an oil burner to scent a room or massaged into the skin. Use in the evening to promote good sleep.

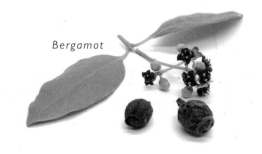

Bergamot

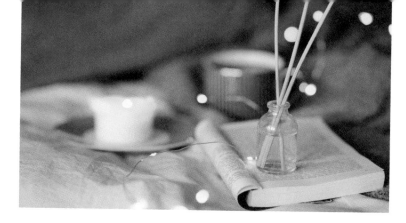

• The fresh and invigorating scent of peppermint is stimulating and uplifting, helping to clear headaches and encourage creative thought. It's a good scent to consider before you practice meditation or yoga, as it can help clear your mind and shake off feelings of sluggishness.

• The earthy aromatic scent of exotic frankincense can help create a sense of calm and spiritual connection, which may help when practicing meditation.

Oil blends for wellness

You can supercharge your self-care routines by using blends of essential oils—combinations of aromatic oils designed with a specific purpose in mind. All of these combinations can be diffused in an electric or candle oil burner, made into roller balls to apply to pressure points on your skin, or used for massage purposes.

To make your own aromatherapy roller balls, look for small, dark-colored glass roller bottles (narrow bottles with a roller ball on the end) and fill them with a carrier oil such as jojoba, sweet almond, or coconut, plus the drops of your selected essential oils. Then apply them to the skin on your pressure points, such as the inside of your wrists or your forehead, when the mood strikes. These little bottles are the ideal size to slip in a purse, pocket, drawer, or to keep on your desk at work. They also make great homemade gifts.

Start by using a combination of two drops of each essential oil, plus the carrier oil where required. If one aroma seems to out-balance the others, adjust the quantities next time. Make a note of what you use so you can re-create your favorite blends.

Oil blend ideas:

• To uplift your mood, combine equal drops of bergamot, mandarin, rose, and chamomile.

• For positivity, combine equal drops of lemon, geranium, jasmine, and rosewood.

• For a clear mind, combine 2 drops each of peppermint, eucalyptus, and rosemary.

• For stress relief, combine 2 drops each of lavender, chamomile, and sandalwood.

• To evoke a feeling of protection and security, combine equal drops of ylang ylang, melissa, sandalwood, bergamot, and geranium.

• To help with the release of emotional baggage, combine equal drops of angelica, lavender, bergamot, melissa, lemon, and chamomile.

• To help boost your energy, combine equal drops of lemon, grapefruit, orange, and basil.

• To boost your physical wellness and ward off germs and bacteria, combine 2 drops each of cinnamon, lemon, rosemary, clove bud, eucalyptus, and orange.

• To cleanse a room of negative energies, combine 2 drops each of tea tree, lemon, and grapefruit essential oils.

COSMETICS AND SKIN CARE

Beauty, especially skin and hair care, is central to the practice of aromatherapy. But while receiving a full body massage from a professional aromatherapist or having an aromatic facial in a beauty clinic is certainly a treat, it is not essential for maintaining a clear and healthy complexion. Many aromatic recipes are simple to make, and regular treatment can easily be carried out at home.

Facial oils

Facial oils are made up in the same way as general massage or body oils, except that the base or carrier oil, as well as the essential oils, can be adapted to the type of skin that is to be treated. Suitable carrier oils include avocado, olive, wheat germ, hazelnut, apricot kernel, peach kernel, borage seed, carrot, and evening primrose, as well as the more basic carrier oils such as sweet almond, grapeseed, jojoba, or sunflower oil. Apart from nourishing and toning the skin, facial oils can also be used for facial massage and local self-massage.

Facial oil recipe:

Mix two parts of a basic carrier oil and one part of a specific carrier oil suited to the skin type, with 0.5–1 percent of an essential oil (or a blend of oils).

Base oil	Percentage	Drops
1 teaspoon	0.5–1 percent	1
1 tablespoon	0.5–1 percent	1–3
2 tablespoons	0.5–1 percent	3–5
⅓ cup	0.5–1 percent	5–10
⅔ cup	0.5–1 percent	10–20

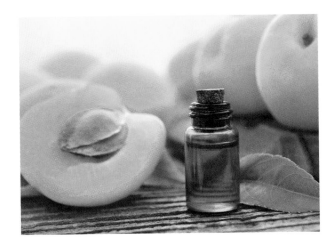

Facial creams

An aromatic facial cream should moisturize, heal, and nourish the skin, trapping the moisture in but also letting the skin breathe. To make a basic cream at home, use the instructions below, based on what is traditionally known as Galen's cold cream recipe.

Cold cream recipe:

Ingredients

3 teaspoons beeswax beads or grated wax

¾ cup almond oil

½ cup rose water

6–10 drops of rose essential oil, or other essential oil according to skin type

1. Put the beeswax beads into a heatproof glass bowl and pour in the almond oil.

2. Place the bowl in a pan of water over a gentle heat and mix until the ingredients are melted together.

3. Warm the rose water in a second bowl or jar, then add to the wax and oil mixture bit by bit, beating all the time.

4. Finally, stir in the essential oil, transfer the mixture to a pot, and put the pot into the refrigerator to set.

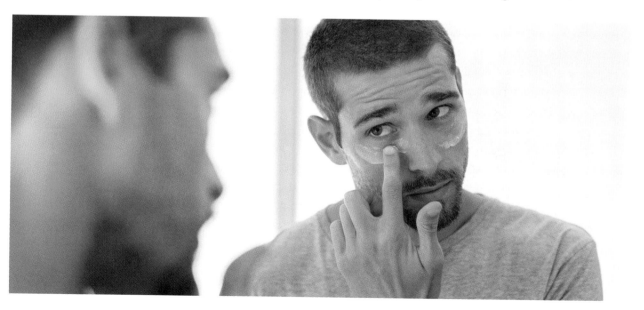

Gels

Water-based gels provide a useful, nonoily medium for the application of essential oils, as an alternative to oils and creams when required. A gel can be used to dilute any essential oils for irritating skin conditions such as eczema or athlete's foot, particularly if the skin is broken or sensitive. Gels are also suitable as a substitute for base or carrier oils for general skin care, especially if the skin is apt to be greasy. The percentage of essential oil to add to the gel base depends on where it will be used and for what purpose. Healing gels may include up to 2.5 percent of an essential oil when applied to the feet, whereas 0.5 percent is enough for application to the face or for general skin-care purposes. A natural soothing and cooling gel can be made with tapioca and water.

Tapioca gel recipe

Use ½ cup water to 1½ teaspoons tapioca. Mix and simmer until the tapioca is dissolved. Strain off the liquid and let it cool to form a transparent gel. Stir in a few drops of essential oil just before it sets.

Masks

Face masks or packs have many benefits—they can nourish, rejuvenate, stimulate, cleanse, or soothe the skin, and generally improve its texture and quality. Masks can be made from a wide range of natural ingredients, including fruit pulp, oatmeal (for allergic and irritated skin conditions), egg yolk (for all skin types), yogurt, honey, and clay. Fruits such as avocado (for dry skin) or strawberry (for oily skin) are extremely nutritious. Powdered oatmeal is also very nourishing and gives the skin a smooth, silken appearance, and brewer's yeast is good for all types of skin. Egg yolks are rich in lecithin, an invaluable skin aid. Natural yogurt contains lactic acid, which is good for large-pored, oily, and blemished skin and to balance combination skin. Honey is moisturizing and slightly antiseptic and can be incorporated into masks to soothe, soften, and nourish the skin— especially dry, sensitive, and mature complexions.

Clay is a useful ingredient for making masks, and is suitable for all but very dry skins. An aromatic clay mask is excellent for the treatment of acne and congested skin conditions, and can nourish dry or mature complexions and help to balance combination skin. However, those with dry, sensitive, or mature complexions should not use a clay-based mask more than once a week because they do have an overall drying effect. Masks are best applied after a bath or shower, when the pores are open and the skin is still warm and slightly damp. Clay cleanses and draws out toxins. It also aids skin regeneration, stimulates the circulation, and soothes inflammation. There are many different kinds of clay available, but green clay is the most versatile, being rich in minerals and a good antiseptic. Fuller's earth is also a good neutral clay base, which is more readily available.

SIMPLE CLAY MASK: Add 2 to 3 drops of an essential oil to 2 tablespoons of wet clay paste, and apply to the skin. Leave in place for 10–30 minutes while you relax. Rinse off with warm water.

ALTERNATIVE CLAY MASK: To make a more elaborate mask, first mix 5 tablespoons green clay powder with 2 teaspoons colloidal oatmeal and keep in a jar. To make the mask, mix 1 tablespoon of the basic mixture with 1 tablespoon runny honey or plain live yogurt, 1 egg yolk, 2 to 3 drops of an essential oil suited to your skin type, and enough water to give a smooth consistency. Apply to the skin and leave for 10–30 minutes—less for dry skin and longer for greasy/blemished skin. Rinse off with warm water. Finish by patting on a floral water.

For oily skin:

• To make a cleansing lotion, mix together 2 tablespoons witch hazel, ½ cup lavender water, 1 tablespoon glycerine, 7 drops each of lavender and geranium oils, 3 drops each of bergamot and sandalwood oils.

• Make a moisturizing oil or cream by mixing 2 to 3 drops each of lavender, geranium, and patchouli or palmarosa oils, 1 tablespoon wheat germ oil, and 5 teaspoons apricot kernel oil or a bland cream. Use in moderation twice daily. Wipe away any excess after 15–20 minutes.

• For a reviving cosmetic vinegar, mix 4 teaspoons cider vinegar with 5 drops of lavender oil, and add 4 tablespoons rose water and 4 teaspoons witch hazel.

• Once or twice a week apply a mask made from 2 tablespoons wet clay paste with 7 drops (in total) of tea tree, bergamot, and lavender oils.

AROMATHERAPY OILS FOR OILY SKIN: Tea tree, bergamot (bergapten-free), geranium, lavender, rosemary, cypress, sandalwood, lemongrass, clary sage, juniper, palmarosa, petitgrain, chamomile (Roman and German), patchouli, lemon eucalyptus, cedarwood.

For dry skin:

• Blend 3 drops each of rose, geranium or palmarosa, and lavender oils, 2 tablespoons of apricot kernel oil, and 1 tablespoon of a rich oil such as avocado, borage, evening primrose, wheat germ, or rose hip seed oil. Use as a moisturizer.

• A good toner or cleanser for dry skin is made by mixing 8 drops each of chamomile, lavender, and sandalwood oils with ½ cup of rose water in a dark, well-stoppered container. After one month, filter (using coffee filter paper), then add 2 tablespoons glycerine and shake well. Use twice daily.

• A mask for dry skin can be made by mixing 2 tablespoons clay, 2 teaspoons honey, 2 teaspoons cornstarch, 1 egg yolk, 1 teaspoon evening primrose oil or rose hip seed oil, and a few drops of rose, lavender, or sandalwood oil. Leave on the skin for 15 minutes, then rinse off with cool water.

AROMATHERAPY OILS FOR DRY SKIN: Rose, sandalwood, neroli, lavender, chamomile, palmarosa, rosewood, geranium, benzoin, myrrh.

AROMATHERAPY FOR AGING SKIN

Cell division slows down with age, and the epidermis (outer layer of the skin) becomes thinner, losing tone and suppleness. Wrinkles develop, and age spots and thread veins are also common. Smoking, drugs, poor diet, too much sun, central heating, and stress can all speed up the aging process.

CLINICAL NOTES: Marguerite Maury demonstrated that essential oils can do much to slow down the effects of aging by encouraging the skin cells to regenerate, as documented in her *Guide to Aromatherapy: The Secret of Life and Youth.*

Methods of use:

• Instead of soaps and alcohol-based products, use a natural toner/cleanser twice daily. In a dark, well-stoppered bottle, mix 7 drops each of geranium and lavender oils and 3 drops each of frankincense and neroli (or petitgrain) oils in ½ cup of rose water. After one month, filter into a similar container (use a coffee filter paper). Add 2 tablespoons glycerine and shake well.

• Regular use on face and neck of an oil or cream containing cytophylactic oils (stimulating new cell growth) is vital. A good basic blend for face and neck is as follows: to 2 tablespoons jojoba, almond, or grapeseed oil (or a bland cream base), add 1 tablespoon wheat germ oil, 1 tablespoon rose hip seed oil (or another rich vegetable oil, such as apricot kernel, avocado, hazelnut, borage, evening primrose, or peach kernel), and 10 to 15 drops (in total) of lavender, rose, neroli, or petitgrain, and frankincense essential oils.

• To treat and help prevent wrinkles around the eyes, apply a little wheat germ oil or rose hip seed oil gently to the area before retiring.

• Gentle facial massage, avoiding the delicate area around the eyes, helps to improve the circulation and muscle tone. Use any of the recommended oils in a light base oil.

• Use a face mask once a week. A basic mask can be made by mixing 2 tablespoons clay, 2 teaspoons runny honey, 1 teaspoon water, 4 to 5 drops (in total) of carrot seed, frankincense, and lavender oils.

Aromatherapy oils: Rose, frankincense, sandalwood, neroli, geranium, lavender, carrot seed, elemi, galbanum, myrrh, palmarosa, patchouli.

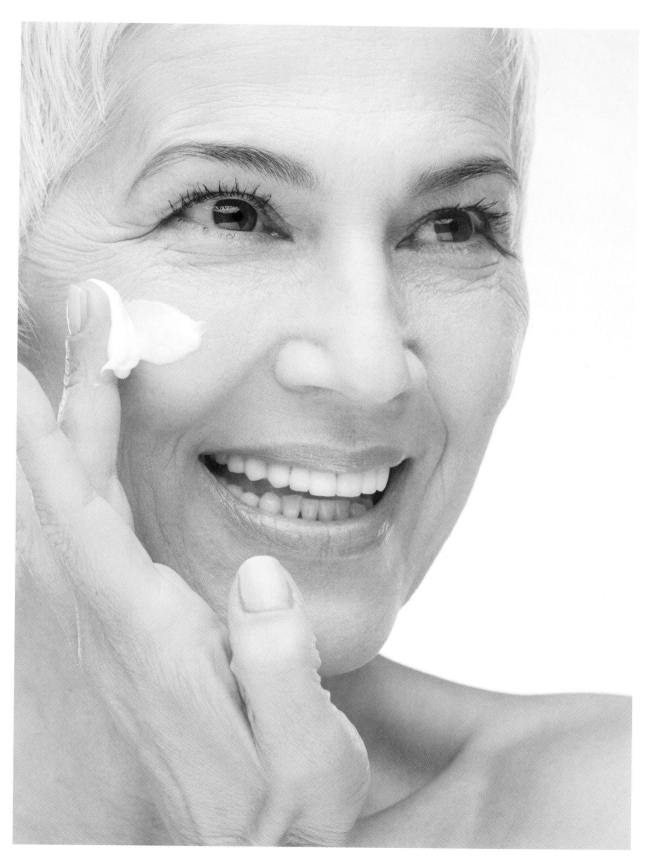

FLOWER WATERS AND STEAMS

It is easy to make flower (or floral) waters at home, and they are beneficial for all types of skin. Simply add 20 to 60 drops of essential oil (or a blend) to an 8-oz. bottle of spring or distilled water, leave it to stand for up to a month, and then filter the liquid using a coffee filter paper. (A more basic preparation can be made without filtering, but this must be shaken before each use.) Even a few drops of essential oil will impart their scent to this amount of water, making it very lightly fragranced. These delicately scented waters can be used to freshen and hydrate the skin, either dabbed on with absorbent cotton or sprayed from a small plant spray. This can be helpful during pregnancy, in hot, dry climates, or simply to help counter the drying effects of central heating.

REFRESHING TOILET WATERS: A variety of essential oils can be diluted in minute proportions with alcohol, cider vinegar, or witch hazel to make toilet waters, eau de cologne, or aftershave lotions. For example, a traditional toilet water called eau de portugal can be made as follows:

Ingredients
20 drops of sweet orange essential oil
5 drops of bergamot essential oil
2 drops of lemon essential oil
2 drops of benzoin essential oil
1 drop of geranium essential oil
1 tablespoon vodka
½ cup spring water

Method
Dissolve the oils in the vodka, then add to the water, shaking well. Leave the mixture to mature for a month at least, then filter and bottle.

TONER/CLEANSERS: Using a flower water as the base, add a little witch hazel, which increases the overall astringency for a greater toning action. For additional moisturizing and cleansing properties, add up to 25 percent of natural glycerine to the mixture. Flower waters that contain a proportion of witch hazel and glycerine will remove oily residues from the skin as well as acting as an astringent and antiseptic. If no makeup (or very light makeup) is worn, they can be used for simple one-step cleansing and toning.

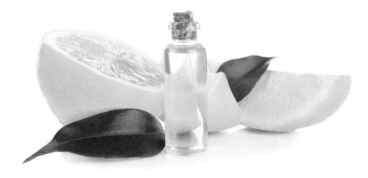

Flower waters that contain a proportion of witch hazel and glycerine will remove oily residues from the skin.

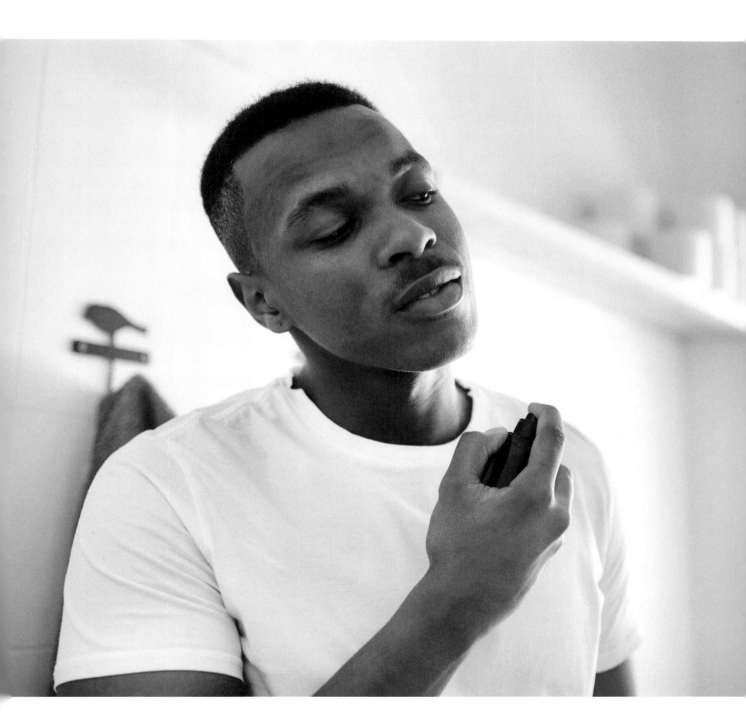

HAIR AND BODY TREATMENTS

Face scrub or exfoliant

To remove dead cells from the surface of the skin and stimulate the circulation, moisten a little medium-ground oatmeal (or colloidal oatmeal—available from pharmacists) in the palm of your hand using a suitable aromatic flower water (see page 168), and rub gently all over the face. For dry or sensitive skins, use ground almonds.

Dry and wet body-brushing

Rub 1 or 2 drops of a chosen essential oil into a dry loofah or a natural-bristle brush to make it smell fragrant. Start by rubbing the feet firmly with the brush, then gradually work your way up the body, concentrating on any congested or fatty areas, such as the hips or thighs. Work up the arms, paying special attention to the backs of the upper arms, up the back from the waist, up over the abdomen, and down the front from the shoulders. Popular in Scandinavia, this technique stimulates the circulation, helps break down fatty deposits, and brings a glow to the skin. Used in combination with other approaches, it is helpful for removing cellulite. For a milder effect, the same technique can also be used in the shower or bath, using a few drops of essential oil on a wet brush, loofah, or sponge.

Aromatic scalp oil preparations

Local massage is effective for conditions such as hair loss and brittle or dry hair, if it is carried out on a regular basis. Massage also stimulates scalp circulation and nourishes the deeper layers of the skin, bringing more nutrients to the follicles and improving the hair. To make a scalp massage oil, mix 3 tablespoons coconut oil and 2 teaspoons wheat germ oil with between 10 and 25 drops of essential oil depending on hair and skin type.

Body powders

Aromatic body powders can be made by mixing about 4 tablespoons unperfumed talc or cornstarch with 5 to 6 drops of essential oils. Seal the mixture in a closed container and let the base absorb the oils for at least 24 hours before use.

Hair conditioner

To make a good hair conditioner to encourage hair growth and improve the quality of the hair structure, mix 12 drops of essential oil with 2 tablespoons of slightly warmed jojoba oil, castor oil, or extra virgin olive oil, and rub this thoroughly into the scalp. Cover the hair with a layer of waxed paper, wrap in warm towels, and leave for an hour. Wash out, applying shampoo before the water, otherwise the hair will remain oily. Repeat weekly.

Hair tonic

Aromatic hair tonics are especially recommended for oily or thinning hair, because they can help to balance sebum levels (the oil produced at the base of the hair) and promote hair growth. Dissolve about 10 drops of essential oils suited to your hair type in 1 tablespoon of cider vinegar and add to ½ cup lavender water. Shake well and massage into the scalp.

Quick scalp rub

A quick method to use for treating the scalp between washes, if required, is to rub about 10 drops of pure tea tree or lavender oil into the scalp using the fingertips. This is beneficial for the treatment of dandruff and as a general conditioner.

Dry shampoo

It is not beneficial to wash the hair too often, as this can strip the hair of its protective acid mantle. When short of time, or between shampoos, simply add a drop of rosemary essential oil, or an oil chosen for its fragrance, to 1 tablespoon of orris root powder or fuller's earth. Part the hair in sections and sprinkle the mixture on. Leave for 5 minutes, then brush out thoroughly.

Aromatic shampoo

Buy a neutral pH shampoo (this is marked on the label) and add your own choice of essential oils to it. Add 1 or 2 drops of essential oil to a capful of shampoo at each wash, or add 10 to 15 drops of your chosen essential oil (or a blend) per ounce of shampoo, and shake well before using.

Aromatic rinse

Add a few drops of a suitable aromatherapy oil, such as chamomile, lavender, or rosemary, to the final rinse water together with 1 tablespoon of cider vinegar. This very effective, yet simple, procedure gives the hair a wonderful shine and maintains the acid mantle of the scalp. It also imparts a delicious fragrance and new vitality to the hair.

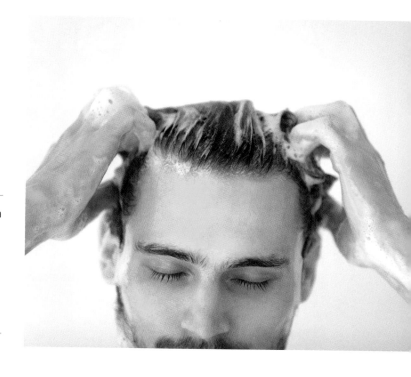

Conditioner for oily hair

Mix 10 to 12 drops (in total) of rosemary, sandalwood, and lavender with 2 tablespoons of slightly warmed jojoba oil (or sunflower seed oil) and massage thoroughly into the scalp. Wrap in warm towels and leave for an hour if possible. Wash out—applying the shampoo before the water, or the hair will remain oily. Repeat once a week.

Aromatherapy oils for dandruff

Tea tree, chamomile, citronella, clary sage, lavender, lemongrass, lemon eucalyptus, rosemary.

AROMATIC BATHING

One of the simplest and most pleasant ways to use essential oils is in the bathtub, where the oils enhance the relaxing effect of a long warm bath, or the stimulating effect of a brisk hot bath or cold dip. The therapeutic effects of bathing have been recognized for centuries. The sophistication of many of the ancient Roman spa bath houses can still be seen, with their hot and cold compartments, steam rooms, and aromatic massage quarters. Very hot baths stimulate perspiration, which is valuable in cases of infectious illness and for encouraging elimination of wastes and detoxification. However, they can also be draining and, in the long run, can cause the skin to lose its elasticity. A medium-hot or warm bath has a soothing and relaxing effect on both the mind and body, while cool or cold water has a more invigorating and stimulating effect. Lukewarm baths are good for lowering the temperature in cases of fever.

Pure essences

This is the easiest and most popular way of using essential oils for bathing. Simply add 5 to 10 drops of your chosen essential oil (or a blend of oils) to the bathtub when it is full, and relax in the aromatic vapors. Use lavender oil for promoting relaxation, rosemary as an invigorating tonic, or marjoram for soothing tired muscles.

Bath bags

Gather a selection of fresh herbs or aromatic flowers together, such as lavender sprigs, rose petals, lemon balm leaves, and chamomile flowers, and tie them loosely in a muslin bag with a piece of string or ribbon. Choose specific herbs both for their therapeutic properties and for their scent. If you wish, add a few drops of a chosen essential oil to the bundle to enhance the fragrance. Then tie the bag to the faucets and let it hang in the stream of hot water while the bathtub is filling.

Bath salts

Epsom salt (magnesium sulfate) and Dead Sea salt are healing substances in themselves, and make an excellent medium for combining with essential oils. Salt contains precious minerals, has an alkalizing effect on the body, promotes the elimination of acidic waste from the muscles and joints, and induces copious perspiration—good for infectious illness, rheumatism, arthritis, and for promoting relaxation. Dissolve one or two handfuls of Epsom salt in boiling water, add a few drops of essential oil, and pour into the bathtub. Alternatively, simply add 5 drops of essential oil to every handful of Epsom salt or Dead Sea salt, pour directly into the bathtub, and agitate the water before getting in.

Moisturizing bath oils

A few drops of an essential oil can also be mixed into a teaspoonful of vegetable oil, such as sweet almond oil, before being added to the bathtub. This helps to moisturize the skin and ensures an even distribution

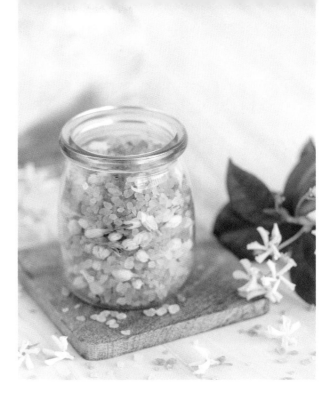

of the essential oil, which is especially important in the case of babies and young children. To make a larger quantity, mix 4 teaspoons of an essential oil (or blend) with ⅔ cup jojoba oil or another base or carrier oil (see pages 116–117) containing 5 percent wheat germ oil, and store in a tinted glass bottle. Add a teaspoonful of this mixture to the bath water when required.

Foot and hand baths

Valuable for warding off chills, for easing arthritic or rheumatic pain, and for the treatment of specific foot complaints, a hot aromatic foot bath can also be very effective for relieving stress and overexhaustion (use lavender and sweet marjoram), and is a quick aid to combating excessive perspiration (use tea tree and rosemary). Simply sprinkle 5 or 6 drops of essential oil into a bowl or basin of warm or hot water and soak feet or hands for about 10 minutes. Alternatively, dilute the essential oils in a teaspoonful of cider vinegar, honey, or a moisturizing vegetable oil beforehand.

Therapeutic hip bath or douche

This method can be helpful in the treatment of urinary or genital conditions, such as pruritus (itching), thrush, or cystitis. The area can be bathed in a hip or sitz bath or a bowl of warm water to which 3 to 5 drops of a suitable essential oil have been added—a mixture of cypress and lavender, for example, can help to heal the perineum after childbirth.

The sauna

In Scandinavia, the sauna is the traditional method of cleansing and toning the whole system. Dry heat and steam are used to open the pores and promote the elimination of waste products. This is followed by a plunge into very cold water that closes the pores, and tones and refreshes the skin. In Finland, where the tradition of the sauna originates, bundles of fresh birch twigs are slapped on the skin, stimulating the circulation and imparting a delicious fragrance. Essential oils that are most suitable for use in the traditional sauna include fresh-scented oils such as pine, juniper, myrtle, eucalyptus, and cedarwood. (Very rich or floral oils such as lavender, ylang ylang, or patchouli are too heady and should not be used.) Add 2 or 3 drops to 2 cups of warm water and throw on the heat source for an aromatic and refreshing steam bath.

CAUTION: Always check with specific safety data before using a new oil in the bathtub, to avoid possible irritation.

USING ESSENTIAL OILS IN YOUR HOME

In addition to natural remedies for health, self-care, and wellness, aromatherapy essential oils can be used for other practical purposes around the home. They offer a more natural approach, which is ideal if you're keen to use more sustainable, eco-friendly, and chemical-free products.

Disinfectants

Many essential oils have natural antibacterial, antifungal, and antiviral properties, so are well suited for use in home cleaning products. Oils such as tea tree, lemon, or lavender can be used for disinfecting clothes and diapers. For washing by hand, add up to 50 drops of essential oil to a bowl of warm water; otherwise add the same quantity to a liquid detergent and use in the washing machine.

For washing tiled floors and kitchen and bathroom surfaces, add up to 50 drops of essential oil to a bucket or bowl of water. If there are very dirty areas, add 1 cup white vinegar to a bucket of warm water, plus 10 drops of tea tree, 10 drops of lemon, and 10 drops of orange essential oils. Vinegar is an effective natural cleaner, but the addition of the essential oils will help improve the smell.

Carpet cleaners

If you have carpets in your home, you can also use essential oils to help clean and freshen them. Mix together 2 cups baking soda with 10 drops of orange and lemon essential oils. Sprinkle the mixture over your carpet, then use a dry brush to brush it in—this ensures that it reaches the base of the carpet. Leave the mixture on the carpet for several hours, then vacuum it thoroughly. The result should be a clean and fresh-smelling carpet.

Perfumes and household fragrance

Some essential oils can be applied undiluted to the skin in minute amounts as perfume. Several essential oils are ideal natural perfumes—either on their own or combined with others. Ylang ylang is renowned as a well-balanced fragrance in its own right; others, such as rose, jasmine, neroli, and sandalwood, are well-known traditional perfume ingredients. Such oils can be dabbed on the wrists or behind the ears, either undiluted or diluted to 5 percent in jojoba or a bland base oil. Always carry out a patch test on the skin before using a new oil as a perfume.

Aromatic oils can be used to scent the hair, linen or clothes, paper, ink, potpourris, or other items, directly from the bottle. Pure essential oils have a totally different quality to synthetic perfumes, since they are derived from natural sources. Artificially made perfumes do not have the subtle balance of constituents and the therapeutic qualities of real essential oils.

Hand sanitizers

Use essential oils to make natural hand sanitizers. Use a base of 2 tablespoons aloe vera gel and add 10 drops of tea tree oil and 7 drops of lavender essential oil. Mix together and add it to a glass bottle.

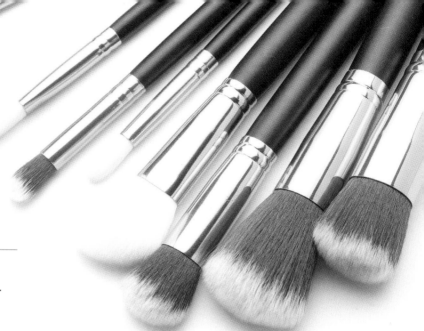

Makeup brush cleaner

Makeup brushes harbor bacteria and are often not cleaned enough, despite being used on a daily basis. Ready-made brush cleaners are widely available from stores, but often contain chemicals. For a more natural approach, you can mix up a batch of homemade makeup brush cleaner. Add 2 tablespoons of witch hazel, 1 tablespoon of white vinegar, ½ teaspoon of olive oil, and 20 drops of tea tree essential oil into a jug. Stir them together well, then place your brushes into the jug. Give them a good wash, making sure that all the bristles are clean. When you take them out, rinse them with water and leave them to dry on a clean towel.

Mold remover

If you have areas of mold in your kitchen or bathroom, for example around taps, in shower trays, in your bath, or lingering on the edges of shower curtains, you can mix up a mold-remover spray. Fill a spray bottle with warm water then add 2 tablespoons of white vinegar, 4 drops of tea tree oil, 4 drops of eucalyptus oil, and 4 drops of rosemary oil. Spray in the areas needed.

Bug-busting oils

If small bugs such as ants are getting under doors and into areas of your home, you could help deter them by using essential oils. It's much more natural than chemical products and won't kill the bugs but ward them off. Cinnamon and lemongrass are two oils that ants aren't fond of. Add 10 to 20 drops of the oils, either on their own or combined, into approximately ½ cup water. Put the liquid into a spray bottle, shake it, and liberally spray the area.

Rodent-busting oils

If mice or rats are a problem in your house, there's an oil they won't like too! Simply put 2 or 3 drops of peppermint essential oil on cotton balls and place them in the areas where you know mice have been and where they might be getting in. They don't like the smell of peppermint, so hopefully it will deter them from being in your home.

Trash can transformer

Trash cans are renowned for getting smelly, even if you religiously use bags and don't put trash directly into the bin. If your trash can aroma is distinctly off, you can freshen it up with a few well-chosen essential oils. Get a couple of cotton balls and add 2 drops of tea tree, orange, lemon, and may chang essential oils to them. Then pop the balls at the bottom of your trash can. They'll help freshen up the scent of your bin. Simply remove them when you empty your trash and replace with new ones.

MORE HOME SOLUTIONS AND IDEAS

Once you've caught the aromatherapy bug, you'll discover there are so many ways you can use essential oils around your home. You don't necessarily need a huge collection of essential oils either, just a few firm favorites will get you started, and you can add to them gradually as your budget allows.

Oils for furniture and wood

A few drops of an essential oil such as cedarwood or rosemary can be used to perfume wooden items such as beads or boxes, or added to furniture polishes. Unfinished woods tend to absorb oils well, but take care to ensure they don't stain. Freshly scented oils such as these can also be sprinkled onto logs before they are burned on an open fire.

Aromatic sachets and pillows

As well as having a pleasing fragrance, lavender oil makes an excellent insect repellent. Lavender has been used for centuries to protect clothes and linen from moths. It imparts a lovely scent when used in aromatic sachets kept in the linen closet or in drawers. Use dried herbs impregnated with a few drops of oil as the stuffing and seal them in small linen or lace sachets, which can be tied at the top with ribbon. Scented pillows can be made for the bedroom in similar fashion—try dried rose petals and rose essential oil for a soft and feminine scented pillow.

Linen refreshers

A few drops of essential oils can be added to unscented laundry detergents, creating a much more natural smell than some artificially fragranced washing liquids. Essential oils can also be added directly into the water as the machine starts its cycle. You can use them with dryer balls too, and this can help the scent set into your clothes more as they dry.

Another idea is to add a few drops of your favorite oils to the outside of wooden clothes pegs (not the part that will clip onto clothes when you hang them up), which will soak up the oils. When the pegs are used to hang out your washing, the aroma of fresh essential oils will also gently permeate your laundry. Good choices of scents include fresh lemon or sweet orange, or floral rose, jasmine, or lavender.

Tip: Terracotta is a highly absorbent stone. If you don't have an oil burner or diffuser, add a few drops of your favorite essential oils onto the rim of a terracotta plant pot instead. It's a quick and easy way of fragrancing a room—and perhaps of also making your houseplants seem more fragrant than they really are!

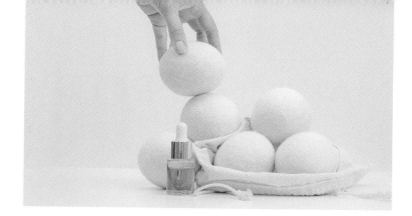

Make your own scented reed diffusers

Reed diffusers are simple ways of enjoying aromatic scents. They're widely available to purchase, but you can easily make your own to enjoy at home or gift to friends. All your need is a small, decorative glass or ceramic jar or mini vase, a set of reed sticks, and essential oils of your choice. If you don't have any suitable jars or vases, have a look in a thrift store as you may well be able to find a pretty vintage vase or jar to use for a sustainable option.

Put 10 drops of your choice of essential oils, either single notes or a blend of oils, into the bottom of the container, then add 3–5 reeds to it. The reeds will soak up the oils and fill the room with a lovely aroma. When you can no longer smell the oils, turn the reeds upside down to refresh them or add more oils. A small reed diffuser can be discreet and can be used in any room of your home, from the bathroom to a living room and bedrooms.

Shoe refreshers

Whether you're a gym bunny, running fan, or simply someone who enjoys wearing clean shoes, you can freshen up all your shoes and those of your family using aromatherapy essential oils. Put 2 drops of your chosen oils on cotton balls and add one into each shoe while they're in your closet. When you come to put them on, take out the cotton balls and you should discover you have nicely scented shoes. For shoes that need deodorizing, use oils such as tea tree, peppermint, or lavender.

Scented paper and ink

An easy way to scent writing paper is to put a few drops of a chosen essential oil onto a ball of absorbent cotton and store this in a sealed box together with the sheets of paper. After about ten days, the paper will have absorbed a good deal of the fragrance. A few drops of aromatic oil can also be dropped into writing ink. Many household items can be scented in a similar manner.

Car air fresheners

If your car could do with freshening up, forget artificial, chemically smelling car air fresheners and make your own using essential oils. There are several ways you can do this, such as by adding cotton balls soaked in essential oils into the car vents, or using the wooden clothes peg method—put a few drops of oil onto the wood, so it absorbs it—and clipping a peg onto the air vent. You could also look for cutout wooden craft shapes at a hobby store. If they have a hole at the top, you can add a piece of ribbon, dab essential oils onto the wooden shape, and hang them inside your car to release a delightful aroma.

MAKING A POTPOURRI

Many traditional dry potpourri mixes displayed in open ceramic bowls in the bedroom or living room are based on rose petals, often with the addition of lavender flowers. However, a great deal of flexibility and individual creativity can be used in choosing plant material and other ingredients. A fresh citrus blend based on herbs such as lemon balm and lemon-scented geraniums together with dried lemon peel and marigold petals can make a refreshing bathroom blend. Spicy mixtures, which are suitable for the kitchen or for festive occasions, may include ingredients such as lemon or orange peel, cinnamon sticks, vanilla beans, whole cloves and other spices, bay leaves, and sprigs of dried rosemary.

Ingredients
20 to 30 drops rose essential oil
20 to 30 drops lavender essential oil
½ nutmeg, grated
½ tablespoon orris root powder
1 cup dried rose petals
¼ cup dried lavender flowers
¼ cup dried mint leaves
decorative rosebuds
small glass mixing bottle
mortar and pestle
small spoon for mixing
glass or ceramic storage jar
decorative bowl

Measure out the essential oils and blend them together in a glass bottle. Put on the lid securely and set aside.

Grind the grated nutmeg and orris root powder together using the mortar and pestle. Add half the total quantity of essential oils and mix with a spoon.

Place the rose petals, lavender flowers, and dried mint leaves in the storage container and add the remaining essential oils, mixing well.

Add the powdered material from the mortar and mix gently, so as not to damage the plant materials. Seal the container and leave to mature for 2–6 weeks in a dark place.

Transfer the potpourri mixture into a decorative bowl or jar and arrange a few tiny rosebuds on top. Later, as the aroma starts to fade, more essential oils can be added to revive the mixture and prolong its life.

Potpourri inspiration
Experiment with your favorite scents to create potpourris for every occasion. The traditional recipe on this page is soothing and relaxing—try blending citrusy scents like lemon verbena, lemon balm, and lemon thyme with marjoram to create an invigorating alternative.

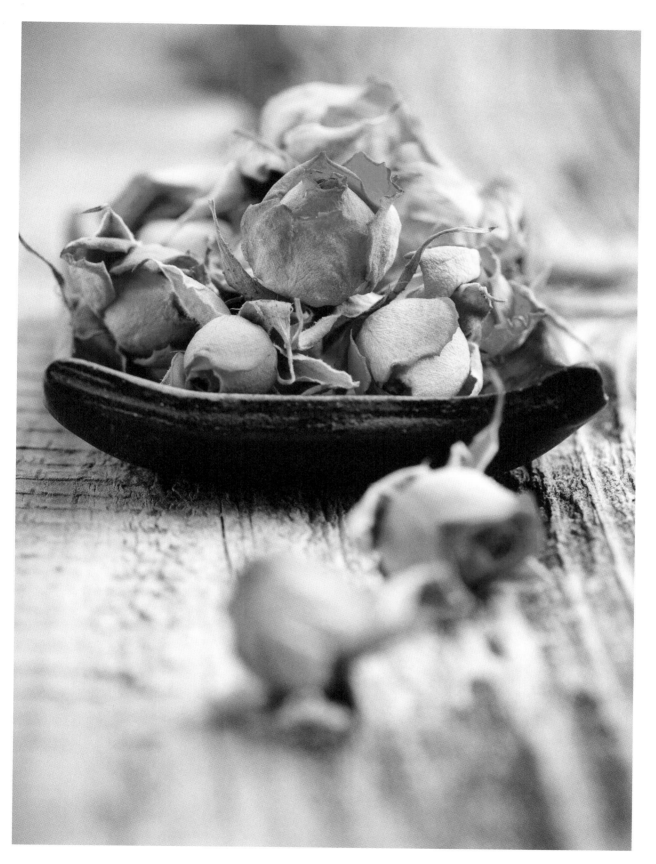

BUYING AND SOURCING ESSENTIAL OILS

When you're buying and sourcing essential oils, you need to ensure you're getting authentic products of the highest quality. Sadly, not all oils are equal, and there are some less than reputable companies peddling so-called aromatherapy oils that aren't the true product. In order to get the best effects and healing outcome from using aromatherapy, you need to make sure that what you're buying is really what you think it is.

What to look for—the contents

Essential oils are 100 percent pure and concentrated, and some may be organic, but there are some products on the market that give the impression of being essential oils when they're not.

The iffy terms to look out for when you're buying essential oils are "fragrance oil," "perfume oil," or, as is occasionally used, "nature identical oil." These descriptions all indicate that an oil is not 100 percent pure or a true essential oil. Instead, they may contain chemicals, additives, or a mix of different types of oils.

What to look for—the bottles

Essential oils should be in dark bottles, such as amber, blue, brown, or green. This is because the oils need to be protected from the damaging effects of sunlight. All good-quality oils are packaged in this way, so any that aren't are unlikely to be top quality.

What to look for—information

Reputable essential oil retailers will be happy to supply details and information about their products, such as where the oils are sourced from and how they're distilled, plus details about their own history in the business and any training and experience they have. Don't be afraid to ask questions; a legitimate company should be happy to provide answers.

What to look for—the price

The nature of essential oils and the fact that the process to obtain oils varies from plant to plant means that the price of products differs too. There are some oils that will always tend to be higher priced than others, such as gardenia, which has to go through a more complicated extraction process. If you find a range of oils where all the oils are priced the same, steer clear, as they may be poor quality.

Where to look

In terms of where best to source essential oils, local health-food stores often stock reputable brands, or you could look online for speciality retailers. If you're unsure whether a brand is reliable or genuine, do a search online and look for any reviews of the company. Most reputable brands will have a web presence of some kind, be it a website or social media channels. Aromatherapy organizations also often provide a list of recommended retailers.

Sourcing and buying aromatherapy accessories

When you begin to look for aromatherapy accessories, you'll realize there's a minefield of products on the market. The same due diligence applies when you're buying accessories, as not all products are worth the money or effective for the required purposes. You want to ensure that the products you're purchasing are good quality, will last, and will do their job in exactly the way you need.

Aromatherapy oil burners

Oil burners are typically made from glazed ceramic or hard stone materials. They can be designed as an all-in-one piece, with a little bowl at the top where a few drops of essential oil are mixed into water, and a hollow underneath where a tea light candle sits; sometimes they're designed in two pieces, with the bowl being removable. To use the burner, you need to fill the bowl about three-quarters full with water, then add a few drops of your chosen oils. Take care not to let the bowl run dry while the candle is still burning, as that's when damage can occur.

When you're choosing an oil burner, look for well-made products that will be resistant to cracks when a candle is burning. Some inferior products have been known to crack after a while from the heat of the candle, so it's better to buy a well-made piece from the outset that will last.

Electric diffusers

Electric oil diffusers do a similar job to oil burners, except for the fact that no burning flame is involved as they plug in to the electricity. This makes them more practical if you have children or pets in your home and if you need to be out of sight of the burner some of the time, as it should be much safer to leave unattended.

The design and style of electric aromatherapy diffusers varies considerably, as does the price, so it's worth researching the options available so you can

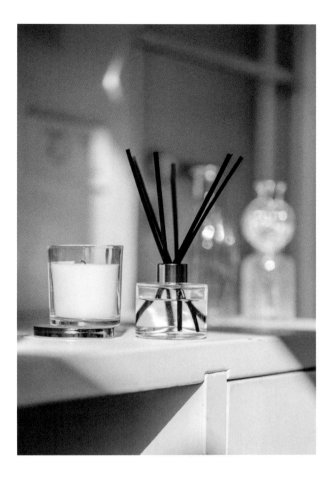

see which would best suit your needs. For example, some designs feature a built-in light in the base, and the oil burner on the top, or color-changing lights, but if it's not something you need then it doesn't make sense to pay for these extra features.

Remember that sometimes a simple oil burner or electric diffuser is all you need. There may be fantastic gadgets that are all singing, all dancing, but when it comes down to it, all you need is something that will effectively diffuse essential oils in a room.

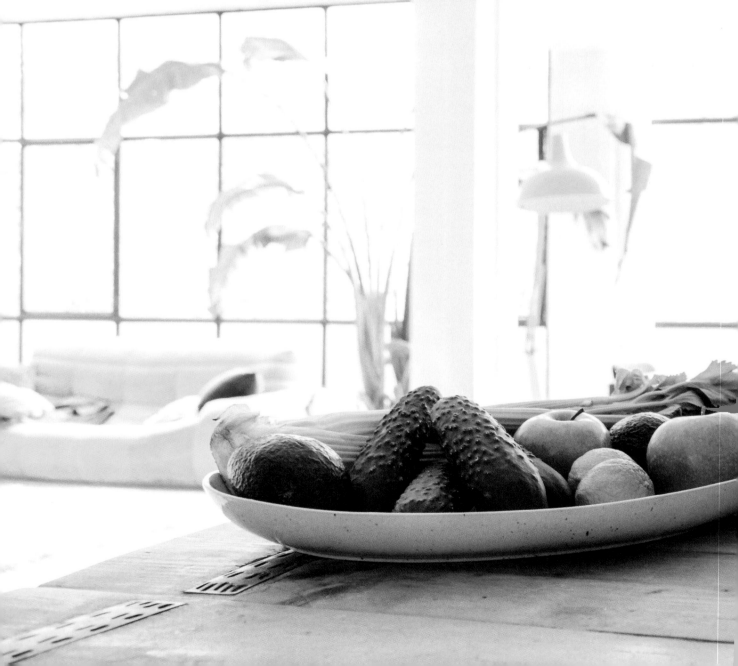

PART THREE

Food and Drink

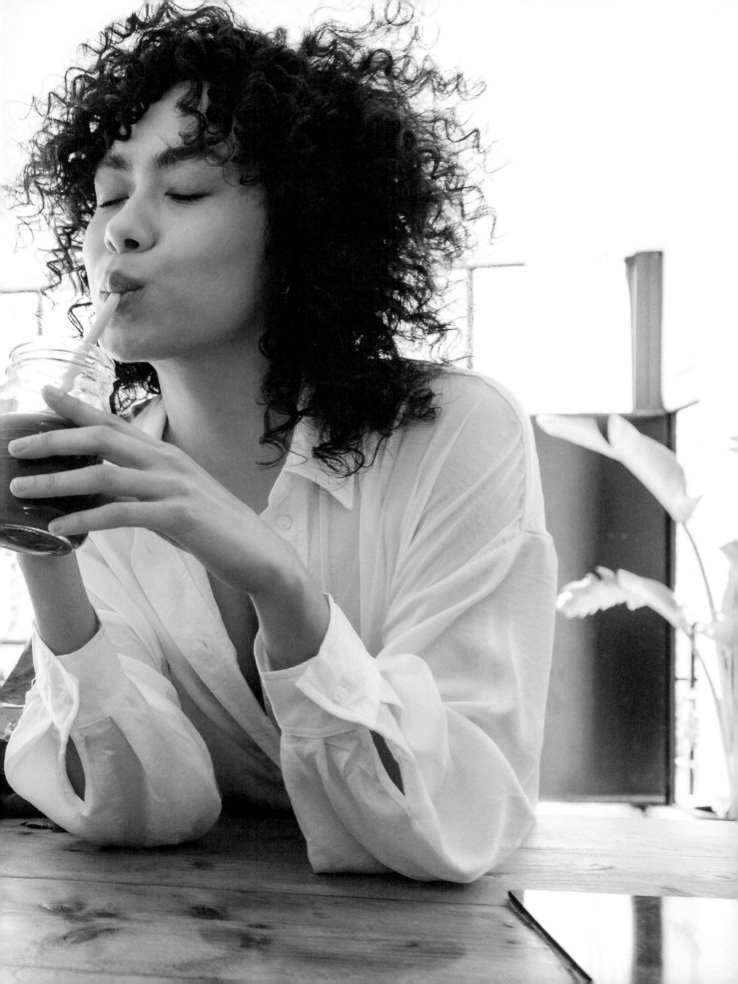

NUTRITION FOR HEALING AND HEALTH

The use of nutrition for health, or nutritional therapy, can help with almost anything, since food is the basic fuel of all the chemical processes that take place in the body. Almost all ill health of body and mind can have a basis in nutritional elements that are missing or insubstantial within the diet—or in unhealthy additions to our diet, such as large quantities of saturated fat, sugar, and salt. All the systems in the body will be improved by a healthy diet. In a fit state, you are much more likely to fight off infection and deal efficiently with any health problems or injury.

A healthy diet

Our daily diet should be made up of complex carbohydrates (5–9 portions), fruits and vegetables (4–9 portions), proteins (3–5 portions), and fat (under 30 percent of total daily calories for a healthy diet). We also need to drink plenty of fluids, particularly water. But eating the right foods doesn't necessarily mean that you are getting enough nutrients. Refining and processing foods takes out much of the nutritional value, and agents used in the growing process place extra demands on our bodies. Before our food reaches the grocery store it may be nutritionally deficient. Therefore, take extra steps to preserve the nutritional content of your food:

• Eat the skins of vegetables.
• Don't cut, wash, or soak fruit and vegetables until you are ready to eat them. Exposing their cut surfaces to air destroys many nutrients.
• Choose brown rice and whole grains.
• Choose fresh fruit and vegetables first, but remember that nutritional value decreases with age. Frozen is a better option if you aren't going to eat the food immediately. Eat raw whenever possible; if cooking, use as little water as possible. If you do boil fruit or vegetables, use the water remaining after cooking in your sauces or gravy.

• Eat organic food whenever possible. It may be more expensive, but it has been grown without the use of pesticides and their chemicals.

Dietary fiber

Dietary fiber, also known as bulk and roughage, is an essential element in the diet, even though it provides no nutrients. It consists of plant cellulose and other indigestible materials in foods, along with pectin and gum. Chewing it stimulates saliva flow, and the bulk it adds in the stomach and intestines

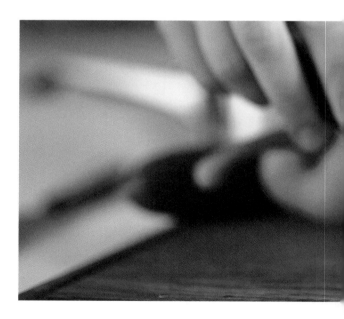

during digestion provides more time for absorption of nutrients. A diet with sufficient fiber produces softer, bulkier stools, and helps to promote bowel regularity and avoid constipation and disorders such as diverticulosis. Other health benefits of fiber include:

• Reduces the production of cholesterol in the body
• May protect against some coronary diseases
• Helps to control diabetes
• Helps to control weight
• Protects against cancers of the colon

The best sources of fiber are fruit and vegetables, whole-grain breads and cereals, and products made from nuts and legumes. An intake of 20–50 grams of fiber per day is ideal. But be aware that a diet too abundant in dietary fiber can reduce the absorption of important trace minerals during digestion. Take a good multivitamin and mineral tablet if you increase your fiber intake significantly.

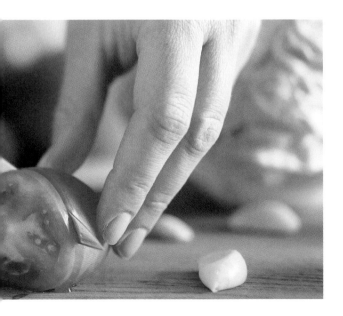

Foods to avoid

Aim to reduce the amount of saturated fat, sugar, and salt in your diet. We all need to consume some fat, yet we need to pay attention to the amount and type of fat we eat. There are two main types of fat: saturated and unsaturated. Too much saturated fat can increase the cholesterol in your blood, which increases your risk of heart disease. Saturated fat is found in foods such as cakes, cookies, French fries, butter, cream, cheese, and fatty meats. Replace these foods with those that contain unsaturated fats, such as oily fish (including tuna, salmon, mackerel, and trout), avocado, and vegetable oils. Trim the fat off meat, drink skimmed milk, replace cream and ice cream with low-fat yogurt, and spread your bread with a reduced-fat spread.

Eating too many foods and drinks high in sugar increases your risk of obesity and related conditions. Swap drinks high in sugars for lower-calorie options. For example, swap a sugary soda for sparkling water with a slice of lemon. Reduce your alcohol intake. Avoid sugary breakfast cereals, cakes, cookies, and pastries. Check the labels of packaged sauces and meals to make sure they are not high in sugar. Too much salt in your diet can raise your blood pressure, which leaves you at greater risk of heart disease or stroke. Even if you do not add salt to your food, there are high levels of salt in many food products, such as breads, chips, cereals, soups, and sauces. Check food labels to help you reduce your salt intake.

VITAMINS AND MINERALS

Micronutrition

Our understanding of vitamins and minerals—and other micronutrients, compounds, and elements—and their role in our body has improved dramatically over the last decades. We now know that "micronutrition"—or the vitamins, minerals, and other health-giving components of our food, such as amino acids, fiber, enzymes, and lipids—is crucial to life, and that by manipulating our nutritional intake, we not only ensure good health and address ailments but prevent illness and some of the degenerative effects of aging.

Vitamins

Vitamins are a group of unrelated organic nutrients which are essential to regulate the chemical processes that go on in the body—such as releasing the energy from food, maintaining strong bones, and controlling our hormonal activity.

Minerals

Minerals are inorganic chemical elements, which are necessary for many biochemical and physiological processes that go on in our bodies. Inorganic substances that are required in amounts greater than 100 mg per day are called minerals; those required in amounts less than 100 mg per day are called trace elements. Minerals are not necessarily present in foods—the quality of the soil and the geological conditions of the area in which they were grown play an important part in determining the mineral content of foods. Even a balanced diet may be lacking in essential minerals or trace elements

because of the soil in which the various foodstuffs were grown. There is some evidence that "subclinical" deficiencies—in other words, a deficiency that is not extensive enough to produce large-scale symptoms—may be the cause of certain forms of cancer, heart disease, weight and skin problems, and a host of other health conditions.

Amino acids

An amino acid is any compound that contains an amino group and an acidic function. There are twenty amino acids necessary for the synthesis of proteins, which are essential for life. These twenty amino acids form the building blocks of all proteins and are involved in important biological processes, such as the formation of neurotransmitters in the brain. There are ten essential amino acids:

- Arginine (essential for children but not adults)
- Histidine
- Isoleucine
- Leucine
- Lysine
- Methionine
- Phenylalanine
- Threonine
- Tryptophan
- Valine

The remaining ten are called "nonessential," which means that they can usually be made by the body from other substances. In some conditions, however, nonessential amino acids are necessary, for example in cases of extreme illness or a very poor diet.

Lipids and derivatives

Lipids are commonly called "fats," and while many fats are now known to be unhealthy, there are many that are essential to body processes and actually work to prevent the effects of "unhealthy" fats in our bodies. Many lipids and their derivatives, including fish oils and evening primrose oil, are used to unclog arteries, and work to retard the effects of aging and to discourage heart disease and cholesterol buildup.

A history of nutrition

Eighteenth century

Although there was not yet any scientific understanding of what a "vitamin" was, in the eithteenth century English sailors were given lime or lemon juice in order to prevent scurvy, a disease caused by lack of vitamin C, which occurred as a result of long periods of time away at sea without fresh fruit or vegetables.

Nineteenth century

In the late nineteenth century, naturopaths drew attention to the use of food and its nutritional elements as medicine, a concept that was not new, but which had not been acknowledged as a therapy in its own right until that time. Naturopaths used nutrition and fasting to cleanse the body, and to encourage its ability to heal itself. As knowledge about food, its makeup, and the effects it has on our body became greater with the development of biochemistry, the first nutritional specialists undertook to treat specific ailments and symptoms with the components of food.

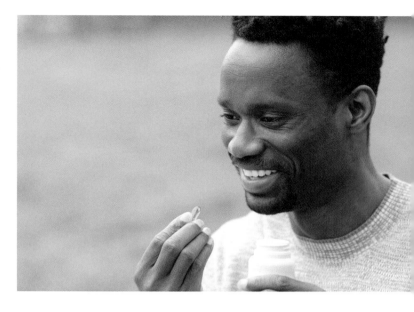

Twentieth century

By the middle of the twentieth century, scientists had put together a profile of proteins, carbohydrates, and fats, as well as vitamins and minerals, which were essential to health. More than forty nutrients were identified, including thirteen vitamins. It was discovered that minerals were needed for body functions, and a new understanding of the body and its biochemistry fed the growing interest in the subject. By the 1960s, physicians began to treat patients with special diets and supplements, prescribed according to individual symptoms, problems, and needs, but while conventional medical physicians discussed nutrition in terms of food groups, nutritionists were prescribing vitamins in megadoses. Other elements and compounds were soon identified as necessary to human life, and we are now able to purchase substances such as amino acids, lipids, and dietary enzymes.

Today

Today, nutrition has changed from a mainly physician-led dietary therapy, also called clinical nutrition, to a more profound theory of health based on treating the patient as a whole (holistic health) and looking for deficiencies that may be causing illness, which are specific to each individual.

WHAT ARE SUPERFOODS?

The term "superfoods" is used to describe foods that are particularly high in nutrients and low in calories, and packed with a great dose of vitamins, minerals, antioxidants, and essential fatty acids—more so than standard healthy foods. They're extra healthy, and ideal foods to include regularly in your diet for their beneficial properties.

Many superfoods are natural and plant-based, although there are other types of food that get the superfood status too, such as some dairy products, meat, and fish. The high levels of antioxidants naturally contained in superfoods are important as they play a key role in helping to neutralize free radicals in the body—without antioxidants, free radicals can cause serious damage to your health. Including plenty of superfoods in your diet can help decrease the chances of suffering from serious diseases and increase the function of your immune system. Plus, many superfoods have lots of other benefits too.

The individual profile of every superfood invariably differs, but on the whole superfoods tend to be associated with health benefits such as:

• Lower cholesterol
• Improved heart health
• Less inflammation
• Improved immune health
• Reduced risk of cancer

They're by no means a magic cure though, and you'll have to do more than eat the occasional superfood to reap the health benefits.

What's more, some marketers tend to use the superfood terminology to try and hike the prices of some foods up. In general, superfoods aren't pricey foodstuffs—a lot of them are well-known foods that have existed in grocery stores for years, not new, rare discoveries. Of course, there are some newer foods that have gained in popularity in recent years and may cost a few dollars more, but they're not necessarily foods you need to eat every week.

When you're out shopping for your superfoods, try and stay away from the hype and shop around. Look for good-quality, organically grown produce and buy local where you can, to cut down on your carbon footprint. To save on cash, where possible buy your own raw ingredients and make your own healthy, home-cooked foods. You could even try growing some of the core ingredients yourself.

Healthy foods versus superfoods

So, what are the differences between healthy foods and superfoods?

Healthy foods are nutritious foods that should form the basis of a healthy diet. They're foods that should be consumed on a daily basis and make up the bulk of your diet.

Superfoods are like extra supercharged versions of the healthy foods you know and love. They're excellent to include in your diet on a regular basis, alongside plenty of other standard healthy foods, and could help kick-start a healthier eating routine.

Superfoods don't instantaneously offer health cures or protect you from illness and disease. In fact, if you only consume them occasionally or on top of a poor diet, you're unlikely to see their true benefits. To get the most out of superfoods, you need to make a conscious habit to eat them regularly. As there's such a variety of different superfoods available, this shouldn't be tricky, and there are a multitude of delicious ways in which you can consume them. Superfoods are excellent for adding to meals such as soups and salads, as well as for making into healthy drinks such as smoothies and juices.

What makes superfoods special?

Both healthy foods and superfoods contain essential nutrients, but superfoods differ as they contain higher levels of key compounds. For example, they may include higher levels of:

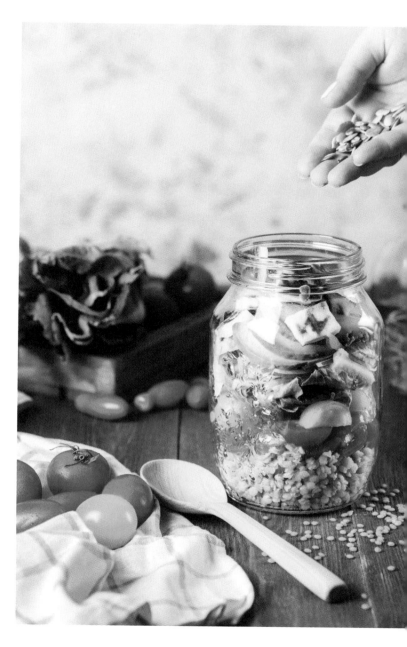

• Antioxidants—natural compounds that help protect cells in your body from becoming damaged.
• Vitamins—organic compounds that help boost your health in many different ways.
• Minerals—essential nutrients such as iron, zinc, and calcium, which play an important role in helping your body function.
• Flavonoids—naturally occurring compounds in foodstuffs such as vegetables, wine, and dark chocolate that can help your body ward off unwanted toxins.
• Healthy fats—fats such as polyunsaturated and monounsaturated, which can play a part in lowering cholesterol and reducing the risk of serious conditions such as heart disease.

• Fiber—fiber is essential for a healthy bowel. Soluble fiber found in legumes, oats, and some fruits can help reduce blood cholesterol levels, while insoluble fiber from whole grains and vegetables help bulk up stools, reducing the risk of constipation and colon cancer.

A TO Z OF SUPERFOODS

Over the following pages you'll discover an A to Z guide to superfoods. It's organized into types of foods, such as dairy, fruits, grains, leafy green vegetables, oily fish, legumes, and nuts and seeds, and offers a comprehensive insight into the most appropriate foods to include in your diet. There's at-a-glance information about each of the foods, then a checklist of what areas of health they're recommended to help with.

In order to have a healthy, balanced diet it's important to regularly consume both healthy foods and superfoods. So, for that reason, the A to Z includes some foods that aren't strictly regarded as superfoods (for example, meats and potatoes) but are an important part of a nutrition-rich diet. The aim is to help you discover the best broad range of foods to consume on a regular basis and develop healthy eating habits that boost your short- and long-term health.

One of the reasons why diets and healthy eating regimes fail is that people get bored eating the same things. But by eating a range of different nutrient-rich foods, you shouldn't get bored and your diet will be full of variety, interest, and flavor. A balanced diet should include:

• Fruits and vegetables—eating a wide variety, and in a rainbow of colors, provides you with the best nutrition.
• Bread, cereals, and potatoes—high-fiber varieties are best for your health.
• Meats, fish, and other high-protein foods—some meats are higher in fat than others, so should be consumed in moderation.
• Dairy products or vegan alternatives.
• Fatty and sugary foods in small amounts.

Water

Water accounts for 50–60 percent of your body weight, but it's constantly being lost every day through sweat and emptying your bladder. That's why it's important to drink plenty of water for your health. Not drinking enough fluids results in dehydration, which can cause symptoms such as headaches, fatigue, and dry skin. As part of a healthy diet and lifestyle, aim to drink at least 40 ounces (5 cups) water every day, with more if you're engaging in physical activities. If you find it hard to get through plain water on its own, try adding some slices of fresh fruit such as lemons and limes to naturally flavor it, or use a fruit tea bag to liven it up.

Water accounts for 50–60 percent of your body weight.

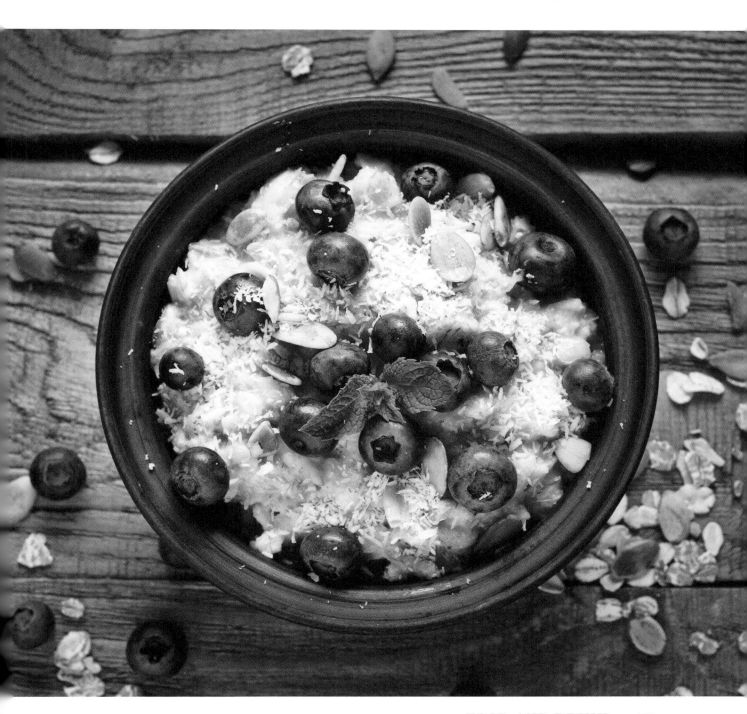

DAIRY

In general, all dairy products are primarily good for quality protein. They provide essential amino acids, many of which are available only from animal protein. They are also a good source of calcium. Fat content is a potential problem, so eat in moderation.

Eggs

As with dairy products, eggs contain an ideal mixture of essential amino acids and are a great source of vitamin B12. The high cholesterol in eggs is at least partially counteracted by the lecithin in the yolk; yet overcooking the yolk will destroy the lecithin. Eggs are an excellent source of nutrition for most, but they they are not suitable for those with an egg allergy or familial hypercholesterolemia. If you suffer from high cholesterol, consult your doctor about egg consumption.

RECOMMENDED FOR HELP WITH

• Cataract prevention • Acne • Immune health

Kefir

A fermented milk drink similar to liquid yogurt, made by adding kefir "grains" to a live culture of cow, goat, sheep, or soy milk. It contains probiotic microorganisms, healthy bacteria that may be beneficial to the gut. Gut-friendly bacteria and yeast consume lactose during the fermentation process, so kefir can be a suitable option for those who are lactose intolerant. It is packed with immune-boosting proteins, essential minerals, and B vitamins.

RECOMMENDED FOR HELP WITH

• Healthy teeth and bones • Immune health
• Possible cancer prevention

Milk

Milk provides a good source of protein, carbohydrate, and fat, except skimmed milk, which contains virtually no fat. Milk contains essential amino acids and calcium as well as lactose. Lactose needs to be broken down by the enzyme lactase in the small intestine. Some people do not have sufficient lactase in their system and therefore find milk difficult to digest. This is known as lactose intolerance. For those who suffer from this (or people who avoid eating animal products), alternative lactose-free options are available, including almond, coconut, and soy milk.

RECOMMENDED FOR HELP WITH

• Prevention of tooth decay • Osteoporosis
• Metabolism

Almond milk

Made from ground almonds, high in immune-boosting antioxidants, and low in cholesterol, almond milk is often used as a lactose-free substitute for cow's milk. It's also dairy-free and therefore suitable for vegans. However, it is lower in protein than cow's milk or soy milk, so you should seek alternative sources of protein if using almond milk as a substitute for these. It is not suitable for anyone with a nut allergy.

RECOMMENDED FOR HELP WITH

• Heart disease • Aging skin • Weight loss
• Possible cancer prevention

Coconut milk

Not to be confused with coconut water, which is simply the juice extracted from the nut, coconut milk and cream are when the flesh of the coconut is mixed with water, the cream rises to the top and is skimmed

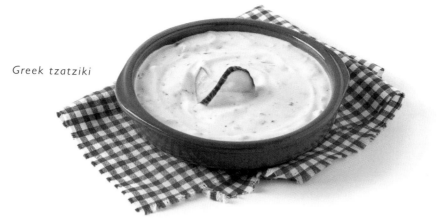

Greek tzatziki

off, and the resulting mixture is sieved to produce coconut milk. A popular alternative to cow's milk for vegans, it is rich in fiber, vitamins, and minerals, and is lactose free, so it is suitable for those who are lactose intolerant. Due to its high fat and calorie content, it should be consumed in moderation.

RECOMMENDED FOR HELP WITH

- Iron-deficient anemia • Improved digestion
- Immune health • Good complexion

Goat's milk

Goat's milk can be a good alternative for those who have an allergy to cow's milk. Goat's milk also tends to be more easily digestible as it contains very little lactose. However, those who are lactose intolerant should check with a nutritionist to determine whether goat's milk is right for them. It's also a good source of essential amino acids, the fundamental building blocks of our tissues, important in the development of the brain and nervous system.

RECOMMENDED FOR HELP WITH

- Lowering blood pressure • Strong bones and teeth

Soy milk

Soy milk is made by grinding soybeans and mixing with boiling water. It's high in health-boosting essential fatty acids, fiber, protein, minerals, and vitamins. A good lactose-free alternative to cow's milk, it contains no cholesterol and is higher in antioxidants. It's also a good source of calcium. Soy milk has been associated with weight loss and reducing the risk of cancer. It also contains phytoestrogens, which have been linked to alleviating post-menopausal symptoms.

RECOMMENDED FOR HELP WITH

- Post-menopausal symptoms • Weight loss
- Possible cancer prevention

Tofu

Tofu, or bean curd, is a soft food made from condensed and curdled soy milk. It is an important source of protein, and has become a popular meat and dairy alternative. Tofu is rich in saponins and contains a plentiful supply of isoflavones, or antioxidants that help to reduce the damage caused by free radicals. Isoflavones may help to reduce LDL or "bad cholesterol" and lower the risk of heart disease. Care is needed if you have an existing thyroid condition as soybeans can affect it.

RECOMMENDED FOR HELP WITH

- Peri-menopause and menopause symptoms
- Heart health • Blood sugar management
- Lowering cholesterol

Yogurt

Yogurt contains essential amino acids, the building blocks of our tissues (in the form of protein), which are important in the development of the brain and nervous system. It's also a good source of probiotic microorganisms, healthy bacteria that may be beneficial to the gut. Yogurt is also rich in bone-building calcium and phosphorus. It is high in saturated fat, so enjoy in moderation, or try Greek yogurt. This contains less sugar, more protein, and fewer carbohydrates.

RECOMMENDED FOR HELP WITH

- Irritable bowel syndrome • Strong bones and teeth • Immune health

FRUITS

Fruits have numerous health benefits, and most are alkalizing foods, which means that they maintain our pH balance. They also contain high levels of antioxidants, including vitamins A, C, and E, and a wide variety of anthocyanins, flavonoids, and polyphenols. However, many fruits provide most of their calories from sugars, so eat them in moderation. Different types or preparations of the same fruit (such as fresh or dried) can have varying nutrients and health benefits.

Apple
Apples are delicious, and rich in antioxidants, vitamins, and minerals. The antioxidants in apples help prevent disease and strengthen the immune system, fighting bone disease and inflammation. Apples are low in calories but rich in fiber, promoting digestion. The carbohydrates and sugar in apples are good for quick energy. Apples have been recommended for acid reflux, and some people swear that eating an apple dispels migraines.

RECOMMENDED FOR HELP WITH

- Immune health • Heart health • Lowering cholesterol • Tissue regeneration • Joint health
- Healthy skin

Apricot
Apricots are small orange fruits that are native to China. They are very low in saturated fat, sodium, and cholesterol, and are a good source of dietary fiber. However, most of the calories come from sugars. Apricots are packed with beta-carotene for heart health and are a good source of vitamins A, C, E, and K, as well as potassium. Apricots provide health benefits for the immune system, vision, skin, and bone strength. The fiber content is good for digestion. Dried apricots are also nutrient-packed and easier to transport, but if you suffer from asthma, avoid those made with sulfites.

RECOMMENDED FOR HELP WITH

- Immune health • Heart and blood health
- Digestive health and bowel regularity
- Healthy skin • Improved vision, reducing risk of macular degeneration • Strong bones • Tissue regeneration

Avocado
Avocados minimize the negative effects of more inflammatory meals and contain healthy fats. They are also extremely low in sodium and cholesterol and a good source of dietary fiber, but high in calories, so should be eaten in moderation. Avocados support the body's absorption of vitamins and minerals and are rich in fatty acids that are crucial to both brain development and heart health. Vitamin K and folate maintain healthy blood cells, and avocados are also believed to promote healthy skin.

RECOMMENDED FOR HELP WITH

- Heart and blood health • Strong bones
- Enhanced brain function • Immune health
- Healthy skin • Digestive health • Developing fetus

Blackberries
Blackberries are rich in antioxidants, very low in sodium, cholesterol, and saturated fat, and are seen as useful for weight loss. Fiber maintains healthy digestion and cholesterol, and the high vitamin C content is great for boosting the immune system.

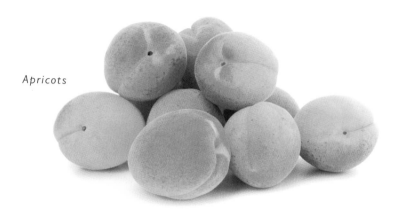

Apricots

• Heart health • Lowering cholesterol • Enhanced brain function • Immune health • Digestive health • Calming diarrhea • Developing fetus

Blueberries

Considered the powerhouse of the fruits, commercial blueberries contain more antioxidants than any other commonly grown fruit—and wild blueberries are even higher in antioxidants than commercial blueberries. They contain optimal amounts of anthocyanins, hydroxycinnamic acids, hydrobenzoic acids, flavanoids, and other phenol-related polynutrients. Blueberries provide a multitude of healing benefits—from brain function, mood, and memory, to heart and skin health, strengthened immunity, bone strength, and purported cancer protection.

Recommended for help with

• Heart health • Healthy blood flow • Enhanced brain function • Strong bones • Eye health • Healthy skin • Immune health • Digestive health • Possible cancer prevention

Cherries

Cherries vary in color from light red to deep purple, but all cherries are rich in antioxidants and loaded with nutrients; sour cherries trump even blueberries in this field. Because of their sweet flavor, they can be substituted for sugar-laden treats. Cherries are high in water and low in calories, which keeps you fuller for longer, and the fiber helps with digestion and weight loss. They contain melatonin, which helps regulate sleep cycles, and the vitamin and mineral content promotes healthy bones and strong immunity. Dried cherries provide slightly less nutrients than raw.

Recommended for help with

• Heart health • Healthy blood flow • Enhanced brain function • Tissue regeneration • Strong bones • Eye health • Immune health

Cranberries

Cranberries were used by Native Americans as traditional remedies and food. They are well known as a remedy for urinary tract infections, but they are also great at maintaining gastrointestinal health and heart health, and preventing kidney stones. Cranberries are high in antioxidants and vitamin C to boost the immune system and fight colds. Dried cranberries are a good alternative to fresh, but have more sugar and less vitamin C.

Recommended for help with

• Immune health • Heart health • Healthy blood flow • Healthy skin • Enhanced brain function • Digestive health • Urinary tract infections • Kidney stones

Goji berries

These little red berries are native to Asia. Part sweet, part sour, they're packed with vitamins and minerals, including iron, vitamin A, vitamin C, and good levels of fiber. Used for centuries in traditional medicine, they've gained a reputation for helping to boost immunity. Goji berries may also play a role in eye health, helping reduce the risk of age-related macular degeneration and preventing oxidative stress. Care is needed if taking prescription medications, as interactions can occur; speak to your medical practitioner for advice.

Recommended for help with

• Immune health • Eye health

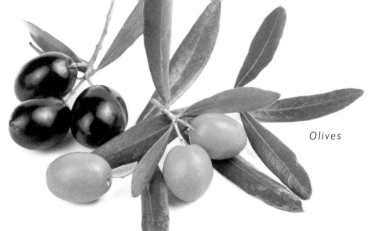

Olives

Grapefruit

Grapefruits come in pink, red, or white, each with varying degrees of sweet or tart flavor. All types are low in calories and high in fiber, as well as providing a wealth of fatty acids, vitamins C and A, and calcium. Grapefruit is known as an immunity-booster, cholesterol-reducer, metabolism-increaser, and potentially a cancer-preventer as well. Some medications, including statins, may not react well with grapefruit; for any concerns, discuss with your doctor.

RECOMMENDED FOR HELP WITH

• Reducing risk of cardiovascular disease • Joint health • Immune health • Enhanced brain function • Weight loss • Easing constipation

Olives

Both green and black olives are high in antioxidants and omega fatty acids and provide fiber and vitamins A and E, protecting against cardiovascular disease, high cholesterol, and arthritis. Green olives contain more sodium, and black olives are slightly higher in calories. Because of the sodium content, olives should be eaten in moderation.

RECOMMENDED FOR HELP WITH

• Heart health • Digestive health • Lowering cholesterol • Skin and eye health • Reducing inflammation and arthritis • Strong bones and tissue • Immune health • Energy levels • Enhanced brain function • Possible cancer protection

Orange

Originating in Asia, oranges are rich in antioxidants, best known as an excellent source of vitamin C. Due to their carbohydrates, they are a good source of energy and help maintain metabolism—a great snack for weight control. Fiber protects against cardiovascular disease and aids digestion. Vitamins A and C and thiamine promote healthy skin and cell regeneration. Like other citrus fruit, oranges are acidic, which can cause damage to your tooth enamel and, in rare cases, trigger an allergic reaction. Consult your dentist or doctor if symptoms develop.

RECOMMENDED FOR HELP WITH

• Immune health and fighting colds and illnesses • Eye and skin health • Reducing inflammation • Lowering cholesterol • Reducing risk of cardiovascular disease • Strong bones and muscles • Energy levels • Enhanced brain function, including memory and mood • Developing fetus

Pineapple

Pineapple is a large tropical fruit that grows in many warm regions worldwide. They are an alkalizing food and are low in fat, cholesterol-free, and provide manganese and vitamin C, exceptional for skin, digestive health, and immunity. They may also reduce the risk of heart disease, stroke, and gout. The enzyme bromelain may treat arthritis, sinusitis, and digestive troubles. The acid can cause a tingling sensation in your mouth. If it is more severe, consult a doctor about possible allergies.

RECOMMENDED FOR HELP WITH

• Immune health • Healthy skin • Heart health • Reducing inflammation from arthritis and gout • Easing sinusitis • Energy levels • Enhanced brain function

Pomegranate

These gorgeous purple-red fruit, and their seeds, pack a considerable amount of nutrients. This superfood boasts an impressive level of antioxidants, plus vitamins C and K, and potassium, for immunity, cellular repair, and blood health, as well as maintaining prostate health. The seeds alone contain fiber, but it is a personal preference whether to eat them alongside the fruit itself.

RECOMMENDED FOR HELP WITH

• Immune health • Heart and blood health
• Improves prostate health in men • Strong bones and muscles • Digestive health • Enhanced brain function • Joint health

Raspberries

Raspberries come in a beautiful array of colors, but red and black are the most common. They are rich in vitamin C and manganese and packed with antioxidants. They are also a good source of fiber, omega fatty acids, and vitamin K. In all, raspberries are good for the heart and blood, as well as important for the immune system and bone strength, and a purifier for the skin.

RECOMMENDED FOR HELP WITH

• Immune health • Digestive health • Weight loss and improved metabolism • Blood and heart health • Strong bones and muscles • Healthy skin
• Energy levels • Enhanced brain function and memory • Developing fetus during pregnancy
• Possible cancer protection • Joint health

Rose hips

Rose hips have many times more vitamin C than oranges, although the amount is dependent on freshness. Rose hips aid the immune system and protect against arthritis. They may disrupt blood sugar regulation in diabetics.

RECOMMENDED FOR HELP WITH

• Skin health and tissue regeneration • Reducing inflammation associated with arthritis • Immune health • Heart and blood health • Bones and muscles • Eye health • Digestive health • Possible cancer protection

Strawberries

Strawberries are an alkalizing food loaded with folate, important for brain function, especially for a developing fetus. Strawberries are also a great source of immune-boosting vitamin C, organ-maintaining potassium, and digestion-calming fiber. Due to potential allergic reactions, some doctors recommend not feeding strawberries to babies.

RECOMMENDED FOR HELP WITH

• Immune health • Digestive health • Heart and blood health • Healthy skin • Enhanced brain function • Developing fetus during pregnancy

Watermelon

Watermelon's high water content means it is a healthy, very low-calorie fruit. It provides vitamins A and C and potassium, as well as moderate amounts of fiber and carbohydrates. The color comes from the compound lycopene, which reduces the risk of heart disease and cancers. The seeds can be roasted for a healthful treat, providing protein and magnesium.

RECOMMENDED FOR HELP WITH

• Heart and blood health • Reducing risk of cardiovascular disease • Strong bones and muscles • Eye health

GRAINS

Over the course of the past 10,000 years, grains—bread, cereals, rice, pasta, noodles—have increasingly been consumed, and even recommended, as the staff of life. Unfortunately, since the twentieth century, genetic modifications have increased the gluten content of wheat. In general, wheat, rye, barley, and spelt contain naturally occurring gluten, and there is good evidence that some oats have been contaminated with gluten. Gluten-free grains include corn, rice, amaranth, millet, buckwheat, quinoa, sorghum, and teff; however, over the past few decades the vast majority of corn has also been significantly genetically modified.

Barley
Barley *(Hordeum vulgare)* is a type of whole grain that is rich in a variety of nutrients and has a slightly nutty, sometimes chewy consistency. It is a great source of fiber, selenium, and manganese and contains lignans, a type of antioxidants associated with reducing the risk of heart disease. It also contains good levels of vitamin B1, magnesium, niacin, and chromium. Due to its high fiber content, eating barley may help to curb your appetite and make you feel fuller for longer, as well as reducing your risk of constipation. The beta-glucans found in barley could help to lower the risk of high cholesterol.

RECOMMENDED FOR HELP WITH

• Weight loss • Constipation • Heart disease
• Lowering cholesterol

Bran flakes
Packed full of fiber. Many breakfast cereals contain bran flakes, which are high in fiber and therefore beneficial for those prone to constipation. However, they also contain gluten and should be avoided by celiacs. Bran flakes are low in fats and sugars and high in immune-boosting vitamin A and metabolism-boosting iron, but these amounts can vary so it's worth checking individual products.

RECOMMENDED FOR HELP WITH

• Lowering cholesterol • Diabetes • Immune health

Black rice
Black rice contains a high level of antioxidants, which help to combat free radical damage to cells, which if left unchecked can lead to disease. Anthocyanins, the antioxidants also found in blueberries, are responsible for the dark-purplish color of black rice. Anthocyanins have been linked to a decreased risk of heart disease and cancer. Black rice is also rich in metabolism-boosting iron and zinc.

RECOMMENDED FOR HELP WITH

• Immune health • Heart disease • Possible cancer protection

Brown rice
A better source of protein than white rice. It is gluten free, making it suitable for those on gluten-free diets. Brown rice takes longer to cook than white rice, but the nutritional benefits are worth the wait. The outer bran and germ layers are where the health-boosting vitamins, minerals, and fiber are stored. As a rule of thumb, the longer the grain, the less sticky and starchy the rice. Long-grain rice is ideal for light, fluffy, pilaf-style dishes.

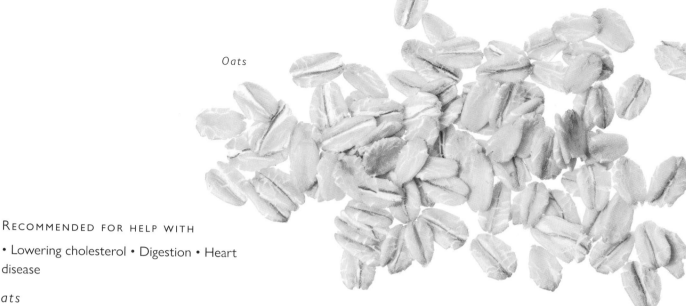

Oats

RECOMMENDED FOR HELP WITH

• Lowering cholesterol • Digestion • Heart disease

Oats

Oats (*Avena sativa*) are a gluten-free whole grain and a good source of carbohydrates and fiber, as well as magnesium, zinc, folate, vitamin B1, and vitamin B5. Along with the B-complex vitamins, these are vital for maintaining a healthy nervous system, building strong bones and teeth, and supplying lots of silicon for healthy arterial walls. They're a nutrient-dense food and, compared to other grains, are packed with more protein. Oats are a good source of polyphenols and antioxidants and contain avenanthramides, which may help lower blood pressure levels. Beta-glucan, a type of soluble fiber, is found in oats, and this is heavily involved in the feeling of fullness when oats are eaten (making them a great breakfast cereal choice) and helping to reduce blood sugar and cholesterol levels. No wonder oats have been the staple food of some of the hardiest peoples, such as the Scottish Highlanders.

RECOMMENDED FOR HELP WITH

• Weight loss • Heart disease • Regulating blood sugar levels • Lowering cholesterol • Lowering blood pressure

Quinoa

Quinoa (*Chenopodium quinoa*) is a nutritious gluten-free grain that originated in South America. It contains more fiber, healthy fats, and protein than other grains and has good levels of magnesium, folate, iron, zinc, thiamine, riboflavin, and vitamin B6. It also contains the plant compounds kaempferol

and quercetin, antioxidants that help protect against infection and inflammation. The three most frequently grown types of quinoa are red, white, and black—black has the lowest fat content and red and black quinoa have higher levels of vitamin E than white quinoa. Quinoa has great levels of fiber, so is beneficial for bowel health. Its magnesium content could help reduce the risk of high blood pressure and cardiovascular disease, and the iron levels support energy and cell function.

RECOMMENDED FOR HELP WITH

• Constipation • Lowering cholesterol • Lowering blood pressure • Heart disease • Eye health • Inflammation • Infection

Wheat germ

Wheat germ comes from the kernels of wheat and is a component of whole-grain wheat. Wheat germ is a good source of fiber, healthy fats, magnesium, zinc, folate, thiamine, and potassium. It's also high in vitamin E, one of the essential antioxidants that helps protect against disease. Wheat germ oil has been linked to helping to control cholesterol.

RECOMMENDED FOR HELP WITH

• Cardiovascular health • Menopause • Lowering cholesterol

LEAFY GREEN VEGETABLES

Leafy green vegetables are rich in many crucial vitamins and minerals, provide an excellent source of fiber, and are low in calories, making them a great addition to your plate. Vital antioxidants, such as vitamin C, vitamin E, beta-carotene, and lutein, are all found in leafy greens, as well as potassium, folate, and vitamin K, and between them they help with a wide range of health conditions. With so many varieties of leafy greens available, there are plenty of chances to get these superfoods into your diet.

Arugula

This zesty salad leaf is an excellent source of nitric oxide, which improves heart health. It's loaded with health-boosting nutrients, from antioxidant vitamin A to immune-boosting zinc. The younger, paler leaves have a more delicate flavor, while the older, darker leaves pack a peppery punch.

RECOMMENDED FOR HELP WITH

• Possible cancer prevention • Liver health
• Gastrointestinal ulcers

Bok choy

Bok choy is a type of Chinese cabbage. It has a mild peppery, sweet flavor and is rich in vitamin A, vitamin C, and vitamin K, and also contains moderate levels of vitamin B6, calcium, and folate. It's a versatile vegetable with high nutrients and low calories that can be steamed, simmered, or stir-fried within minutes. It's best not eaten in large quantities as it contains glucosinolates, which can affect iodine levels.

RECOMMENDED FOR HELP WITH

• Bowel issues • Bone health • Blood pressure
• Heart health • Inflammation

Broccoli

Broccoli is loaded with antioxidants to help protect cells against free radical damage, and sulforaphanes, molecules that may help to combat cancer. Nutrients in broccoli help the body to eliminate unwanted contaminants, resulting in a strong, positive detoxification impact. It's also rich in the flavanoid kaempferol, which lessens the impact of allergy-related substances on your body, providing broccoli with unique anti-inflammatory benefits.

RECOMMENDED FOR HELP WITH

• Possible cancer prevention, especially prostate and colon • Detoxing • Immune health

Brussels sprouts

A great source of digestion-boosting fiber, immune-boosting vitamin C, and various phytochemical compounds, including glucosinolates, which have been linked with protecting against cancer. Just ¼ cup boiled Brussels sprouts contains nearly a third of your recommend daily value of vitamin C, and almost half of vitamin K, which helps with blood clotting and maintaining healthy bones.

RECOMMENDED FOR HELP WITH

• Possible cancer prevention • Immune health
• Detoxing

Collard greens

Collard greens are a great source of phytonutrients—natural compounds that may help prevent disease and keep your body working properly. They're packed with vitamin K—just ½ cup raw collard greens contains a huge 179 percent of your recommended value of this bone-nourishing vitamin. The

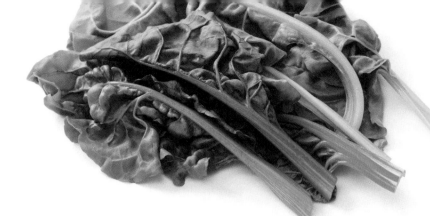

Swiss chard

glucosinolates glucoraphanin, sinigrin, gluconasturtian, and glucotropaeolin provide unique cancer protection too, making collard greens a highly nutritious addition to any diet.

RECOMMENDED FOR HELP WITH

• Possible cancer prevention • Strong bones
• Immune health • Lowering cholesterol

Kale

Green leafy kale is rich in antioxidants and high in calcium. It's also a good source of immune-boosting vitamin C, vision-boosting vitamin A, and vitamin K, essential for blood clotting and bone nourishment. Flavonoids in kale have been shown to have strong antioxidant and anticancer properties.

RECOMMENDED FOR HELP WITH

• Possible cancer prevention, especially prostate and colon • Detoxing • Macular degeneration

Lettuce

A very low-calorie food, lettuce is loaded with vision-boosting vitamin A and vitamin K, essential for blood clotting and bone nourishment, as well as dietary fiber, iron, and energy-enhancing B vitamins. A good rule of thumb is that the nutritional value becomes greater the darker green the leaves, with iceberg at the lower end and green leaf lettuce at the higher end of the spectrum. However, all varieties are low in calories and provide fiber, vitamins, and minerals.

RECOMMENDED FOR HELP WITH

• Digestion • Vision • Immune health

Spinach

Since most people's bodies are far too acidic, alkaline spinach is a welcome addition to any diet. Spinach is full of vitamins and minerals—½ cup raw spinach contains 169 percent of your recommended daily value of vitamin K, essential for blood clotting and bone nourishment, over half of your recommended daily value of vision-boosting vitamin A, and 4 percent your recommended daily value of iron.

RECOMMENDED FOR HELP WITH

• Lowering cholesterol • Vision • Immune health

Swiss chard

Also known as silverbeet or spinach chard, this is a storehouse of nutrients. It's rich in antioxidants and loaded with immune-boosting vitamin C, bone-nourishing vitamin K, and vision-boosting vitamin A, as well as health-boosting flavanoids.

RECOMMENDED FOR HELP WITH

• Lowering cholesterol • Vision • Immune health

Watercress

This aquatic leafy green plant is found near springs and slow-moving streams. It's a close cousin to arugula and cabbage, yet it is often overlooked as a nutritional food source. Watercress is packed with vitamins and contains more vitamin C than oranges—½ cup raw watercress provides 20 percent of your recommended daily value, as well as 18 percent of vitamin A, and a huge 87 percent of vitamin K. It's also rich in iron.

RECOMMENDED FOR HELP WITH

• Lowering cholesterol • Vision • Immune health

LEGUMES

In general, legumes—including peas, beans, and lentils—are high in fiber and protein; however, they are "incomplete" proteins, lacking some essential amino acids. They need to be eaten alongside milk, meat, or egg protein to be complete. Legumes are also high in carbohydrates, which is where most of their calorific content comes from.

Cannellini beans

Cannellini beans are packed to the brim with vitamins, minerals, fiber, and protein. They're a good source of zinc, calcium, selenium, vitamin B6, magnesium, copper, folate, iron, potassium, thiamine, and riboflavin, and have high levels of polyphenol antioxidants that help deal with oxidative stress. Cannellini beans have a slightly nutty flavor to them and are a versatile addition to many meals, including salad, chili, soup, and stew. Dried cannellini beans need to be soaked before they are cooked. Sometimes cannellini beans are known as white kidney beans.

RECOMMENDED FOR HELP WITH

- Constipation • Cardiovascular health
- Weight maintenance

Edamame beans

Edamame beans are one of the newer superfoods to rise in popularity. Now widely available, they are young soybeans that are picked before they get too ripe. They're naturally gluten free, low in calories, and provide a good punch of iron, calcium, and protein. They also contain potassium, magnesium, folate, choline, beta carotene, vitamin K, lutein, zeaxanthin, phosphorous, selenium, and vitamin C. They're a useful source of polyunsatured omega-3 fats and isoflavones, which help lower the risk of cancer. Edamame beans have a mild flavor and can be added to a variety of dishes, including salads, soups, casseroles, and stir-fries.

RECOMMENDED FOR HELP WITH

- Cardiovascular health • Constipation
- Cholesterol • General health • Immune health

Garbanzo beans (chickpeas)

Like other beans, garbanzo beans are rich in soluble and insoluble fiber. Soluble fiber helps with the removal of cholesterol, and insoluble fiber prevents constipation. Garbanzo beans are low in saturated fat and sodium, and a very good source of anemia-

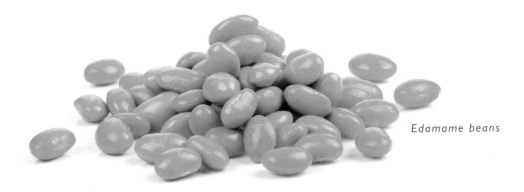

Edamame beans

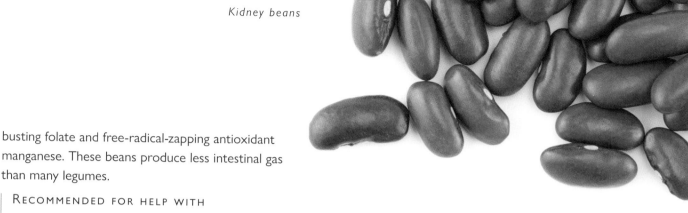

Kidney beans

busting folate and free-radical-zapping antioxidant manganese. These beans produce less intestinal gas than many legumes.

RECOMMENDED FOR HELP WITH

• Constipation • Blood circulation • Lowering cholesterol

Green beans

Also known as French beans or string beans. Low in sodium and very low in saturated fats and cholesterol, green beans are packed with dietary fiber, vision-boosting vitamin A, immune-boosting vitamin C, and vitamin K, essential for blood clotting. They are also a good source of the antioxidants folate and manganese, which help to protect cells from free radical damage.

RECOMMENDED FOR HELP WITH

• Age-related macular degeneration • Blood clotting
• Energy levels

Haricot beans

Also known as navy beans, as they were a staple of the U.S. Navy in the early twentieth century. They are low in saturated fat, cholesterol, and sodium. Haricot beans are packed with fiber and anemia-busting folate. They are also a good source of energy-boosting thiamine (B1). All animals require vitamin B1, which is made in bacteria, fungi, and plants, but a large portion of the nutritional B1 content of foods is often lost due to modern food processing.

RECOMMENDED FOR HELP WITH

• Diabetes • Constipation • General health

Kidney beans

Low in saturated fat, cholesterol, and sodium, kidney beans are packed with protein and digestion-boosting soluble and insoluble fiber. One cup boiled kidney beans contains more than half of your recommended daily value of anemia-busting folate, which contributes to healthy heart and brain function. In common with most legumes, cooking red kidney beans by boiling will considerably reduce the sodium content, which is high in the raw product.

RECOMMENDED FOR HELP WITH

• Heart health • Digestion • Brain function

Peanuts

Low in cholesterol but high in sodium and calories, peanuts are one of the anti-inflammatory and alkalizing legumes. They're a good source of free-radical-zapping manganese and niacin (vitamin B3). Nutritional properties vary according to variety; for example, Virginia peanuts are much more anti-inflammatory than Valencia peanuts. It's worth noting that although they are called "nuts," peanuts are actually legumes and therefore not harmful to nut-allergy sufferers. However, some people do have a specific allergy to peanuts.

RECOMMENDED FOR HELP WITH

• Lowering cholesterol • Bone formation

MEAT

All meats have optimal essential amino acids, including taurine, which is vital for many biological functions in humans. Meats are also one of the best sources of vitamin B12. No plant food contains either taurine or vitamin B12. A couple of servings of red meat in your weekly meal plan as part of a healthy diet can provide your body with many vital nutrients. The white meat found in most poultry is lower in fat than the dark meat, so consider this when choosing your cut. Additionally, baking and broiling are healthier means of cooking poultry than frying.

Beef
Depending on the cut and the preparation method, beef tends to be low in sodium and is a good source of many vital nutrients. However, it is relatively high in saturated fat, which can lead to a buildup of cholesterol in the arteries and a higher risk of heart disease, so should be included in your diet in moderation. As a rule of thumb, the leaner the beef, the lower the levels of saturated fat. Choose lower-fat cuts such as top round, bottom round, eye round, flank, and strip for healthier options. Higher-fat cuts such as ribeye steak contain higher levels of total fat, saturated fat, and calories, which can be difficult for the body to process. Cooking methods impact the level of fat as well. Grilling, baking, poaching, or steaming are healthier options, while frying or roasting increase the fat content.

RECOMMENDED FOR HELP WITH

• Iron-deficient anemia • Immune health • Muscle maintenance

Chicken
Chicken is one of the best sources of complete protein, featuring all essential amino acids. Protein is a building block of bones, muscles, and the components of the body's makeup. The human body requires a large amount of protein, so chicken is a good part of any meat-eater's well-balanced diet. Amino acids are required for cell development and muscle development, and chicken also has a healthy ratio of fats. Breast meat is particularly low in fat; gizzards and giblets are especially high in protein, and liver contains high levels of iron and vitamin B12.

RECOMMENDED FOR HELP WITH

• Muscle maintenance • Energy levels
• Oxygenation of the blood • Possible cancer prevention • Iron-deficient anemia

Duck
Duck is an excellent source of protein, with all essential amino acids and a good ratio of fats. In the United States, mild Pekin or Long Island duck is the most common, while the stronger Muscovy is popular in France. Duck has the reputation of being fatty, but in small portions duck is nutritious and protein-packed. The dark color of the meat comes from high levels of oxygen-storing protein, creating the richer, meatier flavor. Remove the skin or score it before cooking to allow the fat underneath to escape.

RECOMMENDED FOR HELP WITH

• Muscle maintenance • Energy levels • Iron-deficient anemia • Possible cancer prevention
• Oxygenation of the blood

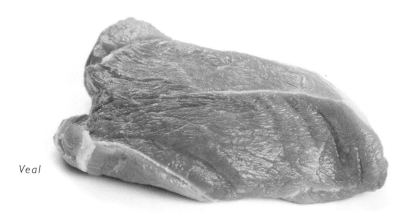

Veal

Liver

Eating liver is not to everyone's taste, but it is packed with protein, essential vitamins, and minerals, and is low in calories, making it a nutrient-rich superfood. Eating liver gives you a good dose of vitamin B12, which is involved in good brain function and maintenance of red blood cells. It is also rich in iron, which helps transport oxygen around the body; folate, which is involved in cell growth; and vitamin A, which is good for vision and the immune system. There's also riboflavin (vitamin B2), copper, and choline.

RECOMMENDED FOR HELP WITH

• Eye health • Brain function • Red blood cell maintenance • Immune health • Liver function • Heart health • Kidney health

Pork tenderloin

Low in sodium and rich in energy-enhancing B vitamins, pork tenderloin is a lean cut, providing a lower-fat alternative to others, such as bacon. It is also a good source of metabolism-regulating selenium and bone-tissue-strengthening phosphorus.

RECOMMENDED FOR HELP WITH

• Nerve function • Energy levels • Immune health

Turkey

Turkey is a lean white meat that can be purchased in many forms. It is a quality protein, with all essential amino acids. Turkey also has a good ratio of fats, and is a great source of tryptophan, which, as a precursor to serotonin, can help with mood and relaxation. Versatile and inexpensive, it has more protein and less fat and cholesterol than other meats. Turkey livers are a particularly good source of vitamin B12.

RECOMMENDED FOR HELP WITH

• Muscle maintenance • Strong bones and teeth
• Improved circulation and blood oxygenation
• Immune health • Possible cancer prevention

Veal

Like pork, veal tends to be lower in fat than beef. It is also richer in energy-boosting thiamine and niacin. Like other red meats, veal is a good source of protein and can contribute to meeting your daily protein requirements. The nutritional value of meats varies according to the type and the cut, while cooking methods impact the level of fat: broiling, baking, poaching, or steaming are healthier options, while frying or roasting increase the fat content.

RECOMMENDED FOR HELP WITH

• Muscle maintenance • Energy levels
• Immune health

Venison

Venison is high in protein and stacked with vitamins and iron. From a nutrient perspective it is similar in some ways to beef, but different in others. Venison is lower in saturated fat than beef. For example, a 4-ounce serving of beef flank steak has more than 8.5 grams of total fat, while an equivalent serving of venison contains only 3 grams of total fat. Both meats provide many other important nutrients, notably iron and complex B vitamins, which are necessary for maintaining healthy energy systems and metabolism.

RECOMMENDED FOR HELP WITH

• Heart health • Energy levels • Immune health
• Iron-deficient anemia

MUSHROOMS

Mushrooms are widely known for their high levels of nutrition and their many health benefits. Low in calories, saturated fat, cholesterol, and sodium, they also contain many vital nutrients, and are being hailed as one of the superfoods.

Morel mushroom

A great source of vitamin D, essential for helping your body absorb calcium, thus supporting bone health. The morel has an intense, woodsy flavor. Dried morels are more flavorful and less expensive than the fresh variety, ideal for cooking. Morel mushrooms are low in calories and a good source of fiber and iron, supporting healthy digestion and oxygenation of the blood.

RECOMMENDED FOR HELP WITH

• Immune health • Digestive health • Metabolism protection

Shiitake mushroom

Great for maintaining a healthy immune system, and also thought to lower cholesterol. These meaty and flavorful mushrooms contain a substance called eritadenine, which encourages body tissues to absorb cholesterol and lower the amount circulating in the blood. Shiitakes are also thought to have antiviral and anticancer effects. Widely available fresh or dried, the dried variety have a particularly intense smoky flavor. Sauté for roughly 7 minutes to get the best flavor while keeping maximum nutritional value.

Shiitake mushroom, raw

Raw shiitake mushrooms are a good source of antioxidant-boosting copper and selenium, as well as metabolism-enhancing B vitamins. Wash raw mushrooms to remove dirt—you may want to chop off the bottom of the hard stem, then slice thinly and sprinkle over salads to add a flavorful nutritional boost.

Shiitake mushroom, dried

A 3½-cup serving of dried shiitake mushrooms provides more than double your recommended daily values of copper and the B vitamin pantothenic acid. Dried shiitake mushrooms also contain even higher levels of niacin, riboflavin, vitamin B6, manganese, selenium, zinc, and dietary fiber than raw. Soak dried shiitake mushrooms in water before using. Chop and use to add depth of flavor to soups, stews, and stir-fries.

RECOMMENDED FOR HELP WITH

• Immune health • Lowering cholesterol
• Possible cancer prevention

Button mushroom, white

Low in saturated fat and sodium and very low in cholesterol. A good source of the immune-boosting B-complex vitamins riboflavin, niacin, pantothenic acid, and folate, as well as antioxidant-boosting copper and selenium. White button mushrooms are the most common and least expensive mushrooms. Their mild taste means they can be used in a wide range of dishes, from salads to sauces, yet their flavor intensifies when cooked, making them ideal for sautéing and grilling.

RECOMMENDED FOR HELP WITH

• Immune health • Digestive health • Metabolism

Low in calories, saturated fat, cholesterol, and sodium, mushrooms also contain many vital nutrients.

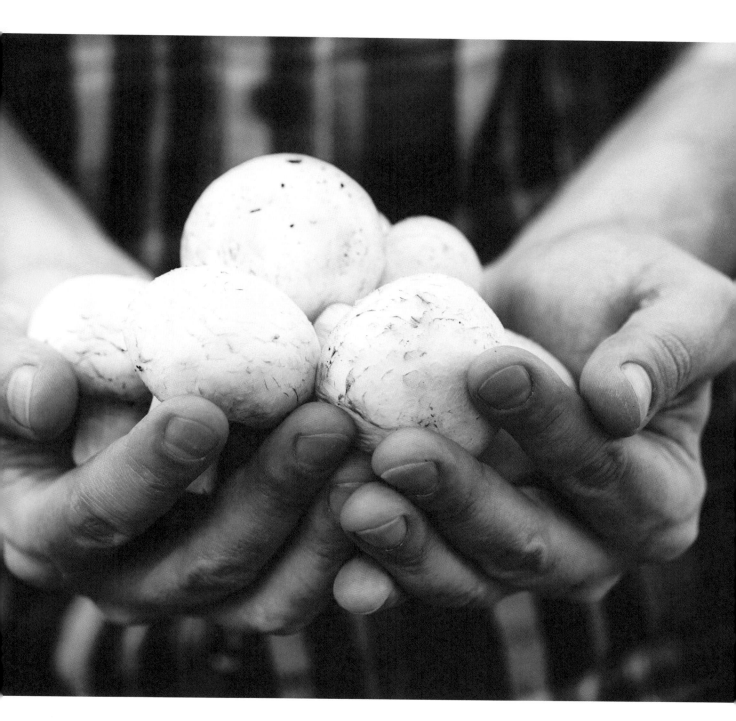

NUTS AND SEEDS

Nuts and seeds are among the nutritional superfoods—packed full of health-giving nutrients such as proteins, healthy fats, and fiber. However, please beware and avoid if you have a nut allergy.

Almonds

Eating almonds five times a week may lower the risk of coronary artery disease by 50 percent. All nuts are good, but almonds and Brazil nuts are the only two that produce an alkaline reaction in the body. Since most people's bodies are far too acidic, almonds are a welcome addition to any diet. They also have more magnesium than other nuts and are an excellent source of monounsaturated fat. And, of course, their excellent taste means that almonds are an all-time favorite. Additionally, almond butter is terrific, either alone or with many other foods.

RECOMMENDED FOR HELP WITH

• Diabetes • Coronary artery disease • Possible cancer protection • Carpal tunnel syndrome

Brazil nuts

Native to the Amazon rain forest, Brazil nuts are one of only two nuts (almond is the second) that produce an alkaline reaction in the body. Since most people's bodies are too acidic, Brazil nuts are a welcome addition to any diet. They are also an excellent source of selenium: just under ¼ cup contains a huge 767 percent of your recommended daily value, making them the highest natural source of this mineral.

RECOMMENDED FOR HELP WITH

• Lowering cholesterol • Reducing the risk of heart disease • Type 2 diabetes

Cashew nuts

Native to the Amazon, these sweet, crunchy nuts are packed with free-radical-zapping antioxidants, energy, vitamins, and minerals—as well as energy-boosting copper and bone-strengthening magnesium. They are low in cholesterol and sodium. Cashews are one of the best legumes, with excellent fat ratios and protein, though with incomplete amino acids. Delicious as a snack, raw, or roasted, and as an addition to salads and stir-fry dishes.

RECOMMENDED FOR HELP WITH

• Lowering cholesterol • Reducing the risk of heart disease • Diabetes

Chia seeds

A super-quality protein and source of fiber, chia seeds are also packed with omega-3s. There may be no other food as rich in overall nutrients and health benefits as chia—the "strength" food of the Aztecs. If I had only one food to eat, I would choose chia! No other food has the overall balance of quality protein, fat, and fiber, and these small black or white seeds pack more energy and value than any other known food. Plus, no other plant protein comes close in terms of the quality of the protein/amino mix. Just ¼ cup of chia seeds contains as much quality protein as a glass of milk.

RECOMMENDED FOR HELP WITH

• Irritable bowel syndrome • Diabetes
• Hypertension • Weight loss

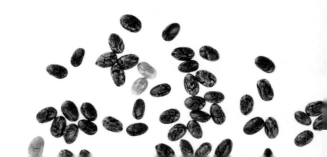

Chia seeds

Flaxseeds

A powerhouse of the seed kingdom, flaxseeds are a great source of fiber, omega-3s, and antioxidants. They make a nutritious addition to everything from muffins, cookies, and breads, to pizza crusts and casseroles. And the good news is that studies suggest that the cooking process doesn't impact the effectiveness of the omega-3 fatty acids, which help to lower LDL or "bad cholesterol" and increase HDL or "good cholesterol" levels in the blood. Flaxseeds are also ranked as the number one source of lignans—phytonutrients that provide both antioxidant and fiber-like benefits to the body. They contain a whopping seven times the amount of lignans as sesame seeds, the closest runner-up in the lignan-rich food stakes.

RECOMMENDED FOR HELP WITH

• Reducing the risk of heart disease and diabetes
• Lowering cholesterol • Colon health • Immune health

Hemp seeds

Technically speaking a nut, but called a seed, hemp seeds come from hemp plants. They have a slightly nutty flavor and are a good source of fatty acids omega-3 and omega-6, protein, B vitamins, zinc, vitamin E, iron, and magnesium. Fatty acids are involved with managing cholesterol and the healthy function of your immune system. Although they are related to the cannabis plant, hemp seeds have no THC in them. Care is needed if you take prescription medications, as hemp seeds may interact—speak to your medical practitioner for advice.

RECOMMENDED FOR HELP WITH

• Immune health • Cardiovascular health
• Lowering cholesterol • Skin conditions
• Brain function

Macadamia nuts

Native to the rain forests of Australia, macadamia nuts are packed with energy and contain high levels of monounsaturated fats, which may help to lower cholesterol. They're also rich in antioxidants, which protect cells from free radical damage. Just under ¼ cup of macadamia nuts contains over half of your recommended daily value of free-radical-zapping manganese.

RECOMMENDED FOR HELP WITH

• Reducing the risk of heart disease and diabetes

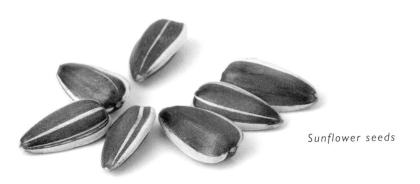

Sunflower seeds

Pecan nuts

These rich, buttery nuts are the most antioxidant-rich tree nut, protecting cells against damage from free radicals. They're also packed with energy and high in omega-6 fatty acids, which can help lower the risk of heart disease. They're popular in sweet desserts, such as pecan pie, but can also be enjoyed as a healthy snack raw or roasted (with or without salt), or as a healthy addition to a range of dishes.

RECOMMENDED FOR HELP WITH

• Reducing the risk of heart disease and diabetes
• Lowering cholesterol

Pistachio nuts

One of the healthiest, lowest-calorie nuts. Pistachios are a good source of "heart-friendly" monounsaturated fats, which help to lower cholesterol. They're packed with antioxidant minerals, such as free-radical-busting manganese and copper, to help protect cells from free radical damage, and crammed with vitamins too—just under ¼ cup of pistachios contains almost a quarter of your recommended daily value of nervous-system-boosting vitamin B6.

RECOMMENDED FOR HELP WITH

• Reducing the risk of heart disease and diabetes
• Lowering cholesterol

Pumpkin seeds

A great source of magnesium and zinc. Eating the entire seed, including the shell, will maximize your intake of zinc. They can also be enjoyed roasted, though it's worth noting that roasted seeds have a significantly higher glycemic load (10) compared to dried seeds (0). It's recommended to roast pumpkin seeds for no more than 15–20 minutes, as after this time unwanted changes occur in the fat structure, altering their nutrient content.

RECOMMENDED FOR HELP WITH

• Reducing the risk of heart disease and diabetes
• Prostate health • Immune health

Sesame seeds

An excellent source of copper and other minerals, sesame seeds are packed with a rich mix of nutrients to maintain healthy bones and muscles, and contribute to good overall health. Sesamin and sesamoli are types of lignan—phytonutrients with antioxidant and anti-inflammatory properties that have been shown to help lower cholesterol. Sesame seeds add a delicate nutty crunch and a nutritional boost to a range of foods, from breads to desserts, and salads to cereals. Sesame seed butter paste is a healthy, nut-free alternative to peanut butter, containing large amounts of omega fatty acids, calcium, copper, and iron.

RECOMMENDED FOR HELP WITH

• Reducing the risk of heart disease and diabetes
• Prostate health • Liver health

Sunflower seeds

A rich source of vitamin E and the B-complex group of vitamins. A handful of these mildly nutty seeds provides a tasty, nutritious, health-boosting snack. Not only do they stave off hunger, sunflower seeds are packed with vitamin E and magnesium, which help keep your heart and bones healthy. Upping your intake of vitamin E can significantly reduce the risk of developing atherosclerosis and boost heart health. B-complex vitamins also provide a boost to the metabolism, ensuring energy levels are well stocked.

RECOMMENDED FOR HELP WITH

- Reducing the risk of heart disease and diabetes
- Possible cancer protection

Walnuts

Walnuts contain valuable and rare nutrients not found in many other food sources, including the tannin tellimagrandin and the flavonol morin. These antioxidant and anti-inflammatory phytonutrients have been linked with a decreased risk of breast cancer and prostate cancer related to walnut consumption. It's thought that walnut skin—the whitish outermost part of the nut—contains many of the key nutrients, so eating the skin is encouraged to gain the full nutritional benefit of these marvelous nuts.

RECOMMENDED FOR HELP WITH

- Reducing the risk of heart disease • Type 2 diabetes • Lowering cholesterol • Boosting memory

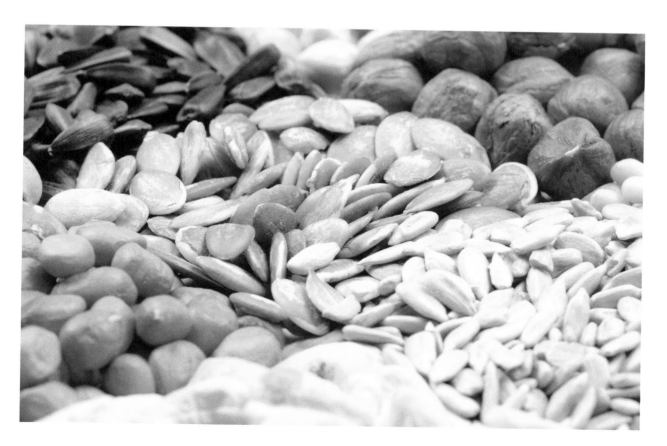

OILS, SEASONINGS, AND SPICES

There are many plant, meat, and fish oils available. Saturated fat in oils is the least healthy, whereas polyunsaturated and monounsaturated fats are considered nutritious. Spices typically originate from the flowers, fruits, nuts, roots, or bark of plants and have many benefits, including their taste!

Canola oil
A vegetable oil that comes from an oilseed plant similar to rapeseed (Brassica napus L.). Canola oil contains low levels of saturated fat, and also contains vitamins E and K, plus alpha-linolenic acid, a form of omega-3. Omega-3 is involved with brain and heart health. Canola plants are often genetically modified to help them fight off diseases, so avoid if this is a concern for you.

> RECOMMENDED FOR HELP WITH
>
> • General health • Brain health • Heart health

Olive oil
A staple of a Mediterranean diet, studies have found that it could help reduce the risk of major disease. Including olive oil in your diet, rather than unhealthy fats, could help lower your risk of heart disease and stroke. High in antioxidants, it can help lower general health risks, and its oleic acid is a natural anti-inflammatory.

> RECOMMENDED FOR HELP WITH
>
> • Heart health • General health • Inflammation
> • Reducing risk of stroke • Cancer prevention
> • Brain function • Diabetes

Allspice
Allspice is thought to aid the motility (or contractions) of the gastrointestinal tract, and promote digestion by boosting the secretions of enzymes in the stomach and intestines. Rich in minerals, a tablespoon of allspice provides 2 percent of your recommended daily values of iron and potassium, contributing to the healthy function of the blood and heart. It's also high in vitamin C, a powerful natural antioxidant that helps the body combat infection.

> RECOMMENDED FOR HELP WITH
>
> • Digestive health • Gastrointestinal issues
> • Cardiovascular health • Immune health

Cinnamon
A powerhouse of the spices, with higher antioxidant properties than almost any other food. For centuries, it's been prized as a spice, a trading commodity, and for its medicinal properties. There are two types of cinnamon: cassia and Ceylon.

> RECOMMENDED FOR HELP WITH
>
> • Brain function • Lowering cholesterol
> • Metabolism

Cumin
Packed with energy-boosting iron, cumin is a peppery little seed with extraordinary health benefits. One teaspoon contains almost a quarter of your recommended daily value of iron. An integral component of hemoglobin, which transports oxygen from the lungs to the cells around the body, iron is particularly important for menstruating women, who lose iron each month during menstruation.

> RECOMMENDED FOR HELP WITH
>
> • Metabolism • Digestive health • Immune health
> • Possible cancer protection for stomach and liver

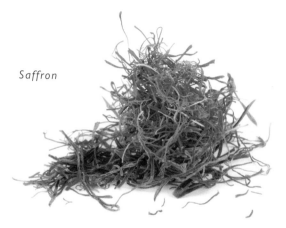

Saffron

Garlic

Garlic has long been celebrated as a king of healing plants, used in traditional remedies for a wide range of ailments, from heart problems to premature aging. It also has a reputation as a natural antibiotic. It packs a flavorful punch, and it's full of nutrients.

RECOMMENDED FOR HELP WITH

• Possible cancer prevention • Lowering cholesterol • Immune health

Ginger root

Long used for its medicinal properties, fresh ginger root has a very high level of antioxidants. Used fresh or dried, it has traditionally been used as a nausea suppressant, including nausea as a result of chemotherapy, morning sickness, and travel sickness. If you experience heartburn or gallstones, consult your doctor before consuming too much ginger.

RECOMMENDED FOR HELP WITH

• Nausea and upset stomach • Improves immune health • Improved circulation • Reducing inflammation and osteoarthritic pain

Miso

Miso is a condiment made from fermented soybeans, its flavor being a salty-savory mix. It contains nutrients including zinc, sodium, vitamin K, copper, manganese, and protein, as well as a small amount of B vitamins, selenium, magnesium, and choline, and heaps of beneficial bacteria. The fermentation process used to create miso is said to make it easier for the body to absorb its nutrients.

RECOMMENDED FOR HELP WITH

• Digestive health • Bowel issues • Immune health

Saffron

Saffron is made from the dried stigmas of the crocus flower. It takes around 4,500 crocus flowers to produce approximately 1 cup of spice, meaning that it's the most expensive of the common spices. It has many health benefits—as an antioxidant, immune booster, and blood sugar regulator.

RECOMMENDED FOR HELP WITH

• Immune health • Skin • Maintaining blood sugar levels

Soy sauce

Very low in saturated fat and cholesterol, and a good substitute for salt, research suggests that soy sauce may not carry the same cardiovascular health risks linked to other high-sodium foods. However, those on a salt-restricted diet or at risk of excessive salt intake should still consult with a health-care provider before using more soy sauce in place of salt.

RECOMMENDED FOR HELP WITH

• Immune health • Digestive health • Blood pressure • Lowering cholesterol

Turmeric

Made from the root of the *Curcuma longa* plant, this is a powerhouse of the spices, used for its anti-inflammatory, painkilling, and antioxidant properties. Just 1 tablespoon of turmeric contains over a quarter of your recommended daily value of manganese, an antioxidant that helps protect cells against free radical damage and promotes healthy skin.

RECOMMENDED FOR HELP WITH

• Inflammatory bowel syndrome • Coronary artery disease • Rheumatoid arthritis • Atherosclerosis

OILY FISH

Oily fish is a healthy, high-protein food and an excellent source of omega-3 fatty acids. Our bodies don't naturally produce these essential fats, so we need to obtain them from food. Omega-3 fatty acids have been linked to a reduced risk of heart disease and play a role in the prenatal development of babies. As part of a healthy diet, it's recommended that you consume at least one portion of oily fish a week.

Anchovy

Anchovies are small, oily ocean fish. They are very nutritious, if eaten in moderation. They contain essential amino acids and are high in selenium, calcium, iron, and potassium, great for healthy eyes, bones, and muscle. Canned or raw, anchovies are high in cholesterol—canned, they are also high in sodium. Anchovies are a great source of omega-3s. If you suffer from gout, watch your consumption. Low in mercury, they can be eaten during pregnancy.

> ### RECOMMENDED FOR HELP WITH
>
> • Metabolism • Stamina • Eye health • Heart and blood health • Possible cancer protection

Herring

Herring contain extremely high omega-3s and are high in protein, but also high in cholesterol. The fatty acids and protein promote healthy brain function and bone strength, and the potassium assists in nerve communication. Herring are rich in iron and vitamin B12, which keep red blood cells healthy. They are considered safe to eat during pregnancy due to the low mercury levels, but the American Pregnancy Association recommends avoiding kippers (smoked herring) during pregnancy due to possible listeria contamination. If you suffer from gout, watch your consumption of this food. Grilling or poaching are the healthiest cooking options; kippers and pickled herring are high in sodium—eat these in moderation.

> ### RECOMMENDED FOR HELP WITH
>
> • Anemia • Cardiovascular health • Strong bones
> • Brain function • Healthy skin • Immune health

Mackerel

Mackerel is an oily fish, and the name applies to several types. Mackerel provides high levels of omega-3—crucial for heart health—and jack mackerel is considered highest of all. Mackerel is a good source of potassium, which, together with the high omega-3, works to control blood pressure, if eaten in moderation. The vitamin B12 strengthens red blood cells. The U.S. Department of Agriculture and American Pregnancy Association recommend avoiding king mackerel during pregnancy due to high mercury levels, but other types can be eaten on occasion.

> ### RECOMMENDED FOR HELP WITH
>
> • Heart health • Reduces risk of cardiovascular disease • Blood health • Reducing blood pressure
> • Enhanced brain function • Strong bones
> • Immune health • Possible cancer protection

Salmon

Salmon meat comes in many varieties, from steaks to raw sushi, and smoked to canned. It is primarily found in the Atlantic and Pacific Oceans, with contention over the best farming and fishing practices. Salmon is full of essential vitamins and minerals: incredibly rich in omega-3 and omega-6, with essential amino acids, low sodium, and high selenium, vitamins B12 and B6, and folate. It is lower in saturated fat than beef.

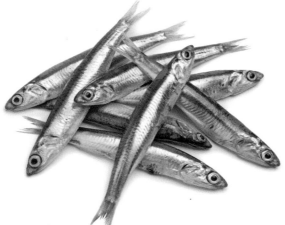

Anchovies

Due to the low purine content, salmon is considered safe in moderation for those suffering from gout. The American Pregnancy Association recommends avoiding smoked fish during pregnancy due to possible listeria contamination, but fresh or canned salmon can be eaten in moderation.

RECOMMENDED FOR HELP WITH

• Reducing risk of cardiovascular disease
• Blood health • Enhanced brain function and memory • Strong bones • Immune health
• Possible cancer protection

Sardines
Sardines are small, oily saltwater fish known to promote heart health, with high omega-6 and omega-3. It is recommended that you look for BPA-free canned sardines (or opt for fresh), as BPA (the compound bisphenol A) is shown to increase cancer growth and diabetes. Sardines are also very high in cholesterol. They are a rich source of protein, vitamins, and minerals, and one of the few natural food sources of vitamin D. Sardines strengthen the cardiovascular and digestive systems and reduce the risk of disease. Sardines are low in mercury and can be eaten in moderation during pregnancy.

RECOMMENDED FOR HELP WITH

• Regulating blood pressure • Blood health
• Enhanced brain function and memory
• Strong bones • Immune health

Trout
Trout refers to a large family of oily freshwater fish, although some do travel to the ocean. Trout are rich in omega-3 and omega-6, as well as amino acids and protein, and low in sodium but high in cholesterol. Amino acids and protein work together to build and repair bones and tissue and maintain organ function. Omega fatty acids work to decrease the risk of heart disease and high blood pressure, as well as helping with brain function. Vitamin B12 helps maintain healthy blood cells. Freshwater trout are low in mercury and can be eaten in moderation during pregnancy.

RECOMMENDED FOR HELP WITH

• Heart health • Strong bones • Tissue regeneration • Enhanced brain function
• Blood health • Energy levels • Immune health
• Joint health • Possible cancer protection

Tuna
Tuna is a saltwater fish with a widespread habitat and a number of species, including bluefin, yellowfin (ahi), bigeye, and albacore. Bluefin tuna is especially high in omega-3 and protein and low in sodium. It is also a good source of vitamins B12 and A. Yellowfin tuna is low in saturated fat and sodium, but high in cholesterol. It is a good source of selenium, niacin, and vitamin B6. Both are protein-rich. Due to the low purine content, light canned tuna is considered safe in moderation for those suffering from gout. The American Pregnancy Association recommends avoiding ahi and bigeye tuna during pregnancy due to high mercury levels.

RECOMMENDED FOR HELP WITH

• Strong bones • Blood health • Anemia
• Immune health • Energy levels • Mood
• Possible cancer protection

SHELLFISH

There are two main types of shellfish: crustaceans and mollusks. Crustaceans have jointed legs and a hard shell—such as crabs and shrimp—while mollusks are soft-bodied invertebrates that largely live in shells—such as oysters and scallops. All forms of shellfish are low in calories and fat, and high in minerals and protein.

Clams

Clams are a type of bivalve mollusk that live in water. They are eaten all over the world, from Italian shellfish pastas to American clam chowder and Indian curries. Clams contain the highest natural source of the amino acid taurine, believed to lower blood pressure and help fat digestion. They are very low in saturated fat, but they are high in cholesterol. Clams are protein-rich and have astoundingly high levels of vitamin B12, plus very high levels of iron and selenium. They are low in mercury and can be eaten in moderation during pregnancy.

RECOMMENDED FOR HELP WITH

• Lowering blood pressure • Anemia • Enhanced brain function • Immune health • Healthy skin • Possible cancer prevention

Crab

Crab is a low-calorie food that is very low in saturated fat and high in protein. Crabs are also very high in sodium and cholesterol. As a result, ensure you do not add extra salt or butter when preparing crab, and limit your intake of this meat. However, crab meat is very high in vitamin B12 (almost twice the recommended daily value) and has high levels of copper, selenium, and zinc. Crab meat is low in

mercury and can be eaten in moderation during pregnancy.

RECOMMENDED FOR HELP WITH

• Reducing risk of cardiovascular disease • Immune health • Strong bones • Energy levels • Enhanced brain function • Developing fetus during pregnancy • Healthy skin • Blood health • Possible cancer protection

Lobster

Lobster is a good source of vitamins and minerals. However, due to its high sodium and cholesterol content, it should be eaten in moderation. Lobster contains essential amino acids and is low in fat. The calcium and phosphorus build strong bones, vitamin B12 works toward brain function and nerve communication, and copper increases energy and assists in cell regeneration and skin health. Lobster has traditionally been considered an aphrodisiac. Because of higher mercury, lobster should be limited during pregnancy. Allergy to lobster and other shellfish is relatively common; if you suffer from any symptoms, get treatment immediately.

RECOMMENDED FOR HELP WITH

• Strong bones • Anemia • Blood health • Energy levels • Immune health • Healthy skin • Possible cancer protection

Mussels

Mussels are an excellent source of iron, vitamin B12, and riboflavin, but also contain other beneficial nutrients, such as niacin, folate, and thiamine. They're naturally rich in omega-3 fatty acids, which are essential for heart health, and their iron and

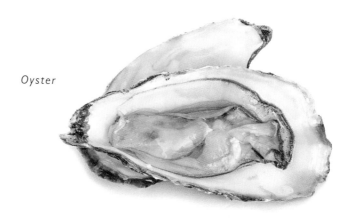

Oyster

B12 levels could aid with anemia and red blood cell production. The protein in mussels is easy to digest and can help build muscle, boost the immune system, and strengthen bones.

RECOMMENDED FOR HELP WITH

• Brain health • Anemia • Heart health
• Blood pressure • Weight loss • Bone health
• Immune health

Oyster

Oysters are bivalve marine mollusks. They are low in fat and contain essential amino acids. They are also a good source of copper, iron, and zinc—the latter of which is especially high in canned oysters. Alongside copper, zinc boosts a healthy immune system, and iron promotes healthy red blood cells. However, oysters are very high in cholesterol and relatively low in protein. Oysters are low in mercury and can be eaten in moderation during pregnancy.

RECOMMENDED FOR HELP WITH

• Strong bones • Blood health • Immune health
• Energy levels • Eye health • Heart health
• Possible cancer protection

Scallops

Scallops are bivalve marine mollusks found in oceans all over the world. They are a lean source of protein, low in calories and saturated fat, making them good for weight management. They are, however, high in cholesterol. They are also high in vitamin B12 and super-rich in fatty acids—in particular omega-6, which is integral to brain and immune system function, and which, with omega-3, reduces the risk of heart disease and high blood pressure. If you suffer from gout, watch your consumption of this food. Scallops are low in mercury and can be eaten in moderation during pregnancy.

RECOMMENDED FOR HELP WITH

• Weight loss • Heart health • Enhanced brain function • Blood health • Immune health
• Joint health

Shrimp

Shrimp are a widespread marine crustacean. The term "shrimp" is often used generally to refer to a number of similarly shaped crustaceans, and sometimes synonymously with "prawn." In North America, "shrimp" is the prevalent term, where they are the most popular seafood; however, in the UK, "prawn" is most often used, especially for larger shrimp. According to the American Heart Association, moderate consumption of shellfish (including shrimp) contributes to a heart-healthy diet. Shrimp contain essential amino acids, including tryptophan, which helps stabilize mood and sleep, as well as selenium, which boosts immune health. However, they are high in cholesterol. If you suffer from gout, watch your consumption. Shrimp are low in mercury and can be eaten in moderation during pregnancy. Allergy to shrimp and other shellfish is relatively common; if you show symptoms, get treatment immediately.

RECOMMENDED FOR HELP WITH

• Heart health • Strong bones • Mood • Blood health • Energy levels • Immune health • Possible cancer protection

VEGETABLES, NON-STARCHY

Non-starchy vegetables contain lower amounts of carbohydrates and calories than starchy vegetables, and are packed with vitamins, antioxidants, and fiber.

Artichoke

Artichokes contain more immune-boosting vitamin C than oranges. They're packed with vitamins and minerals, including vitamin K, essential for blood clotting, free-radical-zapping manganese, and cholesterol-regulating folate. They're also a very good source of fiber: just 1 ounce contains 10 percent of your recommended daily value, helping to maintain a healthy digestive system.

RECOMMENDED FOR HELP WITH

• Immune health • Digestive health

Asparagus

Succulent asparagus spears have been considered a delicacy for centuries. They're loaded with antioxidants, which help protect cells from free radicals. Rich in phytonutrients known as saponins that have been shown to have anti-inflammatory and anticancer properties, asparagus packs a healthy, nutritious punch. Delicious in salads or on its own.

RECOMMENDED FOR HELP WITH

• Possible cancer prevention • Regulating blood sugar levels and blood pressure

Bell peppers

Also known as sweet peppers or capsicums, bell peppers are native to South America but have spread to the rest of the world. Their crunchy, sweet, brightly colored skin makes them a favorite ingredient in a range of dishes. Bell peppers are a great source of antioxidants, compounds that help decrease free radical molecules, which damage cells. Higher-heat cooking can damage some of the delicate phytonutrients in bell peppers, so use lower-heat methods for a short period of time to keep the nutrients intact. Just 1 ounce of red bell pepper contains 16 percent of your recommended daily value of vision-boosting vitamin A, and 80 percent of immune-boosting vitamin C, compared with 3 percent and 35 percent in the equivalent amount of green bell pepper.

RECOMMENDED FOR HELP WITH

• Immune health • Age-related macular degeneration

Burdock root

Burdock root is the tuber of the greater burdock plant. It is high in free-radical-zapping antioxidants, soothing mucilage, and carbohydrate- and fat-regulating insulin. Burdock root has long been used in traditional medicines to help purify the blood due to its diuretic properties. Its soothing, demulcent properties mean it has also traditionally been used to treat throat and chest problems.

RECOMMENDED FOR HELP WITH

• Regulating blood sugar • Mild laxative
• Cardiovascular health

Celery

Since most people's bodies are far too acidic, celery being alkaline is a welcome addition to any diet. Popular for its flavorful leaves and shoots, and crunchy roots, celery is rich in immune-boosting, anti-cancerous antioxidants, which help protect cells against free radical damage; its leaves are a good

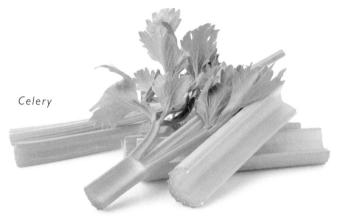

Celery

source of vision-boosting vitamin A. Enjoy celery roots in salads for a healthy, nutritious crunch, or in soups and stews.

RECOMMENDED FOR HELP WITH

• Lowering cholesterol • Reducing anxiety levels
• Immune health

Fennel bulb
Succulent fennel bulb is loaded with free-radical-zapping antioxidants and dietary fiber. Its anise-like flavor makes it a favorite in Mediterranean dishes. Anethole, the essential oil that gives fennel its distinctive flavor, has been shown to have antifungal and antibacterial properties, while heart-friendly potassium contributes to a healthy cardiovascular system, helping to regulate heart rate and blood pressure. Fennel is a flavorful addition to many dishes, from roast chicken to seared salmon.

RECOMMENDED FOR HELP WITH

• Lowering blood pressure • Digestive health

Leeks
Leeks are rich in antioxidants, protecting cells against damage from free radicals. They're also a good source of immune-boosting vitamin C, vision-boosting vitamin A, and vitamin K, essential for blood clotting and bone nourishment. For a healthy cooking option, slice thinly and briefly sauté. As with garlic and onions, allowing leeks to sit after chopping, before heating or adding to other ingredients, enhances their nutritional benefits.

RECOMMENDED FOR HELP WITH

• Lowering cholesterol • Reducing anxiety levels
• Immune health

Tomato
Tomatoes are a nutritional powerhouse. Tomatoes and tomato products, including tomato sauce and tomato juice, are rich in vitamins and antioxidants, including lycopene. Research has shown that diets rich in lycopene may help decrease the risk of heart disease, age-related macular degeneration, stroke, high cholesterol, and certain types of cancer. Cooked tomatoes contain significantly more lycopene than raw tomatoes. However, whether eaten raw or cooked, freshly picked or canned, tomatoes provide a healthy addition to most diets, though high acidic levels may aggravate reflux or heartburn in those prone to these conditions. Include a mixture of cooked and raw tomatoes in your weekly meal plan to reap the most health benefits from tomatoes. Due to their moisture content, tomatoes deteriorate rapidly after being picked. Sun-drying removes the water to preserve the tomato, while retaining the flavor and many of the nutrients. Sun-dried tomatoes are low in fat and high in fiber and immune-boosting vitamin C.

RECOMMENDED FOR HELP WITH

• Lowering cholesterol • Vision • Immune health

Zucchini
Also known as courgette, zucchini is one of the most popular summer squashes in the Americas, low in calories, and high in vision-boosting vitamin A and heart-friendly potassium. The skin is particularly rich in nutrients, so leave it on to reap the full nutritional benefits of zucchini.

RECOMMENDED FOR HELP WITH

• Lowering cholesterol • Vision • Immune health

VEGETABLES, STARCHY

Starchy vegetables are higher in calories than non-starchy vegetables, but their health benefits are enormous as they are rich in vitamins, minerals, and fiber. They are also high-quality carbohydrates, so those with diabetes need to be wary of their intake.

Beet
Beets are a good source of many nutrients, including vitamin C, iron, magnesium, potassium, folate, manganese, and dietary fiber. The nitrates in beets help the body to produce nitric oxide, which improves heart health. Avoid eating beets if you suffer from kidney stones.

RECOMMENDED FOR HELP WITH

• Constipation and diarrhea • Lowering cholesterol • Heart health • Brain function • Immune health • Healthy bones • Healthy skin • Pregnancy • Iron-deficient anemia

Carrot
Carrots are one of the richest sources of beta-carotene, which the body converts into vitamin A. Carrots also have no fat and no cholesterol, which makes them a great choice for anyone watching their weight.

RECOMMENDED FOR HELP WITH

• Weight loss • Intestinal health • Stroke and heart attack prevention • Lowering cholesterol • Heart health • Immune health • Eye health

Cauliflower
Most vegetables that are highly rated for their nutritional value are deep greens or bright reds—but in spite of its pale color, cauliflower is just as jam-packed with nutrients. It is very low in saturated fat and cholesterol, and a good source of both protein and dietary fiber. A real powerhouse for its immune system and anticancer benefits.

RECOMMENDED FOR HELP WITH

• Weight loss • Intestinal health • Immune health • Possible cancer protection • Reducing risk of cardiovascular disease

Parsnip
Parsnips are related to carrots, celeriac, and fennel. They are not a widely used root vegetable in the United States, but are popular as a roasted side dish in Europe. Parsnips are rich in antioxidants and a very good source of potassium, dietary fiber, vitamin C, folate, and manganese. They are also very low in saturated fat, cholesterol, and sodium.

RECOMMENDED FOR HELP WITH

• Digestive health • Lowering blood pressure and cholesterol • Enhanced brain function • Strong bones and teeth

Potato
Potatoes are starchy vegetables that are grown as underground tubers. Potatoes are versatile and when potatoes are cooked with their skins on, they're a good source of vitamins and minerals, including vitamin C, folate, vitamin B6, and potassium, plus fiber. These compounds may play a part in helping to lower blood pressure and reduce the risk of heart disease. Baked potatoes are a filling food, so could help manage weight.

RECOMMENDED FOR HELP WITH

• Lowering blood pressure • Heart health • Weight loss and management

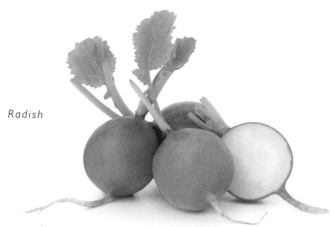

Radish

Pumpkin

Not just a fun Halloween tradition, pumpkin is also a delicious and nutritious food. While fresh whole pumpkin is best, canned pumpkin does still maintain a good amount of vitamins and minerals for a healthy diet. Pumpkin is a low-calorie, appetite-satisfying, alkalizing food that is rich in antioxidants.

RECOMMENDED FOR HELP WITH

• Enhanced brain function • Blood pressure and cholesterol • Strong bones and teeth • Possible cancer prevention • Weight loss

Radish

A healthy, alkalizing food, radishes are often overlooked and relegated to the place of a pretty garnish. But radishes are packed with vitamin C, potassium, and fiber. As a low-calorie food, they are excellent for anyone watching their weight. White icicle radishes provide slightly more vitamin C.

RECOMMENDED FOR HELP WITH

• Digestive health • Lowering blood pressure and cholesterol • Reducing risk of stroke and heart attack • Eye health • Enhanced brain function • Strong bones and teeth • Weight loss

Sweet potato

One of the healthiest of all starchy vegetables, sweet potatoes are delicious and versatile. As mashed potatoes, they require very little butter and milk, making them a healthy alternative. They are loaded with antioxidants and a good source of dietary fiber (especially if you leave the skin on), potassium, and a huge array of vitamins, as well as being low in sodium, saturated fat, and cholesterol.

RECOMMENDED FOR HELP WITH

• Weight loss • Immune health • Digestive health and regularity • Strong bones • Healthy skin • Eye health • Energy levels • Reducing risk of stroke and heart attack • Lowering cholesterol • Possible cancer prevention

Turnip

Turnips are an incredibly nutritious root vegetable that are high in antioxidants. They are also a good source of dietary fiber, vitamins A, C, and K, as well as a range of other minerals. They are low in saturated fat, sodium, and cholesterol. Their greens also provide fiber, folate, and very high levels of vitamin K.

RECOMMENDED FOR HELP WITH

• Immune health • Digestive health and regularity • Strong bones • Healthy skin • Eye health • Lowering cholesterol • Reducing risk of stroke and heart attack • Possible cancer prevention, especially prostate and colon • Weight loss

Winter squash

Winter squash comes in several varieties, and is a healthy, alkalizing food that is versatile and delectable—bake it whole, or make a warming winter soup. Winter squash is full of vitamin A, which improves lung health, and a good source of folate, a beneficial vitamin during pregnancy.

RECOMMENDED FOR HELP WITH

• Lung health • Pregnancy and developing of fetus • Immune health • Digestive health • Healthy skin • Eye health • Lowering cholesterol • Reduce risk of stroke and heart attack

OTHER NOTABLE SUPERFOODS

Apple cider vinegar

Apple cider vinegar is a traditional tonic that is made via a fermentation process. The main active component in apple cider vinegar is acetic acid, or ethanoic acid, which is a short-chain fatty acid. Unfiltered, organic apple cider vinegar also contains what's called "mother"—friendly bacteria, proteins, and enzymes that may provide extra health benefits. It's been associated with lowering blood sugar levels, lowering cholesterol, and helping with various digestive complaints.

RECOMMENDED FOR HELP WITH

• Digestive issues • Weight loss • Weight management • Lowering blood sugar • Lowering cholesterol

Cocoa nibs

Cocoa or cacao nibs are tiny pieces of crushed cocoa beans in a pure format that come from the *Theobroma cacao* tree. They have a strong and bitter dark chocolate taste and, despite being tiny in size, are abundant in nutrients and plant compounds, such as flavonoid antioxidants. They're a good source of protein, healthy fats, and fiber, and rich in various minerals, such as iron, zinc, magnesium, and manganese. Magnesium and manganese both play a role in healthy bones, and the flavonoids may play a part in reducing the risk of heart disease and cancer. As there's no sugar in cocoa nibs, they're a healthier option to consume than milk chocolate.

RECOMMENDED FOR HELP WITH

• Heart disease • Cancer • Weight loss • Weight management

Dark chocolate

Dark chocolate contains high levels of flavonoids and is renowned for its antioxidant effects. Research into the benefits of dark chocolate has found that it's linked to a reduced risk of heart disease and better brain function. Look for options with high percentage levels of cocoa content—anything marked as 70 percent or above will be good. Fair Trade and organic dark chocolate have the added benefits of no chemicals being involved in the growing process of the cocoa.

RECOMMENDED FOR HELP WITH

• Heart disease • Brain function

Green tea

Green tea is made from the unoxidized leaves of the *Camelia sinensis* bush and contains the most beneficial polyphenols and antioxidants. Green tea has been drunk for centuries in some countries and is widely used as a form of medicinal tea in Chinese and Indian medicine. One of the most powerful components is a natural compound called epigallocatechin-3-gallate (EGCG), which is a form of antioxidant that has been linked to anti-inflammatory effects. The tea also boasts benefits for lowering cholesterol, reducing the risk of strokes, and helping with weight loss.

RECOMMENDED FOR HELP WITH

• Lowering cholesterol • Reducing risk of stroke • Weight loss • Inflammatory conditions

Matcha

Matcha is a form of powdered green tea. It comes from the same plant as standard green tea but is grown slightly differently, which results in an

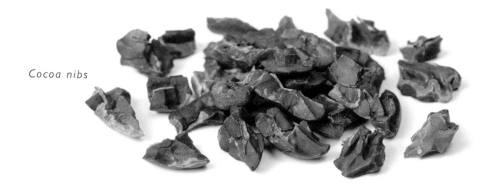

Cocoa nibs

increase in amino acids. Matcha has high levels of antioxidants, which help protect cells from damage, and may play a part in reducing inflammation in your body. It may also help reduce the risk of heart disease and strokes.

RECOMMENDED FOR HELP WITH

• Inflammatory conditions • Heart disease reduction • Stroke reduction • Weight loss

Sauerkraut

Sauerkraut is a form of fermented cabbage that is packed with probiotics, vitamins, and minerals, including vitamin C, vitamin K1, manganese, vitamin B6, iron, folate, copper, and potassium. The probiotics in sauerkraut can have a beneficial effect on digestion and gut health, helping improve the bacterial balance in your body, plus they can help boost your immune system. As it's low in calories and high in fiber, eating sauerkraut may help with weight loss too.

RECOMMENDED FOR HELP WITH

• Digestive health • Gut health • Immune issues
• Weight loss • Brain health

Sea vegetables

Sea vegetables or seaweeds are low in fat and contain essential nutrients, including potassium, iodine, calcium, magnesium, and iron. Nori seaweed is a great source of potassium, iron, and iodine, the latter of which can help maintain hearing. Wakame seaweed is one of the few foods containing iodine, which improves thyroid function and has been linked to the prevention of breast cancer. However, it is high in sodium, so should be consumed in moderation.

RECOMMENDED FOR HELP WITH

• Thyroid problems • Hearing • General health

Spirulina

Spirulina is a blue-green algae that grows in salt- and fresh water. As a dried powder, it is highly nutritious. It has the antioxidant phycocyanin, which gives it its blue-green color, and contains high levels of protein, vitamin B1, vitamin B2, vitamin B3, iron, and copper, plus magnesium, potassium, and manganese. It's also a good source of omega-3 and omega-6 fatty acids. Spirulina is known for its anti-inflammatory properties, and may play a role in lowering cholesterol, helping reduce blood pressure, and maintaining general health.

RECOMMENDED FOR HELP WITH

• General health • Heart health • Immune health
• Cholesterol

Wheatgrass

Wheatgrass is made from the *Triticum aestivum* plant. It comes in a liquid or powdered form, and has antibacterial, anti-inflammatory, and antioxidant properties. Some of the nutrients in wheatgrass include calcium, magnesium, amino acids, protein, iron, enzymes, vitamin A, vitamin C, vitamin E, vitamin K, and vitamin B complex. It helps support the healthy functioning of the liver and helps remove toxic substances from your body, plus it can cleanse your intestines, boost metabolism, and aid digestion.

RECOMMENDED FOR HELP WITH

• Digestive health • Bowel issues • Liver • General health • Cleansing • Weight loss

EATING FOR HEALTH AND WELLNESS

When you think of the term "self-care," what springs to mind? A relaxing massage, time to yourself, or doing a yoga class perhaps? All are perfectly valid, but the chances are you might not have thought of food and nutrition. Yet food and what you choose to eat is a really important part of self-care.

When it comes to managing your self-care regime, nutrition and food should be a top priority. What you eat and drink directly affects your health in numerous ways. On a short-term basis, it can affect your digestion, your mood, and your energy levels, and on a longer-term basis it can boost your immunity, strengthen your muscles, and help your overall health. Your diet should be an integral part of your regular self-care regime. This doesn't mean *dieting* or restricting what you do and don't eat, but rather the choices you make about how you fuel, feed, and nourish your body on a daily basis. It's about learning to love the healthy choices you make and the fact that you're nourishing your body with good-quality, nutritious foods and drinks.

Developing a good relationship with food helps create a better balance in your life and impacts on how you feel in a multitude of ways. Good nutrition can have an impact on how you feel physically and mentally, and how you feel about yourself. It can positively affect your skin, hair, and nails, and help you develop better feelings of self-worth, as well as helping you feel stronger, happier, and more resilient to face life's challenges.

Ways to incorporate good nutrition into your life

Here are some of the ways you can incorporate good nutrition into your life and develop positive food-related self-care habits.

Plan ahead
Making meal plans may sound like a bit of a chore, but planning ahead can help you be much more organized, both in terms of shopping for ingredients and knowing what you're going to have for dinner on any given day. Planning helps you to get a better balance of foods in your diet and prevents impromptu meal choices that may be unhealthy.

Make it a habit to sit down on a Sunday and plan your meals for the week ahead. It will make your shopping easier, as you'll know exactly what you need to buy and, in theory, you won't get distracted too much by other options in the grocery store. It doesn't have to be perfect and neither does it have to be set in stone—you can easily switch around options later in the week if you need to.

Eat regular meals
One of the best ways to support your nutritional self-care is to fuel your body by eating regular meals. Skipping meals takes its toll on your body, resulting in you not functioning at your best. Without regular meals you may experience fatigue, headaches, lack of concentration, or feelings of brain fog, all of which can impact your ability to function. Your body needs a good balance of protein, carbohydrate, and fat from

regular meals throughout the day; this will help keep your blood sugar at a stable level and give you the fuel you need for energy.

Don't rush meals
When you do stop to eat, don't rush your meals. Take time to enjoy them, eat slowly so your body can properly digest everything, and relish the time you get to spend with family or friends eating a meal. Try and avoid the temptation to rush a meal or eat on the go—your digestive system will thank you for it.

Eat healthy fats
Not all fats are bad for you. In fact, you need to include some fat in your diet in order for your body to function properly. Learn to give your body the healthy fats it deserves, such as omega-3 fatty acids, found in olive oil, avocado, oily fish, and nuts.

Be creative with your meals
Eating a variety of different meals keeps things interesting and ensures your body gets a good range of essential nutrients. So, be creative with your meals, experiment with new recipes, and step out of your comfort zone to try new foods.

Drink water
Remember to drink plenty of water. Often thirst can be mistaken for hunger, so rather than reaching for a snack when you think you feel hungry, try drinking a glass of water first.

Cut down on caffeine
Caffeine, which is in drinks such as tea, coffee, soda, and energy drinks, is a stimulant. It gives you a quick burst of energy, but drinking lots of it can affect your sleep—especially when you drink it at night—or

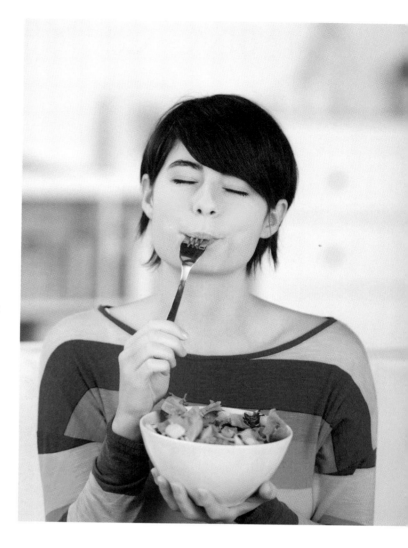

give you withdrawal symptoms if you suddenly stop your regular habit. If you currently consume a lot of caffeine, try and cut down on it slowly, gradually reducing the amount you drink. Swap to decaffeinated options instead, or try herbal teas. Think of your body first before you order that extra-large latte every morning!

TIMING OF MEALS

Far less well publicized than what we eat is the importance of when we eat. The old adage "breakfast like a king, lunch like a lord, and dine like a pauper" is supported by naturopaths and other natural practitioners, who recommend a hearty breakfast, a moderate lunch, and a light dinner, eaten if possible no later than 6:00 p.m.

There are very good biological reasons for this: the human digestive system functions best in the morning, when it produces a good supply of enzymes for the quick and efficient absorption of nutrients. The digestive process gets slower throughout the day, really starting to slow down around 6:00 p.m.; by 9:00 p.m. it is very sluggish indeed. You may feel sleepy after a heavy meal, because the blood goes from the head to the stomach, but still find it difficult to get to sleep because your body has been given an extra task when it should be resting—you wouldn't like to start work at bedtime either! In addition, digestion takes place most efficiently when the body is upright. Although people's body clocks differ, this slowing down of digestion throughout the day seems to be true for everyone. This means that food eaten late in the evening is liable to remain in the stomach half-digested and putrefying all night, affecting both sleep and our enthusiasm for breakfast in the morning. In some cases it can actually cause a buildup of toxins, leading to ill health.

If you habitually sleep badly, a large breakfast may well be the last thing you feel like in the morning. But remember that you are now changing your habits to encourage your body to relax and sleep; how you start the day will affect how you end it. If you try for a three-week period having a good lunch and an early, light dinner, you'll soon find yourself much keener on breakfast.

A hearty and healthy breakfast could include oatmeal, muesli with yogurt and fruit, whole-grain toast with honey, or cheese if you like it. Unfortunately, our social system is not geared to our body clock, and for the rest of the day you may have

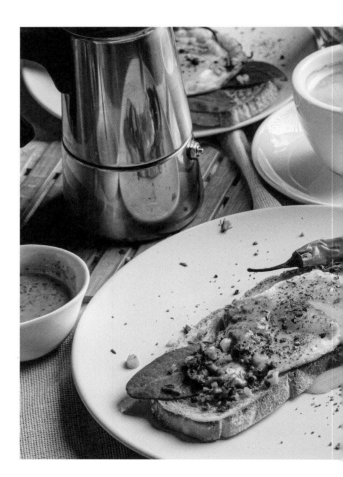

The human digestive system functions best in the morning.

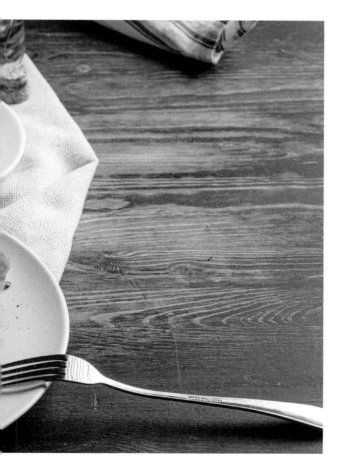

to do some adaptation. The lordly lunch accompanied by a large salad may not be available where you work, and if you have a long journey home, the early, light dinner may present difficulties. Experiment with packed lunches; raw carrots, celery, and apples need scarcely any preparation. If possible, finish your evening meal by 8:00 p.m.

If you are going straight from work to an evening class, have your hot meal at lunchtime and a sandwich or baked potato before the class. And if you're invited out for a late, delicious dinner—keep the portions (and the alcohol) down, relax, and enjoy it! Eating happily is possibly as important as what you eat.

Allergies and sensitivities

If you suffer severely from a food allergy, you will probably already be aware of it. But degrees of allergic reaction vary; some people are sensitive to particular foods without having an out-and-out allergy. Their degree of sensitivity can also vary, with reactions worse at particularly stressful times and unnoticeable at others.

The substances that most commonly cause allergic reactions or intolerance are wheat, eggs, dairy products, sugar, and caffeine, as well as certain chemicals and additives. Very often, people are unaware that something they've been enjoying for years is affecting them badly. This is a common phenomenon known as a masked allergy, when sufferers are actually addicted to the substance that is doing them harm.

It's worth observing your reactions to foods and drinks, particularly those you crave for or consume every day. If you notice that you regularly feel extra hyped up or depressed after any of these, try cutting them out of your diet for a week or two and see whether this makes a difference. If you are suffering from a masked allergy, you may get slight withdrawal symptoms; people giving up caffeine, for instance, sometimes experience headaches and fuzziness for a few days. If this happens to you, tell yourself it's a good sign, showing that your system is cleansing itself of something that was doing it harm. Drink plenty of water to help the process along.

MINDFUL EATING

Our life and well-being rely upon the nourishment we receive. Every mouthful of food we eat is the result of the efforts of the numerous people involved in its growth and the benevolence of nature. For the countless people in our world who face daily deprivation, every meal is a blessing and a lifeline to survival.

For those of us who live with greater abundance and security, food is often taken for granted or has assumed layers of emotional overtone. Moments of mindful eating may be rare in our lives. When we are rushed, food is consumed in haste, something used solely to subdue the distraction of our body's hunger. When our minds are overly full of preoccupation, meals are often eaten habitually, something to get over so we can resume the obsessive thinking we are more interested in. When we are bored, food can become a primary means of distraction. In the midst of distress, food is frequently turned to as a source of comfort. Food can become a substitute for the seemingly impossible task of understanding the source of inner turmoil. Learning to approach eating with care and sensitivity is a direct way of cultivating appreciation and nurturing moments of calm in our days.

Approaching meals with intentional awareness creates a deeper sense of connection with all life and an appreciation of how precious our well-being is. Learning to stop when we eat, to be fully attentive, is a powerful way of introducing moments of stillness and calm into our day. It can be helpful to approach at least one meal a day with the intention of focusing fully upon it, sitting down to eat, and consciously unhooking from telephones, television, or reading.

Approach this as a time of letting go of haste and busyness. Many people find it useful to have one meal a day in silence, allowing their minds and bodies a time of renewal and ease.

Guided meditation for eating

• As you sit down with your food, take a few moments just to consciously relax your body and sit quietly.

• Sense the space around you, listen to the sounds around you, feel the contact of your body with the chair and the touch of your feet on the ground.

• Calmly pass your eyes over the food on your plate. Sense the different textures, shapes, smells, and colors of the food.

• As you move to pick up your fork or spoon, be present within the movement of your arms and hands. Be aware of the sensation of your hand taking hold of your cutlery.

• As you put the food in your mouth, notice the taste as the food contacts your taste buds.

• Chew mindfully, savoring the taste of the food. Notice the moments when your mind is focusing on the next bite, and gently bring your attention back to savor the food you are eating now. You might even experiment with putting your spoon or fork down after each mouthful.

• As you swallow and move to take up the next mouthful of food, stay clearly present with that movement.

• Let the meal from beginning to end be a time of appreciation and sensitivity.

• Notice the changing sensations in your body as they shift from hunger to satisfaction.

• Let the whole mealtime be a dedicated time of calmness and mindfulness.

• Sense within your body when you have eaten enough, and stop at that point.

• As you end your meal, again bring your attention into your body, sensing its ease.

• And again, before getting up, feel the contact of your body on the chair, your feet touching the ground, and the sights and sounds of that moment.

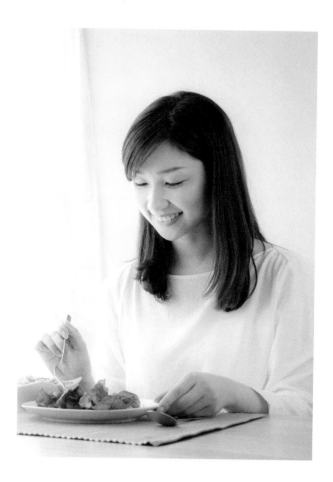

HEALTHY DRINKS

Water is the most common substance on the Earth's surface, covering more than 70 percent of the planet and present in the atmosphere as water vapor or steam. Human beings are comprised of about 75 percent water. Water is necessary for maintaining the correct osmotic pressure in cells, and is needed for many other bodily processes, such as transporting nutrients and waste products around the body in the blood (blood is about 80 percent water). Water that has been cooled or heated to form ice, hot water, or steam can be used to treat minor complaints.

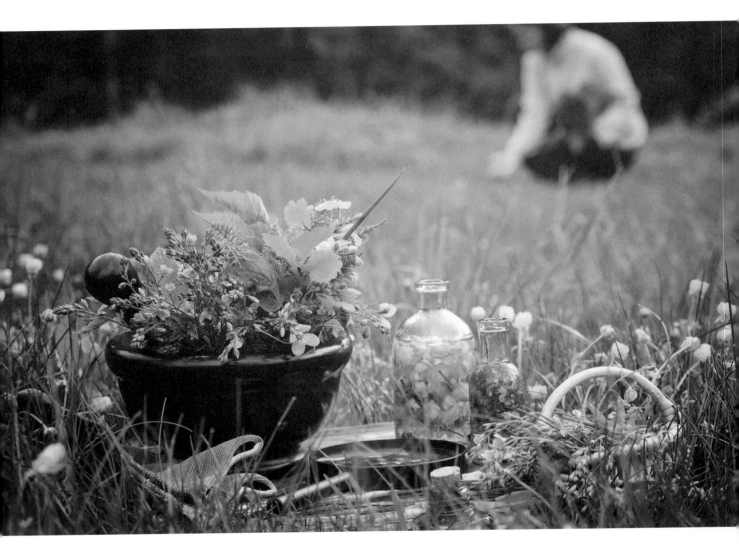

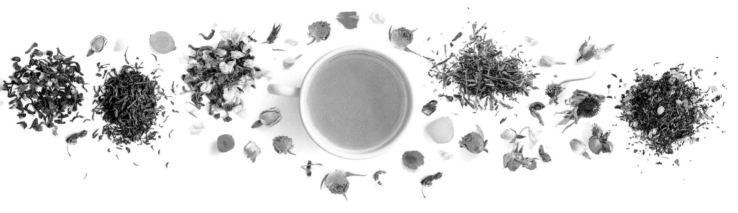

Harmful drinks

Although not harmful in small amounts—approximately one drink per day for adults—there is no nutritional need for alcohol. Soft and energy drinks are nonessential and, in the case of energy drinks, may be harmful.

Herbal drinks

Herbal teas are becoming increasingly popular as replacements for caffeine-containing drinks. There is a good variety of herbal tea bags available, some of them specially blended to help you relax or sleep. They can be quite expensive; it's often cheaper to buy loose herbs from an herbalist (see pages 90–91) or health-food store and experiment with single herbs or mixtures. Herbs can lose their efficacy over time, so buy them in small quantities, keep them in airtight jars, and use them promptly.

Herbal infusions

Herbal infusions are slightly stronger than teas, and can be taken medicinally three times a day. You can make up an infusion of one or more herbs, using 1–2 heaping teaspoonfuls of dried leaves or flowers to a cup of water. Use an herbal infuser or small teapot, and pour the water onto the herbs when just at a boil. Leave to stand, covered, for at least 5–10 minutes before drinking, or up to 20 minutes if you are taking them medicinally.

Chamomile is one of the best-known herbs for calming the nerves, and for settling the digestion. It is said to have cumulative effects, becoming more effective over a period of time. However, some people find the flavor rather bland, and it has the disadvantage of being mildly diuretic. Lime flower (linden) makes a very effective and pleasant-flavored nightcap and is good for headaches, nervous tension, and restlessness. Skullcap is a tonic as well as a sedative, high in magnesium and calcium, which help to strengthen the nervous system. It is not always easy to obtain, and what is often sold as skullcap is another herb called teucrium (wood sage). So get the genuine article, *Scutellaria laterifolia*, from a reputable herbalist.

Passiflora (passionflower) is another good soporific, a constituent of many herbal sleeping pills. Valerian root is also well known as a sedative. It tastes like old socks (and smells worse), but a quantity of it can be mixed with more pleasant-flavored herbs. Valerian has a more "druggy" effect than most herbs, and some people find it gives them headaches if drunk in large quantities, so (unless prescribed by an herbalist) it is recommended not to take it on consecutive days for more than a week or two.

Hawthorn flowers are good for people who don't sleep because they have heart palpitations. Mint is good for soothing the digestion. Lemon balm and vervain are good for depression.

HOW TO INCLUDE MORE SUPERFOODS IN YOUR DIET

Keen to eat more superfoods? There are plenty of ways in which you can get these super healthy foods into your diet.

Add fruit to your breakfast

Get the day off to a good start by including fruit in your breakfast. Add berries, sliced kiwi, or grapes to your cereal or a bowl of natural yogurt. Mix up a fruit smoothie with banana, mango, and passionfruit, or make your own fruit, nut, and seed muesli using a variety of ingredients.

Have a side salad

A side salad is a great way to add a mix of vegetable and fruit to any meal, either eaten with it or as an additional course. You can vary salads so no two are the same, using ingredients such as lettuce, cabbage, carrots, peppers, cucumber, tomatoes, dried dates, and dried apricots.

Try new recipes

One of the best ways of eating a variety of superfoods is to try new recipes. It's easy to get into the habit of having the same meals week in, week out, but varying what you eat will liven things up and give you access to lots more nutrients.

Add vegetables to sauces

Chopped vegetables can be added into sauces such as tomato-based sauces for pasta dishes, to bulk them up. Keep small pieces for texture and interest or blitz them for a smooth finish.

Make soups

Making your own soups is a great way to try out new vegetables and discover what combinations you find most appealing.

Get creative with your baking

Step out of your comfort zone and try out new recipes. Did you know zucchini or beet can be used to make cakes? Do something different and discover new ways to include superfoods in your home baking.

Be adventurous

Set yourself the task of trying a new superfood every week. Are there superfoods you've never eaten before? Perhaps there are foods you think you don't like, but in reality haven't tried for years? Challenging yourself can be motivating and you may discover some new likes and loves along the way.

Benefits of eating a rainbow of foods

When you're choosing what fruits or vegetables to put on your plate, aim to eat a rainbow of different-colored fresh produce every day. This isn't just due to it looking pretty when you dish it up, but for nutritional reasons too. The more variety and the more colors of fresh produce that you consume, the more essential nutrients you'll gain.

As well as vitamins and minerals, plants contain a variety of different phytonutrients. The phytonutrients give fresh produce their distinctive colors but, as we've already covered, they're also packed with health benefits.

Eating a rainbow of fresh foods shouldn't be tricky. On a daily basis, try and include two or three different-colored vegetables or fruits at every mealtime. If you have snacks, add a piece of fruit to it. While it's not essential to eat foods of every single

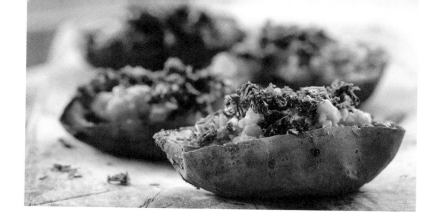

Sweet potato, feta cheese, and crispy kale

color every day, it's highly beneficial to eat colorfully as much as you can.

Below are some of the key phytonutrients found in fresh produce, along with some examples of the fruits and vegetables in that color group that you could eat.

Red

Red foods contain lycopene (tomatoes), anthocyanins (red berries), ellagic acid (such as strawberries, raspberries, and pomegranates).

FRUITS: Raspberries, strawberries, cherries, pink guavas, watermelons, pomegranates, cranberries, red grapes

VEGETABLES: Tomatoes, red peppers, radishes, red onions

Orange

Fruits and vegetables that are orange in color have high levels of carotenoids, such as beta-carotene and alpha-carotene. When beta-carotene is consumed, it is converted into vitamin A.

FRUITS: Cantaloupe melons, mangoes, nectarines, oranges, tangerines

VEGETABLES: Carrots, butternut squashes, pumpkins, sweet potatoes, orange peppers

Yellow

Fruits and vegetables that are yellow contain carotenoids such as beta-cryptoxanthin and beta-carotene, both of which are transformed into vitamin A.

FRUITS: Bananas, lemons, honeydew melons, pineapples

VEGETABLES: Yellow peppers, sweet corn, rutabagas

Green

Green fruits and vegetables get their color from the pigment chlorophyll. Many naturally green foods contain lutein and zeaxanthin, as well as sulforaphane, indoles, and glucosinolate.

FRUITS: Pears, green apples, kiwis, limes, green grapes

VEGETABLES: Spinach, broccoli, zucchini, kale, avocados, celery, lettuce, leeks, peas, green beans, cabbage, sprouts, bok choy, cucumbers, asparagus

Blue and purple

The pigment anthocyanin is responsible for giving blue and purple foods their natural color.

FRUITS: Blueberries, grapes, blackberries, blackcurrants, elderberries, plums

VEGETABLES: Eggplants, red cabbage, beets, purple cauliflower

White and beige

Fresh produce that are naturally white or beige in color get their pigments from anthoxanthins.

FRUITS: Bananas, white peaches, lychees

VEGETABLES: Onions, cauliflower, mushrooms, garlic, celeriacs, turnips, Jerusalem artichokes, potatoes, parsnips

SUPERFOOD SOUPS, STIR-FRIES, AND SALADS

If you're keen to include more superfoods in your diet and eat healthily, homemade soups, stir-fries, and salads are all good options to include on your menu. All of these types of meals are versatile, can involve fresh vegetables, meat, fish, or vegan alternatives, and can be adapted according to the foods you have at home or have easy access to. If you're making a conscious effort to eat healthily, be aware with stir-fries and salads that added sauces and dressings can contain hidden fats, sugars, and calories in them and can jeopardize the healthiness of your plate of food. To be sure of what's in your sauce or dressing, aim to make your own from healthy oils or fresh ingredients. A good option for stir-fries is to use soy sauce, which is a superfood in itself. For salads, you could mix up your own dressing using honey and mustard.

Soups

They can be chunky or smooth, hot or even cold (think gazpacho)—soups are a great way of getting a good dose of superfoods in a tasty and filling meal. A chunky soup can be hearty and warming to consume on a cold winter's day, while a smooth soup can be a lighter option for lunch or as a starter any time of the year. Soups freeze well so can be made in batches then frozen into your desired portion sizes. If you go out to work, freshly made soup makes an ideal packed lunch—just pop it in a thermal flask to keep it warm.

Soup is easy to make in a pan on the stove, but soup-makers are now widely available too and a useful addition to your kitchen if you're short on time and want to make soup quickly. The ingredients can

all be added to the gadget and set to cook, so you don't need to stand over a pan of soup as it cooks. Finish soups with some toasted seeds, such as pumpkin seeds, or a small sprinkle of cheese.

Good superfood combinations to consider for soups include:

• Carrot and sweet potato
• Winter squash (or butternut squash), carrot, and sweet potato
• Lentil and carrot
• Parsnip and apple
• Tomato and red bell pepper
• Watercress
• Broccoli
• Carrot and orange
• Sweet potato and miso
• Chicken and mushroom
• Leek and potato
• Spiced cauliflower
• Fennel, pea, and lemon

Stir-fries

Despite the name and the frying aspect, stir-fries are a healthy option. The art of stir-frying involves cooking fresh vegetables, meat, or fish in a wok at a hot temperature, while constantly stirring it. Only a small amount of oil is needed, so the amount of fat is relatively low. Stir-fries are quick to cook too, especially when all the ingredients are in small pieces, so they're a good choice when you don't want to spend too much time in the kitchen.

The idea with a stir-fry is that you have small pieces of tender, crunchy vegetables alongside a protein of your choice, or just vegetables if you

Fennel and orange salad

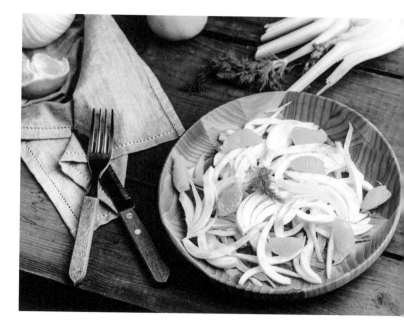

prefer. Some good choices of vegetables to add to stir-fries include:

• Bean sprouts
• Peppers
• Water chestnuts
• Bok choi
• Carrots
• Peas
• Edamame beans
• Mushrooms
• Shredded cabbage
• Broccoli
• Zucchini

Salads

Salads are primarily made from fresh raw vegetables or fruit, with added cooked meat, fish, seafood, or vegan alternatives. Salads are super versatile and can be eaten as a side dish or a main meal, and you can be creative with the combinations of foods you use. Elevate a basic salad with the addition of a few dried fruits (such as dates, sultanas, or dried figs), raw nuts, or a sprinkling of seeds.

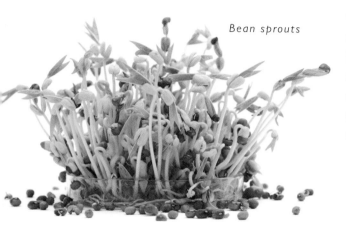

Bean sprouts

Examples of some of the foods that you can add to a salad include:

• Arugula
• Lettuce—add lots of different types and colors
• Watercress
• Avocado
• Celery
• Tomato—a mix of red and yellow tomatoes adds color
• Cucumber
• Radish
• Scallion
• Beet

As a bit of a change, or for a lunch on a colder day, try a warm salad. Cook lentils or mixed beans along with a mix of vegetables such as chopped tomatoes, slices of zucchini, diced onion, chopped peppers, butternut squash, and mixed herbs, and serve with a portion of quinoa or brown rice. Aside from the quinoa or rice, this will freeze, so you could batch-cook more than you need and have extra portions ready to thaw when you need them.

SUPERFOOD SMOOTHIES AND FRUIT JUICES

Drinks such as smoothies and fruit juices are a great way to get a dose of superfoods. If you're not a great fan of eating breakfast, a homemade smoothie can provide you with a portion of nutrients to get your day off to a good start. They're a good option for children too, especially fussy eaters, as all kinds of fruits and vegetables can be added to drinks! By making your own you can be sure of exactly what ingredients are going into the drinks. Take care if you're purchasing ready-made smoothies or juices, as they can have hidden fats and sugars.

In the case of smoothies, you retain the fiber, which can make the drink more filling. Juicing on the other hand doesn't involve the pulp, simply the juice, and results in a very concentrated and nutrient-high drink. It can take a lot of fruit or vegetables to make a small amount, though, and you do need to be aware that juices can have high sugar levels, even when freshly squeezed.

Both smoothies and juices can be garnished with fresh fruits, vegetables, herbs, and spices. Milk, yogurt, tofu, nut milks, or other nondairy alternatives add a creamy texture to smoothies and make them more filling.

There are lots of combinations you can try and we encourage you to be adventurous and creative. Here are some ideas to get you started.

Beet and ginger smoothie
This rich-colored smoothie creates a fruity smoothie with a zingy punch.

1 beet
1 apple
⅔ cup blueberries
1 tablespoon grated fresh ginger
1¼ cups water
Peel and chop the beet and the apple. Add all the ingredients into a blender and blend until smooth.

Matcha green tea smoothie
This smoothie is a great way of using up ripe bananas and can be vegan-friendly, if desired. Add the matcha powder first, before the liquid ingredients, as it will prevent unwanted clumping.

1 ripe banana, fresh or frozen
½ cup milk or dairy-free alternative
½ teaspoon matcha powder
1 teaspoon honey
Put the chopped banana and matcha powder in your blender and combine, then add the milk and honey. Blend until smooth.

Mango lassi
Mango lassi is a drink that originated from northern India and was made following Ayurvedic medicine principles to help aid digestion after a meal. It's similar to a smoothie as it contains milk and yogurt, but the spices add an Indian twist.

3–4 chopped ripe mangoes, either fresh or frozen
2 cups plain natural yogurt
½ cup milk
1 tablespoon runny honey
Juice of 2 limes
Ground cardamom—crush the seeds from 1–2 pods
Crushed or cubed ice

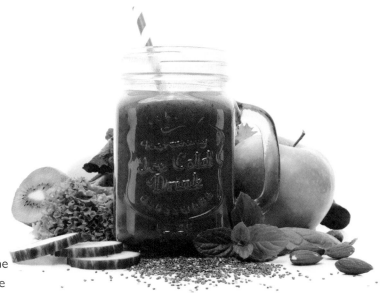

Put the mango, yogurt, milk, honey, and ice into a blender or smoothie maker and blend for up to 2 minutes, or until blitzed. Add the lime juice and the cardamom, then pour the drink into glasses. Sprinkle a tiny pinch of ground cardamom on top to serve. The ice helps the drink become more smoothie-like and it's delicious served cold on a hot day. If you're not a fan of cardamom, try other ground spices such as nutmeg, cinnamon, saffron, or turmeric.

Fresh green juice
This green juice contains nutrient-rich fruits and vegetables and is a light and refreshing drink.

1 cup spinach
Juice of 2 limes
1 cucumber, chopped
A small piece of fresh ginger, finely chopped
1 apple, chopped
Put all the ingredients in your juicer and juice. Add ice if desired. If you don't have a juicer, you could blitz the ingredients in a blender.

Vitamin C booster juice
This tasty juice is packed full of vitamin C, and the mint gives it an extra twist.

4 large kiwi fruits, chopped
1 large apple, chopped
Approximately 1 cup fresh mint
Add all the ingredients to your juicer, then serve with ice.

Apple and blueberry booster
This tasty juice is good to drink when you're feeling tired and need a boost. It contains a good dose of nutrients, including vitamin C, folate, and fiber, plus an interesting twist.

1 apple, chopped
¾ cup blueberries (fresh or frozen)
1 small bulb of fennel, trimmed and cut into pieces
1 teaspoon lemon juice
Put the apple, blueberries, and fennel into your juicer and juice, then stir in the lemon juice.

More combinations to try

Smoothies
Mixed berries • Strawberry, banana, and orange • Carrot, banana, and pineapple • Mango and pineapple • Mango, pineapple, and coconut • Kale, avocado, and lime • Watermelon, apple, and banana • Avocado and mango • Raspberry and coconut • Blueberry and tofu • Fig and honey • Raspberry and lychee

Juices
Lime and basil • Carrot and pineapple • Cucumber, melon, and lime • Orange, lemon, and lime • Watermelon and apple • Spiced apple (try ginger or cinnamon) • Pomegranate, strawberry, and lemon • Spinach, carrot, and kale • Apple and kale

GROWING YOUR OWN SUPERFOODS

Growing your own superfoods is perfect if you love having access to the freshest fruits and vegetables. It also gives you the opportunity to have full control over the growing conditions, ensuring no chemicals or pesticides are added, resulting in fully nutrient-rich foods.

You don't need to have a huge garden to start growing your own food. A small bed of soil will do fine, even in among your flower beds, or you could use pots to grow some produce on your patio or balcony. A window box or hanging basket is sufficient for growing some foods too, such as strawberries.

Preparing your soil

Most fruits and vegetables grow well in soil that's good quality, well drained, rich, and balanced. Ideally it should be a spot in your garden where it's not too shady. Dig over your vegetable patch before planting anything and, if necessary, add some store-bought all-purpose compost to improve the quality.

Growing from seed

The cheapest way to grow your own foods is to sow them from seed. Traditionally, you sow seeds in drills or straight lines. Mark a straight line across the soil and use the end of a garden tool, such as a spade, to make a ridge in the soil where the seeds will be sown. Follow the instructions on the seed packets, as some may need to be sown deeper than others.

The spacing of the seeds is important, so make sure you follow the instructions on this, as if you plant seeds too close together, you'll end up with smaller crops. When all the seeds are planted, push the soil back over the seeds, gently press down the surface, and water the soil. Before you

finish, remember to put a plant marker in to tell you what you've planted and where they are!

Take care when you plant seeds out, as putting them in the ground too early, when they could be prone to frost, will hinder their ability to grow. Some plants, such as tomatoes, bell peppers, and eggplants, are best started off inside in pots, before being transferred to the garden. A few days before you plant them out, it's a good idea to acclimatize them to being outside by putting them out during the day.

Buying plug plants

If you don't want to grow from seed, then you could buy plug plants instead. Plug plants are ready-grown young plants that are at the right stage to be planted in the garden. It's a bit more expensive than growing from seeds, but if you don't have room inside to grow lots of seeds, it can be more convenient. If you're unsure if all your seeds will grow, it's also useful to have the backup of some plug plants.

TIP: Plant marigolds among your vegetables to ward off unwanted pests and attract beneficial insects.

Choosing what to grow

If you're new to growing your own fresh fruits and vegetables, then it's a good idea to opt for easy-to-grow options first. Choose produce that you know you enjoy and will eat, as well as anything that you'd

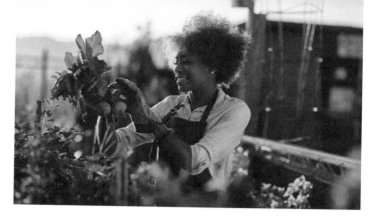

like to try. When you've had a bit of experience, you can move on to something a bit more adventurous. If you're already experienced with gardening, then it's worth considering which superfoods are most expensive or hard to find and focusing on growing them. That way you can save some money and enjoy the experience of growing them yourself.

It's not unusual to find yourself with a glut of one particular crop. So, if you have friends or family who also grow their own, or perhaps have an allotment, then you can share and exchange produce and you can all gain access to a better variety.

Easy vegetables to grow

Some of the easiest vegetables to grow include:

• Zucchini and marrows—look for the compact and bushy varieties, as these are good for containers and small plots.
• Lettuce—small varieties such as Little Gem don't need much space.
• Broad beans—there are dwarf varieties available for small spaces and they have the benefit of not needing to be staked.
• Salad leaves—choose green and purple varieties for the most nutrients; if you keep cutting and eating them, they'll keep growing.
• Cherry tomatoes grow well in baskets and containers, as well as in garden plots.
• Radishes—sow them regularly (for example, every two weeks) so you have a ready supply for salads.
• Potatoes—seed potatoes can be planted in the ground, or in bins or potato bags, half full with compost to start with. When green shoots begin to

appear, cover them over with more soil and repeat until the bag or bin is full. Harvest when the foliage dies back.
• Peas—add canes to support your peas. The more you pick the ripe pods, the more pods will grow. Peas are delicious eaten fresh from the pods.
• Scallions—easy to grow in pots, or in vegetable plots, and perfect to add to salads and stir-fries.
• Runner beans—these climbing beans need support from canes, but grow well throughout the summer.

Easy fruits to grow

• Strawberries grow well in hanging baskets, containers, and window boxes—just make sure the birds don't get them first!
• Raspberries—there are summer and autumn varieties available.
• Blueberries grow well in containers—look for a self-pollinating variety, as these need only one plant to produce fruit.
• Blackberries grow well and don't need much attention or care.
• Goji berries grow well in sunny positions and are rich in nutrients.
• Figs grow against a wall or in containers. The roots of fig plants can spread, so it may be worth planting the roots in a bucket to restrict them.
• Currants—black, red, or white currants are great for making jams and jellies, or adding to fruit salads. Add netting to protect them from birds.
• Apples—ideal if you have a sunny spot in the garden; prune the tree well each winter to encourage crops. Dwarf versions can be grown in pots.

BUYING AND SOURCING SUPERFOODS

Now that you've discovered the benefits of superfoods, here are some ideas for buying and sourcing them so you've always got plenty of choice for meals.

Fresh produce

Where possible, try and source your fresh fruits and vegetables from local growers, as this cuts down on the amount of airmiles and is more sustainable. Town, community, and neighborhood markets or local farm shops are a good place to shop, and will allow you to make contact with local suppliers.

Many places have fruit and vegetable box schemes, where you sign up and have a box of fresh produce delivered every week. Sometimes you're able to customize your choices, while in other cases you get what's available—this provides a nice surprise element that makes you really think about and plan your meals for the week, plus it adds to the variety of foods you eat. It also helps you eat more naturally and in season with fresh produce, a habit that's easily lost when buying from grocery stores.

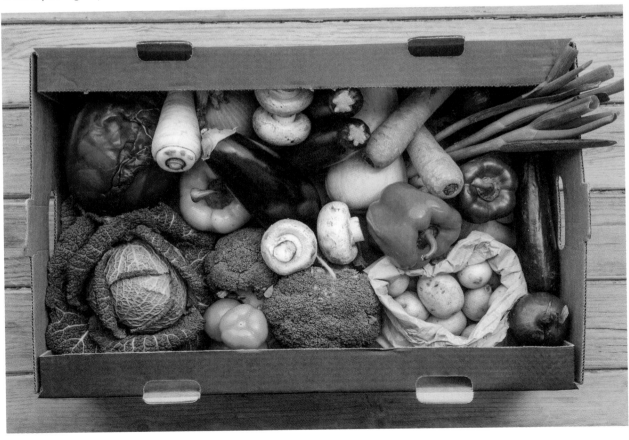

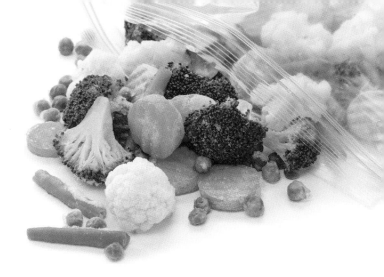

Frozen foods

While fresh is always best, frozen foods are a good alternative, and it's handy and convenient to be able to stock up your freezer with frozen fruits, vegetables, meat, and fish. In general, frozen foods tend to retain most of their nutrients, so they're still a healthy choice. Sometimes salt, sugar, or other flavorings are added to frozen foods, so check the labels to be sure.

Frozen foods allow you easy access to produce that would otherwise be out of season, enabling you to continue getting the key nutrients in your diet. They're also quick and easy to use, as you don't have to spend time peeling, chopping, or preparing; instead, it's just a case of opening a package.

Frozen vegetables are ideal for adding to soups, stews, chilis, casseroles, or to serve as a vegetable side with a variety of meals. Frozen berries, bananas, and other fruits are a useful ingredient to add to smoothies, make desserts with, or serve as fruit salads. If you have your own glut of homegrown produce, or are given windfalls by neighbors, freezing them is a good option.

Frozen fish and meats are useful to have in stock ready to defrost to use for meals. You can buy ready-frozen strips of meat that are useful for a quick stir-fry, or you can buy fresh and freeze it yourself.

Canned foods

Some superfoods are available in canned form too, and it's always useful to have a selection of items in your cupboard at home, ready when needed. Canned fruit and vegetables still count toward one of your five a day and, like frozen foods, most nutrients are preserved. For example, the levels of minerals, protein, and fat-soluble vitamins are relatively the same for canned foods. However, as the method of canning involves a high heat (this helps kill bacteria and improve longevity), some water-soluble vitamins, such as the B vitamins and vitamin C, may be reduced. As a bonus, though, the heating process does result in items such as canned tomatoes having more lycopene—a beneficial antioxidant—than fresh tomatoes. Once foods are canned, they should last on average one to five years, and sometimes longer, so you've got plenty of time to use them!

All sorts of foods are available in cans, including fruits, vegetables, meat, seafood, beans, and coconut milk. Aside from being convenient and involving far less preparation than fresh produce, canned goods also tend to work out cheaper, which is useful if you're on a budget but still want to eat healthily.

How to save money

Some of the more unusual superfoods, or newer and more hyped choices, may end up being expensive to buy and not cost-effective if you're feeding a family. It's always useful to look for discount offers, coupons, or saving vouchers that you could put toward buying the items. Newly released products, for example, often have promotional offers to help sales. Depending on the longevity of the item, you could stock up and freeze the extras for another day.

If practical and you have the space, buying in bulk might help you save money on groceries too.

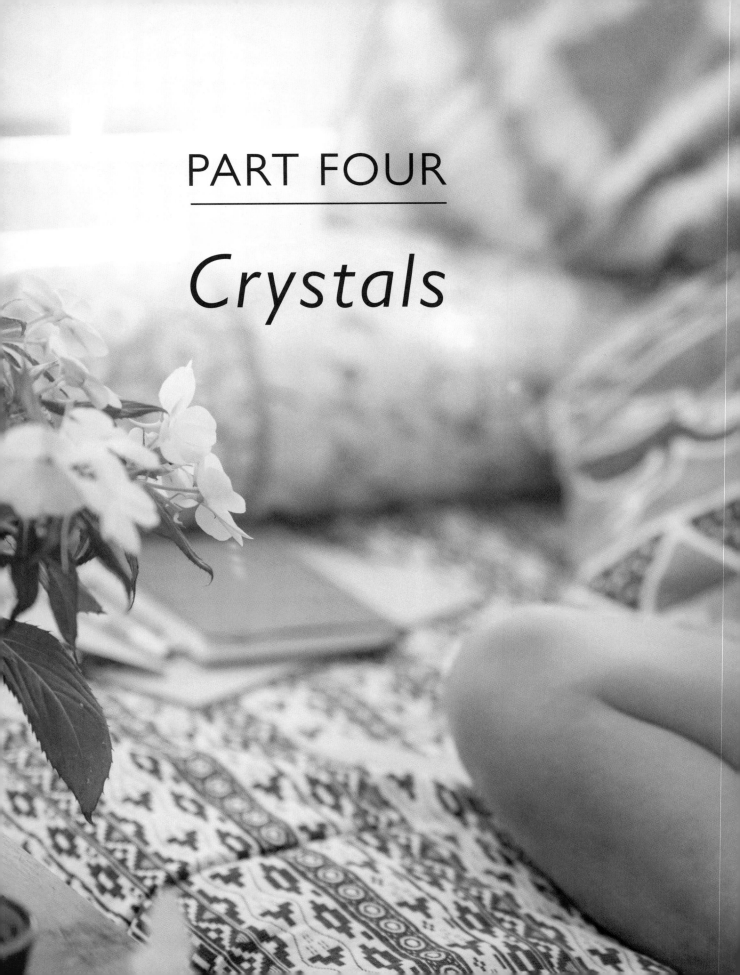

PART FOUR

Crystals

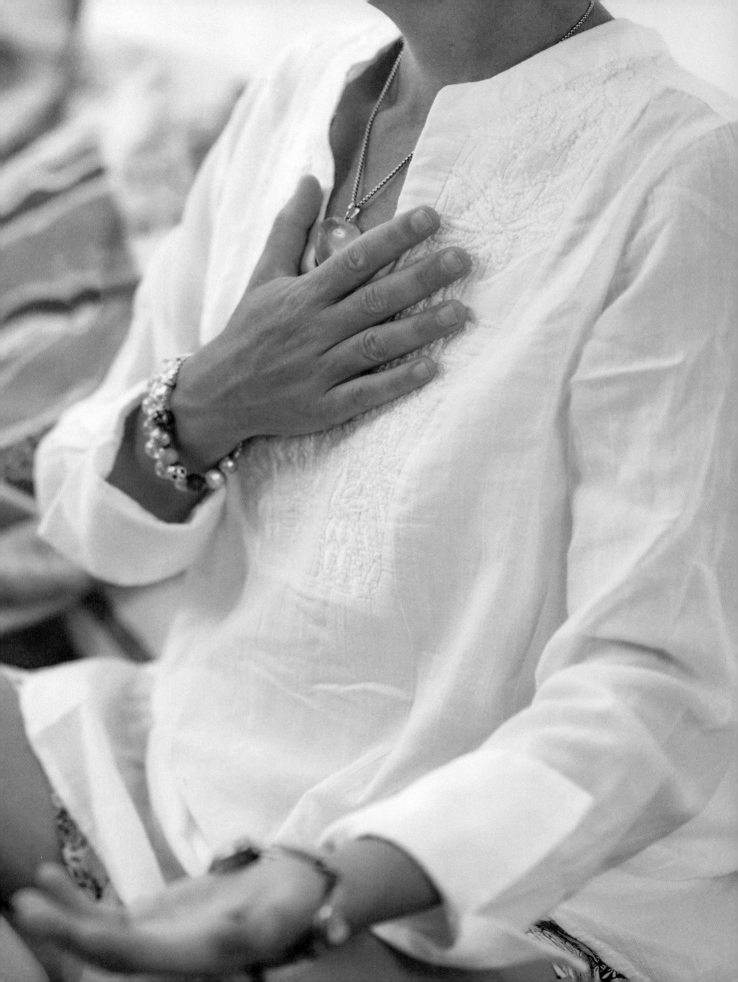

INTRODUCTION TO CRYSTALS

Crystals form in the earth over hundreds and thousands of years and are prized for their beauty, unique qualities, and healing powers. They have been used for centuries in various cultures and traditions, for both decorative and healing purposes. For example, the ancient Egyptians used crystals such as lapis lazuli and turquoise in jewelry; the Romans wore protective amulets made out of crystals; and there's even a mention in the Bible of the High Priest of the Israelites wearing a breastplate studded with crystals. The ancient Greeks rubbed crushed hematite crystals onto the bodies of soldiers to protect them in battle, and in India the Vedas Hinduism scriptures include details of their healing properties as part of Ayurvedic medicine.

Crystals today

As you can see, the idea of harnessing the power of crystals isn't new. Even today, crystals are used in numerous ways that you may be unaware of. In modern technology and medicine, for example, crystals are used for their piezoelectric properties—or the ability to produce electricity and light via compression. Quartz crystals can be found in electronic products such as watches, radios, computer chips, and sonar devices, and they're used in ultrasound machines in hospitals. In terms of health, crystals offer a holistic way of adding an extra dimension to your healing. Used alongside conventional medicine, crystals can help the mind and spirit and provide an uplifting way of rebalancing your well-being.

Understanding crystal vibrations

All crystals have a unique energy or vibration and can absorb, focus, store, transmit, and transmute electromagnetic energy.

Crystals are formed from an organized structure of repeated geometric molecular patterns, and it's this structure that gives them a strong vibration. It's not just crystals that have a vibrational frequency—humans do too. But while the vibration of crystals remains strong, constant, and powerful, due to their unique structure, our vibrations can go up and down and be influenced by a range of factors. For example, your mood and how you feel can be affected on a daily basis by other people, by social media and what's in the news, by your past memories, daily experiences, and a host of other factors. That's one reason why crystals can be so beneficial to use, as the vibration of crystals never ebbs, but always flows.

Of course, this vibration can be dulled by dust, dirt, overuse, and negativity, but cleansing and purifying crystals can bring them back to their full potential. Each crystal has a different type of vibration or frequency. Their energies depend on factors such as the type and color of the crystal, and the size of the piece. It can be hard to get your head around the idea of vibrational frequencies. But as Albert Einstein said, "Everything is energy and that's all there is to it. This is not philosophy. This is physics."

The Romans wore protective amulets made out of crystals.

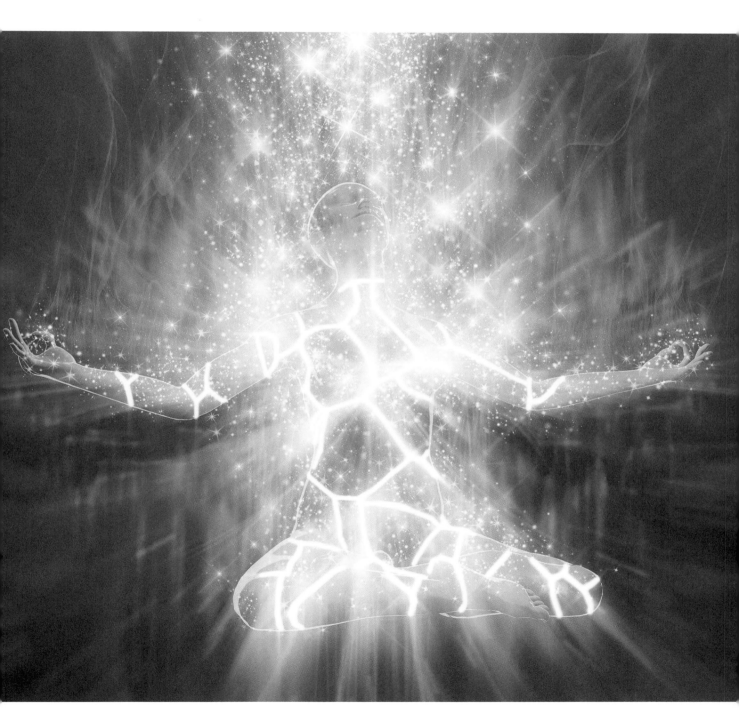

HOW TO USE CRYSTALS FOR HEALING AND HEALTH

Crystals can be used as a form of holistic healing. They're not an alternative to conventional medicine—especially treatments, therapies, or medications prescribed by a doctor—but they can be used alongside it to add an extra dimension of support and healing.

Crystal remedies work differently than conventional medicine, focusing on subtle energies and vibrations, and working on the emotional, mental, and spiritual levels. They can be used to help balance and strengthen the chakras and the aura, which can reflect back on your physical health. There are various ways in which you can use crystals, including:

• Placing crystals directly onto your body, at points of pain or discomfort.
• Placing crystals around your body.
• Wearing crystal jewelry.
• Creating crystal grids or layouts and using the dowsing method over them.
• Placing crystals onto or near your chakras to unblock and rebalance them.
• Making an indirect crystal gem elixir and bathing in it, spraying it around you and your aura, or putting it directly onto your skin.

• Using a crystal wand, point, or crystal egg to gently massage points on your body, such as reflexology or acupuncture points.

Balancing crystals on your own body can be tricky, so they can be temporarily held in place using medical tape. If you're going to try placing crystals directly onto or around your body, aim to keep them in place for a maximum of 10–20 minutes. The energies of crystals are all different, but some can have powerful effects, so it's important not to overuse them without professional advice and guidance. If at any time you feel uncomfortable while using crystals, stop immediately and remove them. Depending on the crystals you've used, you might feel slightly spaced out or tired after using crystal remedies. If possible, take it easy and drink plenty of water to hydrate yourself. If you have any concerns about using crystals, always consult a qualified crystal therapist.

How to choose the right remedy for you

Choosing the right remedy to use isn't always straightforward. Sometimes there are multiple underlying causes of symptoms—some that you're able to identify, and others you're unaware of. A headache, for example, can be caused by eyestrain, alcohol, or stress, so focusing on the underlying cause may be helpful.

When you're choosing which remedy to try, be honest with yourself and think about how the ailment

could have been caused. If your headache is down to stress, try some of the crystals that can be used to ease stress (see page 296). If you have a crystal pendulum, you could use the dowsing method to try to find the right crystal for you.

If you don't find the perfect remedy for your ailment right away, be patient and try again. Not every crystal works in the same way for everyone, and it can be a matter of trial and error to find the

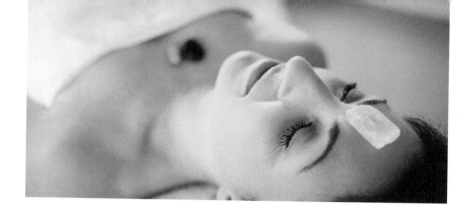

right one for you. Plus, crystals work through subtle vibrations and energies and it's possible you might not immediately notice benefits, but they do become apparent at a later stage.

On the following pages there are some suggestions for crystals that can help common ailments. Each condition included has some of the key crystals listed, along with ways in which they could be used or chakras on which they could be placed.

Crystals work in mysterious ways, so enjoy using them and letting them work their magic on you.

When to seek help from a qualified medical practitioner

Crystals are great to use in conjunction with other treatments, medications, and therapies in a holistic manner, as they can add an extra dimension to mental, spiritual, and emotional healing. But you do need to keep in mind at all times that crystals are not an alternative to conventional medicine and should never be regarded as one. Always consult a qualified medical practitioner first for any health or medical conditions. This is especially so if you:

• Experience sudden, unexpected symptoms for the first time
• Experience new symptoms for an existing condition
• Have an existing condition that suddenly worsens
• Need first-aid treatment
• Are experiencing a medical emergency

• Have sudden pain or discomfort in your chest that doesn't go away
• Experience breathing difficulties
• Have sudden severe pain anywhere in your body that doesn't go away
• Suddenly lose the feeling in your arms or legs for no apparent reason
• Suddenly develop a rash, particularly if it's red-hot, rapidly spreading, and doesn't fade if you press the side of a clear glass against the skin

Always follow any medical advice you've been given by a medical practitioner, take medicines as prescribed, and take a full course of antibiotics, even if the condition seems to improve before the end of the course of medication.

When to seek help from a professional crystal therapist

There are times when making contact with a professional crystal therapist or crystal healer could be beneficial. As a result of their training, they'll have more in-depth knowledge about certain crystals and could have ideas as to treatments, layouts, or grid combinations that could work effectively for you. Some crystals are best used and handled by a professional, as they can potentially be toxic and could cause you more harm than good if you're unaware of their true properties.

Make sure that you ask a crystal therapist in advance what training and qualifications they have, plus how long they've been practicing. Some might use crystals alongside other holistic health treatments. Most professional crystal therapists will charge an hourly fee for a consultation.

THE DOS AND DON'TS OF USING CRYSTALS

As you can see from the previous pages, there are many important factors to keep in mind on your journey with crystals. These considerations should not be ignored and, ultimately, they will only benefit the relationship you have with your crystals, and are key to maintaining your general health and well-being. To summarize some of the important information, here are some useful dos and don'ts to keep in mind as you explore and work with healing crystals:

Do:

• Enjoy experimenting with crystals and learning about the many different types.

• Put crystals in your home, car, and workplace, as it's good to have the energies around you.

• Learn to be guided by intuition and tune in to crystal vibrations when choosing and working with crystals.

• Remain positive and open-minded when working with crystals; the results may surprise you.

• Make indirect crystal gem elixirs, as they offer a safe way of harnessing the power of crystals.

• Remember to cleanse and purify your crystals after use. This keeps them in tip-top condition and ensures all negative energies are removed.

• Take care to look after delicate crystals, as some can be more fragile than others.

• Reach out for additional help and advice from a crystal therapist or medical practitioner when you need it.

Don't:

• Use crystal remedies for serious conditions before seeing a medical practitioner.

• Use crystals as an alternative to proper first-aid treatment.

• Rely on the crystals to heal all physical, mental, or emotional ailments.

• Give up—if one crystal doesn't work for you, try another one.

• Worry about the size of crystals or not being able to afford large specimens—even small stones can be powerful!

• Abandon prescribed medications or therapies in favor of only using crystals instead—they work better in harmony with other treatments, rather than as an alternative.

• Leave small crystals in accessible places if you have children or animals in your home—they should not be put in mouths or swallowed.

• Leave crystals unattended in direct sunlight— they run the risk of being a fire hazard if the direct rays of the sun shine onto them.

It's not just crystals that have a vibrational frequency—humans do too.

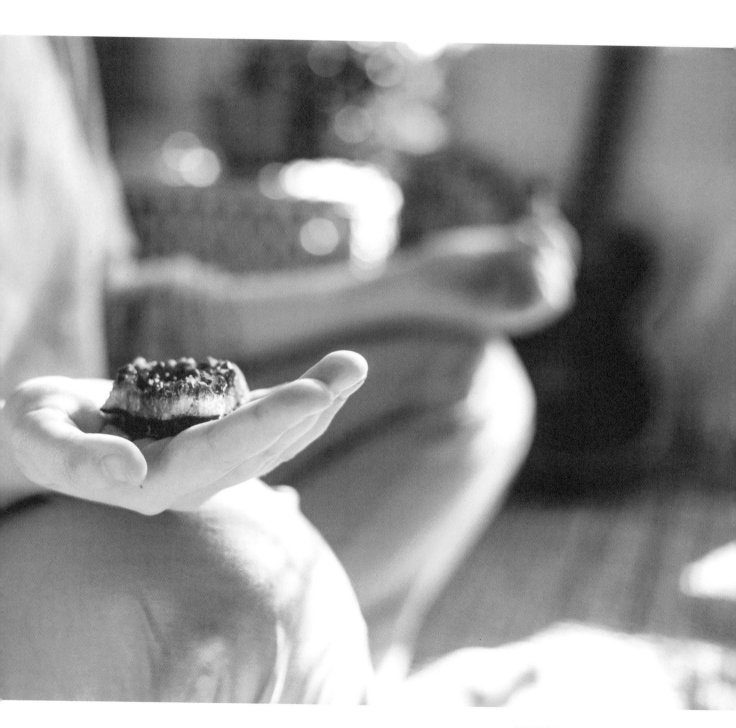

MAKING CRYSTAL ELIXIRS

Experienced crystal healers and therapists may sometimes make crystal elixirs, which can be applied externally to the skin or, in some cases, consumed. Crystal elixirs are made in two main ways: indirectly and directly. The indirect method, which is the safest and recommended way to try, involves filling a large glass bowl with water (ideally pure spring water), then placing a smaller glass bowl containing the crystals into the larger bowl.

Once the crystal bowl is inside the water bowl, it should be left for a few hours. The idea is that the water will become infused with the healing vibrations of the crystals. If you wish, you can cover the bowl with plastic wrap or a glass lid and place it outside in the moonlight or sunlight.

When the crystals have finished infusing, you can decant the water into a bottle to use for healing purposes. A dropper glass bottle made from colored glass is useful, or you could fill a spray bottle.

How to use crystal elixirs

Indirectly made crystal elixirs are best used freshly made. You can use your homemade elixirs in number of ways:

• By putting a few drops (4–6 drops) of the water under your tongue every few hours.
• By directly dabbing a few drops of the water onto your skin. (Note: if you have sensitive skin, do a small patch test first.)

• By spraying the water around you, to clear and clean your aura or to banish unwanted negative energies from a room.
• By adding the crystal elixir to a bath.

If you visit a professional crystal healer, they may prescribe a crystal elixir that will last for a longer period. This is because the elixir will be preserved in alcohol, such as brandy or vodka.

Crystal elixirs—direct method safety warning

The direct method of making a crystal elixir involves immersing crystals into water directly.

As tempting as it may be to try this approach, it's very important not to attempt making direct method crystal elixirs without having been properly and professionally trained in crystal healing. This is especially so in the case of crystal elixirs that are consumed, as well as those that are applied directly onto your skin.

Not all crystals are capable or safe to be made into elixirs. For example, some crystals don't react well when they come into contact with water. More importantly, some crystals—such as dragon's blood, which contains lead, and malachite, which has traces of copper—contain toxic elements. The toxicity can be transferred into the water and could be highly dangerous and poisonous if consumed.

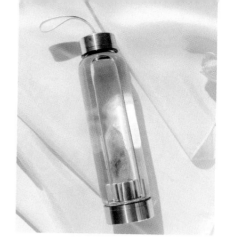

Special crystal water bottles

Look for specially designed crystal water bottles, which can provide a great alternative to the indirect method. These bottles are usually made of plastic or glass and look very much like a normal water bottle. However, they are designed with a special inner compartment where small crystals can be placed.

The main bottle is then filled with water and it can be drunk from safely, as there is no direct contact between the crystals and the water. Most bottles are sold complete with the right-sized crystals to place in the compartment, such as quartz, rose quartz, and citrine.

Essential crystal self-care toolkit

As a beginner, it can be hard to know which crystals are best to buy first, especially when there's such a range of choices out there. Plus, buying lots of crystals can become expensive. Tumbled crystals are great for beginners, so if you're just starting out, here are some ideas for a basic self-care crystal toolkit.

• Amethyst—a stone that soothes and balances, and also amplifies the energy of other crystals. Useful for times of stress or worry.
• Black tourmaline—an essential stone to help keep you grounded in any crystal work.
• Blue lace agate—calm and soothing, blue lace agate is a gentle stone to work with.
• Carnelian—an energizing and stimulating crystal that's useful for chakra balancing.
• Citrine—useful for attracting all forms of wealth into your life, as well as to dispel anxiety.
• Clear quartz—for purifying, healing, and balancing. Use with the higher chakras to open the mind.
• Green aventurine—a good stone to encourage spontaneity, making time for others, and for chakra work.
• Lapis lazuli—a beautiful blue stone that helps promote communication and openness.

• Moonstone—a calming stone for times of emotional stress and a useful aid for a good night's sleep.
• Obsidian—good for helping you find direction and having the courage to do so. Useful for the root chakra.
• Red jasper—a good stone to help enhance the spiritual in your life and for working with the chakras.
• Rose quartz—a soothing stone of love that's good for all types of relationships and helping you love yourself more.

This selection of crystals gives you a good balance of different colors, so you could use them to work with the chakras. They're all easy stones to get used to, with many having calming and relaxing energies. If you can afford to buy multiples of one type of crystal, always choose clear quartz, as this is used on grid layouts to help amplify the effect of other crystals.

An extra you might like to consider is selenite—either a piece, small slab, or bowl made from selenite. Selenite has the natural ability to cleanse and charge other crystals, so this can be very useful to have as a beginner.

PURIFYING AND PROGRAMMING CRYSTALS

Purifying your crystals

In order for your crystals to be in prime condition for use, you'll need to purify and cleanse them first. This is especially important when you first buy crystals, or after you've been using them for a while. Purifying crystals helps rejuvenate their energy and remove negativity, as well as revive their color, sparkle, and shine.

There are several methods you can use to purify crystals:

• Running water—hold your crystals under running water for a few minutes, then leave them to dry naturally or pat dry with a towel.
• Still water—place your crystals in a bowl of still water. As an optional extra, add a teaspoon of salt. Leave them to cleanse for up to an hour.
• Sunlight—place your crystals in sunlight to purify them. Be aware that some crystals, such as quartz, could be a fire risk if left in direct sunlight, even on a windowsill, so avoid leaving them unattended.
• Moonlight—place your crystals outside or on a windowsill to charge them by moonlight. This is especially good in the light of a full or new moon.
• Incense—burn incense sticks, such as sandalwood, or a traditional sage smudge stick, and let the smoke waft over your crystals to purify them.
• Earth—bury your crystals overnight in soil (outside in your garden or inside in a plant pot) to help them reconnect with the earth.

CAUTION

Some crystals, such as selenite, fluorite, calcite, and azurite, are water soluble, so are not suitable for water cleansing. As a general rule, any crystals that are rated five or below on the Mohs' hardness scale should not come into contact with water. Plus, crystals that contain minerals such as hematite and magnetite should not be purified with water as they contain iron ore and iron oxide, which will rust when in contact with water.

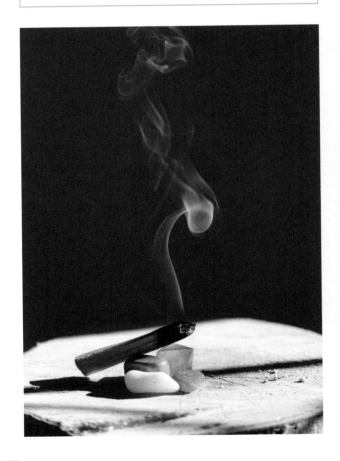

Programming your crystals

Once your crystals are purified and cleansed, it's time to program them. The idea of programming your crystals is that you're getting them ready for the special purpose you want them to serve. Each crystal has its own individual strengths and abilities, and some can have more than one benefit.

By programming a crystal, you clearly set your intention for the specific purpose for which you want to use the stone. Programming helps the crystal energies to focus on specific intentions, goals, or desires, which is said to enhance its vibrations, ability, and power.

Step-by-step guide to programming crystals
First, spend a few quiet moments holding each crystal and connecting to its energy. Look at its color and appearance, touch it, and notice how it feels in your hands. You can do this as part of a mindfulness or meditation exercise if you wish.

Next, set your positive intention for how you want to use the crystal. Choose one specific intention or purpose for your crystal. For example, if you want to use a crystal to help attract prosperity into your life, state that. If you're seeking help with dealing with a health condition, be specific about the exact condition or symptoms. Form the intention into a single sentence—you may find it helpful to write this down. Once you have your sentence, say it out loud while holding the crystal. For example, a quartz crystal can be beneficial for dispersing negativity and helping you feel more energized. So, you could program a quartz crystal with the words "I program this crystal to boost my energy and disperse negativity from my life."

In the case of a citrine crystal, which is associated with manifesting abundance, you could program it with the words "I program this crystal to manifest more money into my life."

Repeat the process and reprogram your crystals frequently, especially before and after using them.

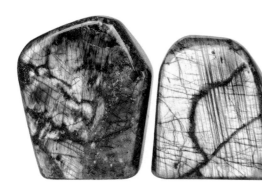
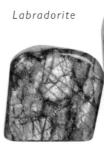

Labradorite

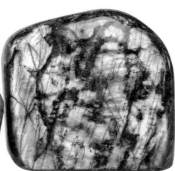

CRYSTAL LAYOUTS AND THE CHAKRAS

You can use crystal layouts to effectively treat and rebalance your chakras. One of the benefits of crystal layouts, especially if you're new to working with crystals and subtle energy healing, is that they work on all the chakras at once. The chakras are interdependent, so if one chakra is out of balance, it can affect all of the others too.

A crystal layout is, as the name suggests, simply a way of laying out your crystals. In this case, crystals that correspond with each of the chakras are placed on or around your body.

Basic chakra body layout

For this chakra body layout you'll need to lie down. So, first find a quiet and comfortable place on the floor or on a bed and lie flat on your back. If it's chilly, get a blanket to keep you warm and turn off your cell phone so you're not disturbed. If you're not comfortable with complete silence, find some calming music to have on in the background. Dim the lights and have essential oils or scented candles burning in the background.

There's no set time limit for how long you should do your crystal layout—anything from 5 to 20 minutes is sufficient. But the longer you practice, the more you're likely to feel the benefits. As a beginner, it's helpful to note down how it makes you feel and whether there are any particular areas of your body that feel different afterward. It will help you get to know how you respond to certain crystals.

Chakra crystal layout

You'll need to choose seven crystals that represent the colors of each of the chakras. If you don't have many crystals, use what you have available. However, a good starting point for a chakra crystal layout includes crystals such as:

• Root chakra—smoky quartz, red jasper, black tourmaline, bloodstone.
• Sacral chakra—carnelian, orange calcite.
• Solar plexus chakra—citrine, yellow calcite, yellow jasper.
• Heart chakra—rose quartz, green aventurine.
• Throat chakra—blue lace agate, angelite, lapis lazuli, turquoise.
• Third eye chakra—amethyst, sodalite, iolite.
• Solar plexus chakra—clear quartz, moonstone, selenite.

Once you have chosen your seven crystals, lay them out on and around your body as follows:

• Root chakra—place the crystal on the floor or bed, between your legs.
• Sacral chakra—place the crystal between your hip bones.
• Solar plexus chakra—place the crystal between your lower ribs and belly button.
• Heart chakra—place the crystal in the middle of your chest, level with your heart.
• Throat chakra—place the crystal on your throat.
• Third eye chakra—place the crystal in the middle of your forehead, between your eyebrows.
• Crown chakra—place the crystal on the floor or pillow, by the top of your head.

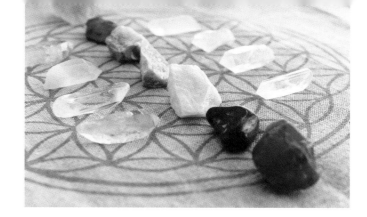

If you're worried about the crystals falling off, you may wish to use surgical tape to gently stick them in place while you're performing the layout.

When the crystals are in place, close your eyes, relax, breathe deeply, and allow the crystals to do their work. You might find it beneficial to say an affirmation to confirm to the crystals that you're open to healing. For example, you could say, "I am open to the healing power of these crystals."

Creating crystal grids

Crystal grids are a special technique you can use to amplify the power of crystals. A grid is an arrangement of crystals in a geometric pattern that is designed with a particular intention in mind. When a selection of crystals is brought together and used in a grid, the individual energetic properties of the crystals are magnified, producing a more powerful effect. Some simple grids to start with include:

• A circle, with one focus crystal in the center. A circle grid represents unity, wholeness, and protection.

• A square, with one crystal in the center and four more positioned in each corner of the square shape. A square grid can be beneficial for helping set and maintain boundaries.

• A triangle, with one crystal in the center and three more on the points of the triangle. A triangle grid shape helps represent structure and order.

• A spiral-shaped grid, which represents reaching out, expanding, and growing.

• A five-stone cross grid, with one crystal in the center, and the other four around it, positioned in the north, south, east, and west points. This can be used to enhance physical and spiritual connections.

The key to a successful grid is to choose the appropriate grid layout, a clear purpose, and the right crystals to achieve this.

How to use your crystal grid

To set up your crystal grid, follow these steps:

• Set your intention for the grid. For example, do you want to focus on creating energy, building emotional strength, or improving communication?

• Select a focus stone suitable for the outcome you're seeking, plus some active or anchor crystals for the key points on the grid. Additional stones can be added as amplifiers between the main crystals.

• Choose a grid layout and decide where you're going to position it. Ideally, it needs to be located where it won't be disturbed but is easily accessible.

• Cleanse and purify your crystals using a method of your choice (see page 260).

• Start by placing your focus crystal in the center of your grid, then add the active stones in their positions. Finally, add any amplifiers between them.

If you've set a clear intention for your grid, it should start to function as soon as it is laid out. But you can make it more powerful by activating all the crystals.

• Use a clear quartz crystal wand and move it clockwise in a small circle over the central stone, while stating your intention for the grid. Repeat the action on the active crystals, going back to the focus stone after each active crystal. You may be able to feel subtle energy changes as you move over each stone.

MEDITATING WITH CRYSTALS

Meditating with crystals is an ideal way to get to know your crystals and learn to attune to their energy. Meditation is the practice of sitting quietly and stilling the mind. Small crystals can be held in your hand while you meditate, while larger crystals can be placed in front of you to look at and meditate on.

Meditation is accessible for anyone—you don't need any specialty training to do it (although you can learn it via classes if you wish). You just need to find some time to yourself where you can sit quietly, breathe deeply, and be calm. Think about whether you could make meditation part of your regular self-care routine, as regular practice can be beneficial.

Getting started

Before you meditate, cleanse and purify the crystal you're going to use. Set the mood by turning off your cell phone so you're not disturbed, then find somewhere warm and comfortable to sit. If you sit on a chair, have your back straight and feet flat on the floor.

Start by closing your eyes and taking a few deep breaths, then breathe slowly for 2–3 minutes. Hold your crystal in your hands and state your intention to connect with it.

As you hold your crystal, let your body and mind attune to the subtle vibrations of the crystal. Use the time to soak up the crystal energies. You might feel sensations in your hands, see colors in your mind, hear sounds, or receive messages.

Sit holding the crystal for as long as you feel comfortable, then thank it for connecting to you. When you finish, jot down a note of how you felt.

It can take time and practice to learn to quieten and still your mind, and it's not a skill that comes naturally to everyone, so be patient. Remember, though, there's no right or wrong way to meditate.

Crystals to meditate with

Any type of crystal can be used to meditate with, especially when you're getting to know a new stone. However, there are some crystals that are naturally regarded as being ideal meditation companions.

Clear quartz—associated with the crown chakra, it is a good balancing crystal to use for meditation; ideal for beginners. Quartz can help you maintain balance, raise your vibrations, and open up to energies.

Selenite—like clear quartz, selenite is also associated with the crown chakra. This calming and cleansing crystal can help to clear your mind and improve your clarity. Try starting the day with a selenite crystal meditation.

Rose quartz—this pink stone is associated with the heart chakra and has properties of love, compassion, and forgiveness. It can help promote feelings of peace and love as you meditate.

Amethyst—an amethyst crystal is associated with the third eye chakra and is a good crystal to meditate with if you're seeking to boost your

Enjoy the chance to sit and spend some time with a crystal in your hand.

intuition. The calming and healing properties can promote inner peace and reduce stress. Try ending the day with an amethyst meditation.

Smoky quartz—associated with the root chakra, smoky quartz is a good choice to use if you want to feel more balanced. If you're stressed, this crystal can help promote feelings of grounding, plus it can dispel negative energy.

Mindfulness with crystals

If you find meditation tricky, try mindfulness instead. Rather than trying to clear and empty your mind of thoughts (which often causes more thoughts to appear!), hold a crystal and focus on the stone. Explore the size and shape of it, look at its structure, angles, and facets, learn how it feels in your hand, and see how the light shines through it. Enjoy the chance to sit and spend some time with a crystal in your hand. Observe how it makes you feel and how you feel about the crystal. Do this regularly with all your stones, and you may find that you feel more at one with all of them. Practicing mindfulness is a great way to get to know your crystals better and to inspire you as to how you could use them more for healing and crystal layout work.

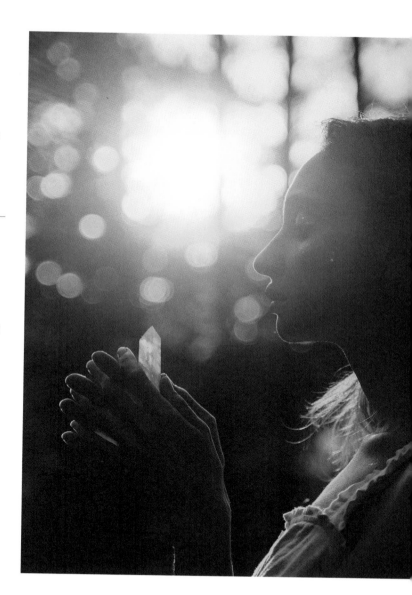

CREATING A CRYSTAL ALTAR FOR YOUR HOME

A crystal altar is a sacred space where you can display your favorite crystals, healing tools, and other items that have special meaning for you. It is the ideal place to put the crystals that you're currently working with, or have set intentions for, and to sit near when you're meditating or practicing mindfulness.

Altars have featured for centuries in religious, spiritual, and cultural belief systems, but today they're a sacred space used for much more. You might like to think of your altar as reminiscent of a 3D vision board—a display that will inspire, uplift, and motivate you when you look at and interact with it.

There's no right or wrong way to create a crystal altar. First, simply find a free space to use, such as a windowsill, shelf, mantlepiece, empty fireplace, or tabletop. Ideally, it should be a location where it won't be disturbed, and you can leave it permanently set up. Clean and clear the space, so it's clutter- and dust-free.

Next, choose the crystals you'd like to display on your altar and cleanse and program them. It could be the crystals you're currently working with, your favorite gems, or larger display pieces, such as chunks of amethyst, rose quartz, or agate geodes.

Also, think about other items you'd like to include, such as shells, flowers, pinecones, acorns, pebbles, driftwood, favorite quotes, photos, or pieces of artwork that you find inspirational. Take time to place your chosen crystals and items on your altar until you're happy with how they look.

Once your crystal altar is created, enjoy it! Sit by it, light some candles, meditate, connect with the crystals, and soak in the energies. It's your special place.

Crystal pendulums and other crystal rituals

A pendulum is a divination and dowsing tool that consists of a symmetrical, weighted object hung from a cord—specially cut crystals can be used for this purpose.

Using a pendulum enables you to tap into your intuition and higher guidance and get answers to simple yes or no questions, such as which crystals to use in grids or layouts, how long to leave them in place, or what chakras need rebalancing. The idea is that the crystal pendulum acts as a receiver and transmitter of information and moves in response to your questions. It's often described as being like bringing together the rational and intuitive sides of you—or the left and right brain—so that you can make well-rounded decisions.

Cleansing and programming your pendulum
Any crystal can be used as a pendulum, but a good starting point is clear quartz. First, you'll need to cleanse and purify your crystal, then charge it with your own energy. To do this, simply hold the crystal in your hands, sit quietly, and state your intention to

charge the crystal with your energy. If you like, say a prayer or ask spirit guides or guardian angels for their support and guidance. A short meditation while holding the pendulum can also help attune you to its energy.

The pendulum works by moving in certain directions—small circles or side to side. In order to understand and use your pendulum effectively, you'll need to ascertain which movement represents a yes answer and which a no. Hold your pendulum cord between your thumb and forefinger, with any excess cord wrapped lightly around your index finger. Still the pendulum by running your hand down the length of the cord, bringing it to rest with the tip of the crystal in the upturned palm of your hand.

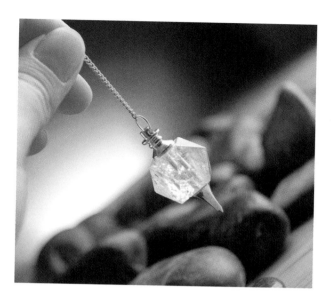

How to use your pendulum

Start by asking a simple question with an easy yes or no answer. For example, "Is my name X?" Relax and watch the pendulum move. Be patient—the first time you do this, you might need to repeat this step several times before you're sure of the response. You may find your pendulum moves in clockwise circles for yes and back and forth for no, but everyone is different and the way it moves may be unique to you. If at any time the pendulum moves in an indistinct way, then it might be a signal of a "maybe" answer. Try again with a more specific question and see if you can achieve a definite response.

Once you've ascertained how the pendulum moves in response to yes or no, try it again with another question. Be sincere about what you ask and treat your pendulum with respect.

Crystal rituals

Many crystal aficionados have crystal rituals they use to enhance various areas of their life. Rituals needn't be complex—just spending a few minutes a day to stop, connect, and set intentions can be beneficial. Here are some examples of popular crystal rituals:

• Sleep ritual—hold a celestite crystal before you go to bed to clear your mind, prepare your body for sleep, and enhance a calm state.

• Home-protection ritual—black tourmaline has energetic shielding properties. Place a piece of tourmaline inside your front door, or outside in a sheltered porch, and imagine it forming a protective shield around your house.

• Stress-release ritual—hold blue lace agate stones in each hand and state the intention that it will release stress and fill your body with calming vibes.

• Manifestation ritual—hold a piece of citrine and set it with the intention to promote manifestation of prosperity into your life. Also try putting small citrine tumbled stones in your wallet to promote wealth.

CREATING CRYSTAL CHARGING STATIONS

Some crystals have a unique ability to purify other crystals. For example, crystals can be placed onto selenite to become purified. Look for selenite carved in the form of round plates, long bars, or bowls, as these are designed so that you simply place your crystals onto or into them and leave them to purify.

If you have a crystal geode or a crystal cluster, such as quartz, you can place your crystals on or inside them for cleansing. Carnelian is also a good purifying crystal. Keep a piece of carnelian in a bag of tumbled gemstones to keep them cleansed and purified, ready for use.

Create your own crystal purifier

One nice idea that is not only practical but also looks really attractive as a decorative accessory in your home is to create your own crystal-purifying station.

Find a suitable empty, clean glass container to use, such as a round bowl or an empty terrarium (normally used for plants) and fill the base with Himalayan pink salt. Himalayan salt is a form of fossilized sea salt, which has traces of minerals in it that gives it a delicate pink color. Salt is traditionally used for purification purposes and it can work as a means of cleansing crystals too.

Once you have a good layer of salt in the base

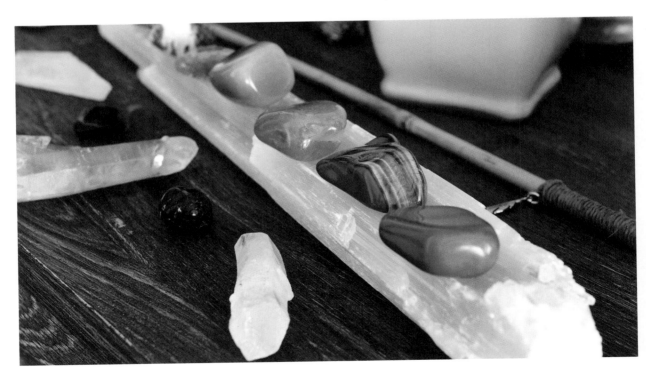

Take care not to place your purifying station in direct sunlight.

of your container, place your chosen crystals inside, onto the salt, to purify and recharge. Position your charging station where you can see it and where you can access your crystals easily when you need to.

Take care not to place your purifying station in direct sunlight, though, as the crystals could catch the sun's rays and become a fire risk.

Cleaning and caring for crystals

Crystals that are out on display in your home or regularly in use will inevitably get dusty. In addition to your crystal-purifying practices, it's a good idea to clean crystals in other ways to help keep them in good condition.

For example, dust is drawn to collect on the surface of crystal clusters and geodes, such as quartz, citrine, or amethyst, and can get between the points. If the dust is left there, over time you'll notice the color and shine of the crystal has dulled, plus it won't be as powerful for healing purposes. Crystals can also pick up sticky residues—for example, from sprays or perfumes.

Crystal points and tumblestones can easily be cleaned with a duster—simply wipe clean the surface. For crystal clusters, use a small brush such as a toothbrush, paintbrush, or makeup brush to remove excess dirt and dust. Any sticky residue can be wiped off with a damp cloth.

Storing your crystals

It's lovely to keep some crystals out where you can see and admire their beauty, whether at home or work. But if you're building up a large collection of different crystals for healing purposes, you're likely to need to think about storage options too.

Crystals can be delicate, so it's important not to put them all together loose in one bag or box, where they could knock against each other. You don't want your treasured stones becoming cracked, broken, or damaged.

As a rule of thumb, crystals that are rated hard on the Mohs' scale shouldn't be stored loose with softer stones.

Look for storage boxes that are split into compartments or consider wrapping your delicate crystals in tissue paper, bubble wrap, or fabric.

You could arrange your crystals alphabetically, by color, by shape, or by purpose—the choice is yours.

CHOOSING AND BUYING CRYSTALS

The practicalities of buying crystals

When it comes to buying crystals, ideally the best method is to choose them in person. This enables you to look at the array of crystals available, touch and feel the crystals, sense their energies, and use your intuition to feel which crystals are calling at you to buy them.

Look for specialty crystal stores, or fairs or events near you, and go along to buy your crystals. It might help to equip yourself with a shopping list of crystals you're interested in, as this can target your buying and prevent you from getting carried away with spending! Though you should always be aware of crystals that are cheap—they may be cheap for a reason and come from nonethical sources (see "Ethical considerations," right).

If you can't find any specialty crystal stores in your area, the next best option is to buy online or by mail order. There are a variety of specialty websites selling online, and you may find that you get more choice and better access to rarer crystals by purchasing in this way.

Many specialty online crystal retailers are passionate about their job, going the extra mile with providing exact photographs of the crystals you're buying, rather than just a general image of ones you might receive. This can help considerably with giving you a clear idea of what you're purchasing. It's also worth looking for websites that use videos to share their crystals or sell via social media, such as Instagram or Facebook live events, as such experiences provide a more personal shopping style.

If you're unsure which crystals to purchase, why not try using your pendulum to dowse? Use it in front of, or over, a picture of a crystal and be guided as to whether it's right for you or not. Sometimes the results may be surprising, but you may later discover why that crystal was right at that particular time.

Ethical considerations

Sadly, not all mines around the world operate ethically. There are issues regarding how the crystals are mined, whether they are regulated or not, and how workers are treated. In a world where ethical issues are increasingly high on the agenda, it's good to factor in these concerns when you're buying and working with crystals.

Mining practices

In the case of diamonds, an international certification scheme exists to ensure that standards are met in the mining process, giving consumers knowledge when they buy. As yet, there's nothing similar for crystal mining, but perhaps there should be.

Mining practices across the world differ to a huge degree, and it's often very hard to know exactly how the crystals you're buying were obtained. Though some countries do have regulations in place, such as the Fair Labor Standards Act (FLSA) in the United States, so you can be assured that if you buy gemstones sourced in the United States, the miners should have been treated well.

Crystal miners

Some of the countries rich in crystals are relatively poor, so don't have the ability to mine with machinery, maintain good work conditions, or pay appropriate wages.

For example, in countries such as Madagascar,

> *A reputable seller who cares about ethics will do their best to source their products with care.*

where the earth is abundant with crystals such as tourmaline, citrine, labradorite, carnelian, rose quartz, and amethyst, the majority of mining is done by hand, rather than by machine. There are some reputable mines, but others are less so and, as a result, many of the workers are paid minimal fees for backbreaking work and long hours.

Ask before you buy

If you're concerned about where your crystals come from and whether they were ethically mined, look for companies that specify details about where the crystals they sell are obtained from.

A reputable seller who cares about ethics will do their best to source their products with care. They'll build relationships with their suppliers, and maybe even individual mines, and be happy to share their knowledge with their customers.

Some sellers will give details about the country and area the crystal originated in, while others will give specific details about exactly which mine it was from. The more details available for you to peruse when purchasing, the better informed you'll be about whether the crystals you're buying are ethically sourced, and the easier your choice will be.

You can ask for details at crystal stores in person, or online. If you're not keen on buying crystals online (many people like to hold them first) and don't have a store near you, look for gemstone fairs and events, where you can meet numerous sellers and select the ones that have the best ethical practices.

DIY crystal hunting

Another way to be sure of where your crystals have come from is to hunt for them yourself!

This doesn't mean randomly digging for crystals wherever you are, but rather going to a commercial mine where you can pay to hunt for crystals. There are various mines offering this service in the United States and it can be a fascinating insight into the process involved, as well as highly rewarding when you find your own crystals.

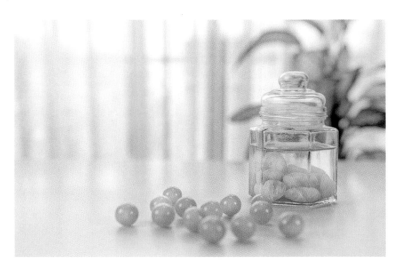

A TO Z OF CRYSTALS

AMAZONITE

APPEARANCE This green-blue or green mineral is often found as prisms, chunks, or tumbled stones. It ranges from translucent to opaque.

RARITY Sources of amazonite include Russia, Mongolia, China, South Africa, and the United States. It may be bought as cabochons, carvings, and jewelry.

FORMATION Amazonite is a potassium feldspar, its main ingredients being potassium, silicon, aluminum, and oxygen. Its color is formed from a complex combination of traces of other elements, including possibly lead, copper, rubidium, and iron.

ATTRIBUTES Amazonite soothes the mind, spirit, and body; easing stress, emotional turmoil, and intrusive or circular thoughts. It encourages us to find respite in our day, taking time to meditate, breathe, or walk in the fresh air. It also helps us to talk about our worries—and find the right people to share them with.

HEALING ACTION Amazonite is considered safe to handle, but observe the precautions below. Hold over the throat chakra to voice your fears and anxieties both calmly and freely. Meditate with amazonite to find relief from stress or a whirring, too-busy mind.

CARE Keep amazonite away from children and pets. Amazonite contains traces of lead and copper, both of which are toxic. Do not use in gem elixirs or breathe in dust. Wash hands after handling. Amazonite scores 6–6.5 on the Mohs' scale. Clean in warm, soapy water with a soft cloth.

AMBER

APPEARANCE Usually golden-yellow to red-brown, smooth, and translucent. It can contain plant or animal material, such as ancient insects.

RARITY Common sources of amber include Kaliningrad, Russia; Kachin, Myanmar; and the Dominican Republic.

FORMATION Amber is not a mineral: it is fossilized tree resin. Millions of years ago, resin-coated logs—sometimes with insects trapped in the sticky resin—were carried by rivers to coastal deltas, where they were buried by sediment. Over time, the amber and the surrounding sediment hardened.

ATTRIBUTES Amber's warming, brightening energy helps us to find joy in the everyday. It encourages loyalty and partnership, strengthening our bonds with the people who are most important to us, whether they are friends, children, or life partners. For those who feel prickly or insecure in social situations, it encourages friendliness and affability. Some say that amber eases problems of the bladder and kidneys.

HEALING ACTION If you are suffering from low mood, meditate with amber regularly. Wear amber jewelry to feel open and at ease in the company of others. To strengthen your bond with a life partner, place in the love and marriage corner of the house, which is at the back right if you enter by the front door.

CARE Amber has a hardness of just 2–2.5 on the Mohs' scale, so it should be protected from scratches. Avoid extremes of heat and prolonged exposure to sunlight. Wipe clean with a damp, soft cloth. Do not soak. Do not use in gem elixirs.

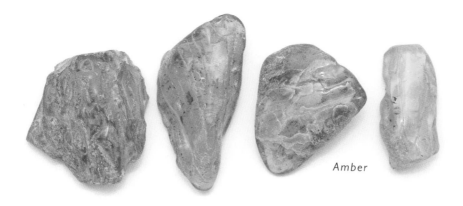

Amber

AMETHYST

APPEARANCE Amethyst is a variety of the mineral quartz that ranges from pale lavender to deep purple. It grows as six-sided prisms ending in six-sided pyramids. It is also often found as geodes, which are clusters of small crystals that grow within hollow spherical rocks.

RARITY Prior to the 1700s, amethyst was considered a precious stone. Today, after numerous deposits were found in Brazil, South Korea, the United States, and elsewhere, it is priced as a semiprecious stone.

FORMATION Clear quartz is made of silicon and oxygen, but amethyst is tinted by natural irradiation and impurities of iron and other transition metals. Geodes form when cavities in volcanic rock are filled with hydrothermal fluid rich in silicon and oxygen.

ATTRIBUTES Like all varieties of quartz, amethyst is an amplifier of energy. However, this variety is also soothing and balancing. It calms overactive, overstressed, and overworked minds. It eases the heart at times of grief and loss. Some crystal therapists claim that amethyst can help rejuvenate the body during convalescence.

HEALING ACTION To ease a stressed or busy mind, place at the crown chakra. To relieve stress or to recover from loss, wear as a pendant, earrings, or ring. Sleep with an amethyst geode by the bed to help with insomnia, night waking, and troubled dreams.

CARE Amethyst scores 7 on the Mohs' scale, which makes it suitable for regular wear as jewelry. However, its color can fade if it is overexposed to light. Do not inhale amethyst dust, which can cause silicosis. Clean in warm, soapy water with a soft cloth.

AMETRINE

APPEARANCE Ametrine, also known as trystine or bolivianite, is a combination of amethyst and citrine, which are both tinted varieties of quartz. While citrine ranges from yellow to orange to brown, amethyst is lavender to deep purple. Citrine grows as six-sided prisms and also inside geodes, which are hollow, spherical rocks.

RARITY Natural ametrine is rare, found only in Bolivia. Lower-priced ametrine specimens may be artificial, formed either from partially irradiated citrine or from differentially heat-treated amethyst.

FORMATION Pure quartz is made purely of silicon and oxygen atoms. Both citrine and amethyst contain traces of iron, with citrine containing oxidized iron, and amethyst containing nonoxidized iron. The different oxidation states occur when there are variations in temperature across the crystal as it grows.

ATTRIBUTES This combination crystal combines the best of both amethyst and citrine. While amethyst calms and balances, citrine clears the mind. Ametrine is ideal for those suffering from burnout, anxiety, and stress. It also encourages us to seek harmony and agreement with others.

HEALING ACTION Meditate with ametrine at times when familial relationships or friendships are stormy. Wear ametrine as a pendant to calm and soothe in the workplace or when faced with challenging people and intolerance. Sleep with an ametrine geode by the bed to aid an unbroken night's sleep.

CARE Ametrine scores 7 on the Mohs' scale. Wash in soapy water with a soft cloth. Do not inhale ametrine dust, which can cause silicosis.

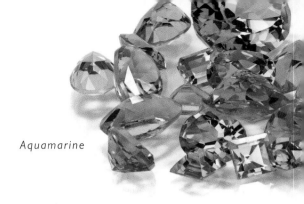

Aquamarine

ANGELITE

APPEARANCE This mineral is commonly medium-light to pale blue, but some crystals may be whitish. Flecks of red hematite are occasionally seen. When well-formed crystals are found, they are orthorhombic.

RARITY This crystal is easily bought. First found in Peru in 1987, angelite is now sourced in Mexico, Egypt, Libya, the UK, Germany, and Poland. Well-developed crystals are rare; the mineral is usually found as a mass.

FORMATION Also known as blue anhydrite, angelite is composed of anhydrous (without water) calcium sulfate ($CaSO_4$). It is an evaporite mineral that forms as the result of gypsum losing all hydration.

ATTRIBUTES Angelite facilitates contact with angels and spirit guides, while helping the birth of psychic gifts. It has a peaceful, soothing vibration, alleviating psychological pain, as well as tension headaches. It helps the user to gain understanding of others and of the universe. It encourages open communication, acceptance, and forgiveness.

HEALING ACTION Placed or held at the throat chakra, angelite may have a powerful effect on communication. To aid the channeling of psychic gifts and the process of grieving, place at the third eye and crown chakras. While attempting communion with spirits, use an angelite pendulum.

CARE With a hardness of 3.5 on the Mohs' scale, angelite is easily damaged and must not be exposed to water. Do not use in gem elixirs as it is soluble in acids and may react dangerously to stomach acid. If necessary, wipe clean with a soft cloth.

AQUAMARINE

APPEARANCE Aquamarine is a turquoise to pale-blue variety of the mineral beryl. A deep-blue beryl may be known as maxixe. Aquamarine is transparent to translucent. It grows in hexagonal crystals, but may also be found as plates, grains, and chunks.

RARITY Gem-quality aquamarine is priced as a semiprecious stone. Common sources are the United States, Brazil, Colombia, Tanzania, and Kenya.

FORMATION Aquamarine crystals are often found in granitic rocks. Beryl is composed of beryllium, aluminum, silicon, and oxygen. Pure crystals are colorless, but aquamarine is tinted by traces of iron.

ATTRIBUTES The ancient Romans believed that aquamarine could protect from the dangers of sea travel. Some say it truly does ease seasickness. This protective crystal gives us strength in the face of emotional and psychic attack. It helps us to see our way through stormy times, safe in the knowledge that better days will come.

HEALING ACTION For emotional and spiritual strength, wear at the heart chakra. When times are hard, meditate with aquamarine to gain strength, perspective, and optimism. A cluster of aquamarine crystals will collect positive energy and is well placed in the self-cultivation corner of the home, which is to the left of the front door.

CARE Aquamarine scores 7.5–8 on the Mohs' scale. It contains beryllium, a known carcinogen, so do not inhale its dust. Clean with warm, soapy water and a soft cloth.

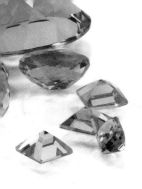

BLACK OBSIDIAN

APPEARANCE A smooth, translucent, volcanic glass, black obsidian is a mineraloid rather than a mineral. It is often found as sharp-edged chunks.

RARITY Obsidian is widely available from stores and may also be collected in areas of rhyolitic eruptions, particularly Argentina, the Canary Islands, Chile, Greece, Iceland, Italy, and the United States.

FORMATION Obsidian forms when lava rich in lighter elements—such as silicon, oxygen, aluminum, sodium, and potassium—cools rapidly, giving no time for crystal growth. This accounts for obsidian's glass-like texture.

ATTRIBUTES Ancient peoples used obsidian for cutting tools and weapons. For a modern user, obsidian aids emotional and mental clarity. If you are well supported by friends and professionals, it is a powerful tool for the examination of past trauma. Jet-black obsidian is not a gentle stone, so should be handled with care and wisdom. Crystal therapists advise that obsidian can speed healing after an injury or surgery.

HEALING ACTION An obsidian pendant may open the door to success in exams or further studies. Placing an obsidian knife on your desk will encourage creativity. Used during meditation, obsidian encourages truth-seeking and clearness of vision. Avoid placing obsidian in the bedroom if you are troubled by repetitive night thoughts.

CARE Obsidian is brittle and amorphous, so is prone to fracturing. It scores 5–6 on the Mohs' scale. Do not breathe in obsidian dust, as it contains silicon, so can cause silicosis. Clean in lukewarm, soapy water with a soft cloth.

BLACK ONYX

APPEARANCE Onyx is translucent to opaque. It may be pure black or display parallel white bands. Traditionally layered white and black, onyx was intricately carved into cameos so that the white layer formed a raised image against the black base layer.

RARITY Black onyx is a fairly common rock. The term "onyx" is sometimes used in a descriptive rather than scientific sense to describe parallel-banded alabaster or obsidian, so ensure you are buying genuine onyx. Some black onyx specimens are artificially colored.

FORMATION Onyx is a form of chalcedony, a cryptocrystalline (with microscopically small crystals) blend of the silicate minerals quartz and moganite.

ATTRIBUTES This rock offers strength and courage. When we feel we lack the willpower to carry on, black onyx can bolster us. It also offers the wisdom to know what is best said and left unsaid, revealed or kept secret. It is said to protect and nourish the digestive system, pancreas, and gallbladder.

HEALING ACTION If training for a marathon or studying for exams, wear black onyx on your body for willpower and the belief that you will triumph through hard work. If you suffer from bad dreams or night terrors, place black onyx under your pillow.

CARE Onyx is durable, with a hardness of 6.5–7 on the Mohs' scale. Do not inhale onyx dust, which can cause silicosis. Clean in warm, soapy water with a soft cloth.

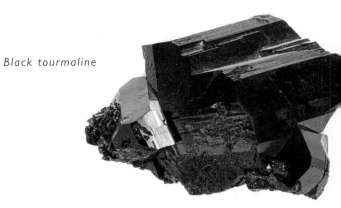

Black tourmaline

BLACK SPINEL

APPEARANCE Spinel takes its name from the Latin word for "spine," due to its pointed crystals. It is often found in eight-sided shapes or flat, triangular plates. Specimens range from transparent to opaque.

RARITY Transparent spinel is priced as a semiprecious gemstone, but tumbled opaque stones are far more common.

FORMATION Crystals of spinel grow in igneous and metamorphic rocks. Spinel is formed from atoms of magnesium, aluminum, and oxygen. Spinel and ruby are often found together, with ruby formed mainly from aluminum and oxygen.

ATTRIBUTES All varieties of spinel offer hope in times of difficulty, with black spinel having particular resonance with material concerns, such as financial problems, house moves, and legal issues. It opens the door to fresh energy and ideas when they are needed the most. On a physical level, it is also said to be highly reenergizing, particularly after periods of overwork.

HEALING ACTION While lying down, place spinel on the root chakra to open the door to hope. If positioned on the third eye, spinel can help with problem-solving. Sleep with tumbled spinel under your pillow to awake refreshed and to be able to find new routes around old obstacles.

CARE This strong crystal scores 7.5–8 on the Mohs' scale. It can be cleaned with warm, soapy water and a soft cloth.

BLACK TOURMALINE

APPEARANCE A translucent to opaque crystal, black tourmaline is often found in columnar, radiating, or needle-shaped forms that are triangular in cross section.

RARITY This semiprecious stone is widely available in specialty stores. Crystals are often mined in Africa, the United States, and Brazil.

FORMATION Tourmaline is a boron silicate mineral. Brownish-black to black tourmaline is often known as schorl, while dravite (named for the Drava district of Austria) is dark yellow to brown. Both varieties are rich in iron and sodium. Schorl forms in the igneous rock granite, while dravite is more common in metamorphic rocks such as marble and schist.

ATTRIBUTES Black tourmaline offers both spiritual grounding and protection. It frees us from fear and allows us to look deep inside ourselves, for the negative emotions and motivations that we find difficult to confront. Due to its iron content, opaque black schorl has high magnetic susceptibility. This makes it a powerful crystal to work with when clearing blockages and dispersing negative energy. It is also said to expel toxins and reduce bloating.

HEALING ACTION A black tourmaline wand can help when seeking a solution to a seemingly impossible problem. Gardeners may find that black tourmaline wind chimes help their plants to flourish. Place a black tourmaline paperweight on your desk to balance the left and right brains.

CARE Tourmaline rates 7–7.5 on the Mohs' scale. Clean in warm, soapy water with a soft cloth. Do not inhale tourmaline dust, which can cause silicosis.

BLUE APATITE

APPEARANCE Crystals sold as blue apatite are often fluorapatite, a common member of the apatite group. Transparent to opaque, this variety of apatite grows as chunks and hexagonal prisms.

RARITY Gem- or collector-quality blue apatite crystals are often sourced from Brazil, Russia, Madagascar, and the United States. Opaque crystals take a lower price.

FORMATION Apatite is a calcium fluorophosphate. Its most important deposits are in sedimentary rocks formed in marine environments.

ATTRIBUTES This shade of apatite encourages communication. It gives self-confidence during spoken and sung performances, as well as social and professional interaction. Blue apatite also frees us to speak from our hearts, with both honesty and kindness. Some believe that apatite improves problems of the throat and neck.

HEALING ACTION If you work in a job where communication is key, place blue apatite in your office. If you feel there is something that must be spoken, yet you cannot find the words, meditate with blue apatite placed on the floor before you.

CARE Blue apatite scores just 5 on the Mohs' scale, so it should be treated with care. Apatite is toxic, so do not use in gem elixirs and wash your hands after handling. Do not immerse in water. If necessary, wipe clean with a damp cloth.

BLUE LACE AGATE

APPEARANCE This variety of agate has a lace-like pattern of frills, eyes, bands, or zigzags. While most lace agate is dusty blue and white, Mexican crazy lace agate exhibits red, yellow, or white patterns.

RARITY Many specimens of blue lace agate are sourced from Namibia. It is often bought as tumbled stones.

FORMATION The blue lace agate found in Namibia is around 50 million years old, but it grew in fractures in igneous dolerite rock that is far older. The seams filled with silica-rich fluid, which slowly crystalized. Agate is a translucent form of quartz and chalcedony, which is itself composed of fine intergrowths of quartz and moganite. Both these minerals are composed of silicon and oxygen atoms, but have different molecular structures. Variations and inclusions in the silica create patterns and swirls of different shades and crystal structures.

ATTRIBUTES When life is busy and stressful, this variety of agate helps us to find peace and inner calm. Like all forms of agate, it stimulates the mind. It encourages dreams and daydreams that shed light on our true needs and goals. Some crystal therapists say that blue lace agate relieves throat problems, as well as relaxing muscle tension of the head and neck.

HEALING ACTION Meditate with blue agate at times of stress. Position on the third eye chakra to open the mind to its full potential. Place under the pillow for lucid and revealing dreams.

CARE Agate rates 6.5–7 on the Mohs' scale. Do not inhale agate dust, which can cause silicosis. Clean in warm, soapy water with a soft cloth.

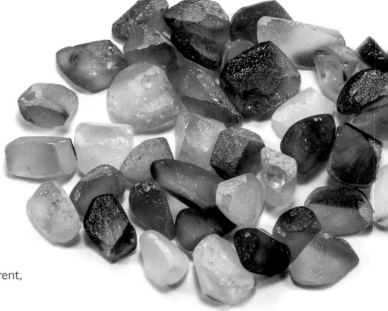

Blue sapphires

BLUE SAPPHIRE

APPEARANCE Sapphire is the name for any gem-quality corundum crystal that is not red, with those crystals named "rubies." A precious stone of great beauty, a blue sapphire is vividly colored. When polished, sapphires are transparent, but they are otherwise cloudy.

RARITY Blue sapphire is easily obtained as an uncut stone, but is expensive. Sapphires are mined in Myanmar, Thailand, India, Sri Lanka, Kenya, Madagascar, the Czech Republic, Brazil, Canada, and Australia. High-quality faceted sapphires are valuable.

FORMATION Sapphires are a variety of the mineral corundum, an aluminum oxide. Corundum forms deep underground under intense heat and pressure. The blue coloration is caused by trace amounts of iron and titanium.

ATTRIBUTES All sapphires are wisdom stones, but blue sapphires—in common with other blue crystals and stones—are particularly useful for encouraging psychic knowledge and spiritual truth. Blue sapphire encourages the user to stay on the right spiritual path, works against negative energy, and encourages self-expression. Blue sapphire is said to regulate the action of the body's glands.

HEALING ACTION The throat chakra is the right position for encouraging self-expression. When placed or held on the third eye chakra, blue sapphire unlocks psychic abilities, enhances learning, and helps to heal wounds from past lives. Place under the pillow to stimulate lucid dreaming. Wearing sapphire jewelry can help mild depression and dispel anxiety.

CARE Sapphire scores 9 on the Mohs' scale, so is very durable. Clean with warm, soapy water and a soft cloth. However, cavity-filled, fracture-filled, or dyed gems should be cleaned only with a damp cloth. Do not use them in gem elixirs.

When polished, sapphires are transparent, but they are otherwise cloudy.

Carnelian is tinted red by traces of iron oxide.

CARNELIAN

APPEARANCE Carnelian, also called cornelian or sard, ranges from orange-brown to brown-red. It is translucent and may have a waxy appearance.

RARITY Most carnelian is mined from India, Indonesia, Russia, Germany, or Brazil. High-quality crystals are priced as semiprecious gems.

FORMATION Carnelian is a form of chalcedony, which is composed of fine intergrowths of the silicon dioxide minerals quartz and moganite, the two forms differentiated by their crystal structures at the microscopic level. Carnelian is tinted red by traces of iron oxide.

ATTRIBUTES This mineral promotes energy and effort, both physical and emotional. It has particular resonance with business pursuits, allowing us to see the right course of action and giving the courage and conviction to pursue it. Carnelian discourages the will to fail. It is also said to improve stamina and muscle strength.

HEALING ACTION When energy is at a low ebb in midwinter, wear carnelian close to the skin for a much-needed boost. To aid success in business, position in the wealth corner of the house, which is at the far left if you come in by the main entrance. Place carnelian under your pillow if you are kept awake by imagining failure.

CARE Carnelian scores 6–7 on the Mohs' scale. Salt water can cause carnelian to fracture. Clean with warm, soapy water and a soft cloth. Do not inhale carnelian dust, which can cause silicosis.

CELESTITE

APPEARANCE Usually obtained as a blue crystal, celestite may also be colorless, white, yellow, or red. The transparent crystals are usually pyramidal or granular, but geodes and plates are found. Celestite may also be called celestine.

RARITY This crystal is readily available as small pieces, tumbled stones, and clusters, but may be expensive. It is found in small quantities in Libya, Egypt, Madagascar, Peru, Mexico, the UK, and Poland.

FORMATION Composed of strontium sulfate ($SrSO_4$), celestite is often found in sedimentary rocks, with angelite and gypsum commonly nearby.

ATTRIBUTES A sister stone to angelite, celestite (from the Latin *coelestis*, meaning "heavenly") also aids contact with the spiritual realm, while encouraging clairvoyance, dream recall, and artistic abilities. Its high, uplifting vibration heals the aura, promotes mental and emotional balance, disperses worries, and encourages peaceful communication. Some crystal therapists say it helps with conditions that affect the nerves, such as neuralgia.

HEALING ACTION Placed or held at the throat chakra, celestite promotes communication. When placed on the crown chakra, celestite allows access to the higher chakras, particularly the soul star, to encourage psychic hearing, clairvoyance, and intuition. Leave a celestite cluster in your healing room or bedroom to aid both mental clarity and to encourage calm and positivity.

CARE Celestite scores only 3–3.5 on the Mohs' scale. To prevent loss of color, do not place in direct sunlight. Do not place in water, which may cause disintegration. Wipe clean with a soft cloth.

Azeztulite is the trade name for a milky quartz found in North Carolina.

CHALCEDONY

APPEARANCE Transparent to opaque, chalcedony is usually white to gray. It is a microcrystalline mineral, so its individual crystals are not visible. It can often be found in geodes, lining the cavity with rounded bumps.

RARITY This is a common mineral, found in a wide range of environments worldwide. Colorful varieties of chalcedony, such as agate and jasper, are popular among collectors and craftspeople.

FORMATION Chalcedony is composed of intergrowths of two silica minerals, quartz and moganite, which are chemically identical but distinguished by their different crystal structures. Chalcedony often forms in vugs inside igneous rocks.

ATTRIBUTES This crystal brings the mind and spirit, body and emotions, into harmony. It helps us to hear the promptings of our emotions. It helps us to see when the body is trying to tell us that our spirit is troubled. It wards off psychosomatic symptoms, such as sore necks, headaches, or stomach disorders caused by stress.

HEALING ACTION If suffering from stress-induced irritable bowel syndrome, place on the lower abdomen. Position on the crown chakra to tune in to the voice of the body. Place chalcedony in the knowledge and self-cultivation corner of the home, which is to the left as you enter by the front door.

CARE Chalcedony scores 7 on the Mohs' scale. Do not breathe in chalcedony dust, which can cause silicosis. To clean, dip in lukewarm, soapy water. Do not soak as chalcedony is mildly soluble in water, particularly hot water.

CHRYSOPRASE

APPEARANCE Specimens vary from deep green to apple-green and turquoise, and from opaque to translucent. They are often small and tumbled.

RARITY This relatively common semiprecious stone is usually sourced from Tanzania or Poland, but a few specimens may be from Russia, Australia, or the United States.

FORMATION Chrysoprase is a form of chalcedony, which is composed of fine intergrowths of the silicon dioxide minerals quartz and moganite, the two differentiated by their crystal structures at the microscopic level. Chrysoprase is colored green by tiny quantities of nickel. The stone is formed during the weathering of serpentinite rocks, which are usually greenish and slippery feeling.

ATTRIBUTES As with other forms of chalcedony, such as carnelian, chrysoprase has resonance with business pursuits. Yet where carnelian encourages drive and ambition, chrysoprase encourages lateral thinking and creativity. It enables us to accept advice from others and to listen to other viewpoints. Chrysoprase is said to settle hormonal imbalances.

HEALING ACTION Position at the heart chakras to accept the kindly advice of others and to awaken empathy even with those we find challenging. Place in the wealth corner of the home; at the far left if you come in by the main entrance, to encourage solutions to business or career issues.

CARE Chrysoprase scores 6–7 on the Mohs' scale. If dropped, it may fracture into sharp-edged pieces. Since it is porous, avoid contact with chemicals. Clean with warm, soapy water and a soft cloth. Do not inhale chrysoprase dust or use in gem elixirs.

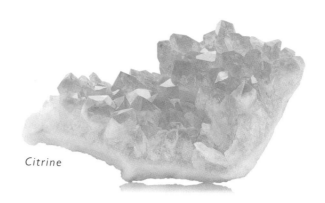

Citrine

CITRINE

APPEARANCE This variety of quartz ranges from yellow to orange to brown. It grows as six-sided prisms ending in six-sided pyramids, as well as in clusters inside geodes, which are hollow spherical rocks. A natural citrine has a cloudy appearance, while a heat-treated amethyst or smoky quartz may display faint internal lines.

RARITY Natural citrines are rare, with most specimens sourced from southern Brazil. Many citrines are artificially heat-treated amethysts.

FORMATION Citrine contains silicon and oxygen, with traces of iron causing its yellow tint. Citrine geodes form when cavities in volcanic rock are filled with hydrothermal fluid rich in silica.

ATTRIBUTES Traditionally, citrine is called the "money stone," due to the belief that it will bring wealth. Although no crystal has that power, citrine does enhance the forward-planning and self-belief that aid success in business. Citrine helps with concentration and clears the mind, helping us to overcome self-doubt, confusion, anxiety, and phobias.

HEALING ACTION To dispel anxiety that is causing difficulties with eating, place at the solar plexus chakra. Meditate with citrine if money worries are disturbing your peace. To help with planning and book balancing, place a citrine geode in the wealth corner of the house or office; at the rear left if you come in by the main entrance.

CARE Citrine scores 7 on the Mohs' scale. Wash in warm, soapy water with a soft cloth. Do not inhale citrine dust, which can cause silicosis.

CLEAR QUARTZ

APPEARANCE Pure quartz is colorless and transparent. Quartz crystals often grow as six-sided prisms ending in pointed pyramids. They may be found as single crystals, twinned crystals, or clusters. If a crystal is white and translucent to opaque, it is known as milky quartz. Azeztulite is the trade name for a milky quartz found in North Carolina.

RARITY Common worldwide. More regularly shaped, transparent crystals take a higher price.

FORMATION Pure quartz is made of silicon and oxygen atoms. Quartz is a common rock-forming mineral, found in felsic rocks such as granite. Milky quartz is caused by tiny bubbles of gas or liquid that were trapped during crystal formation.

ATTRIBUTES Clear quartz is a powerful amplifier of energy. It heightens our awareness of this world and others, while attuning us to notice changes in our own physical and mental state. Quartz purifies, heals, and balances. Some crystal therapists say that it stimulates the immune system. Milky quartz is valuable for situations where a gentler energy is needed.

HEALING ACTION Place at the higher chakras to open the mind to endless possibilities and to reach for true enlightenment. When working with quartz wands, turn their points toward yourself to draw energy inward. Turn wands outward to direct the way to new possibilities. Clear quartz is an ideal crystal for scrying.

CARE Quartz is named for the Germanic word for "hard." It scores 7 on the Mohs' scale. Do not inhale quartz dust as it contains silicon, which can cause silicosis. Clean in warm, soapy water with a soft cloth.

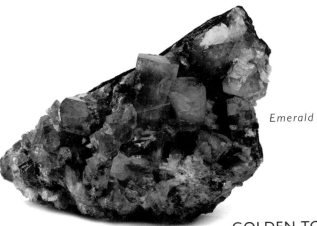

Emerald

EMERALD

APPEARANCE It ranges from vivid blue-green to yellow-green. Crystals grow in hexagonal prisms.

RARITY Transparent, high-quality emeralds are rare and valuable, but clouded or opaque specimens are readily available. Emeralds are mined across the world, with the two biggest producers being Colombia and Zambia. Note that only emeralds with a vivid hue earn the name: paler crystals must be known as "green beryl."

FORMATION A variety of the mineral beryl, emerald grows in metamorphic rock as well as in cavities and along fractures in granite. Beryl is composed of beryllium, aluminum, silicon, and oxygen. Pure crystals are colorless. Emerald is tinted by traces of chromium and sometimes vanadium.

ATTRIBUTES Emerald helps us to nourish our relationships through love, good communication, and empathy. It helps us to be true to our emotions, escaping coldness, hypocrisy, and pretense. It is said to help with recovery after illness, particularly viruses.

HEALING ACTION To focus on the needs and lives of those we love, meditate with emerald. Position on the heart chakra to awaken honest emotions and the ability to express them. To focus positive energy on your relationship with your spouse or partner, place an emerald crystal in the back right of the home, if you enter by the front door.

CARE Emerald scores 7.5–8 on the Mohs' scale, but crystals usually contain a high quantity of inclusions, giving them low resistance to breakage. Clean with warm, soapy water and a soft cloth. Care must be taken when handling. It contains beryllium, a known carcinogen, so do not inhale its dust.

GOLDEN TOPAZ

APPEARANCE Ranging from yellow to golden-brown, gem-quality topaz is transparent. It commonly forms prisms that terminate in pyramids.

RARITY Relatively common but popular for jewelry, topaz is priced as a semiprecious stone. Much yellow topaz comes from Brazil, Mexico, Russia, or Germany.

FORMATION Topaz is a neosilicate mineral that forms in silicon-rich igneous rocks, particularly granite and rhyolite. The presence of iron results in golden-yellow crystals.

ATTRIBUTES Golden topaz enhances motivation. Whether we are training for a race, studying for exams, or trying to maintain a healthy diet, topaz bolsters willpower as well as the self-belief that tells us we can and will meet our goals. This crystal encourages us to listen for the voices that empower us rather than to focus on negative words. It is also said to strengthen the muscles, ligaments, and tendons.

HEALING ACTION If your goal is a healthier lifestyle, place golden topaz at the solar plexus chakra for the strength, energy, and confidence to keep working. Wear golden topaz jewelry to foster self-assurance and fortitude. If you are working toward a career goal, place golden topaz in the career area of the home, which is just inside the front door.

CARE Although topaz scores 8 on the Mohs' scale, making it very hard, its crystals have a weakness in their atomic bonding along a certain plane, where it has a tendency to break if struck with enough force. Clean in warm, soapy water with a soft cloth.

Green fluorite has particular resonance with our closest relationships.

GREEN AVENTURINE

APPEARANCE A form of translucent to opaque quartz that appears to sparkle or glitter. This is known to mineralogists as aventurescence, from the Italian words meaning "by chance."

RARITY Much green aventurine is sourced from India. It is often carved into beads, cabochons, and artworks.

FORMATION A metamorphic rock composed of quartz (silicon dioxide) with flake-like inclusions of chrome-rich fuchsite, which also give its green shade.

ATTRIBUTES This is an ideal stone for someone ambitious and go-getting, as it encourages us to seize the day and to spot opportunity wherever it arises. Aventurine also encourages us to nourish our relationships, finding moments to feed them and enjoy them. It is said to aid the absorption of vitamins and minerals in the intestines.

HEALING ACTION If you feel you are losing touch with friends or family, wear green aventurine to encourage yourself to make time for them. Meditate with this stone to find joy in the moment. If you are striving for a career goal, place green aventurine in the career area of the home, which is immediately inside the front door.

CARE This rock has a hardness of around 6.5 on the Mohs' scale. Abundant inclusions can lower its hardness further. Do not inhale dust from aventurine. Clean in warm, soapy water with a soft cloth.

GREEN FLUORITE

APPEARANCE Fluorite often forms well-defined cubes and octahedrons. It is also found as columns, fibers, and chunks. Many crystals fluoresce in ultraviolet light. It is transparent to translucent.

RARITY Sometimes called fluorsoar, it is widespread worldwide, but specimens suitable for decorative rather than industrial use are less common and may be priced as a semiprecious gem. Green fluorite may be sourced from South Africa or Namibia.

FORMATION This mineral forms in igneous rocks, such as granite, particularly as a result of hydrothermal activity. Pure fluorite, composed of calcium and fluorine, is colorless. Impurities, natural irradiation, and structural defects (called "color centers") can tint it any shade.

ATTRIBUTES All varieties of fluorite help us to make positive changes in our lives. Green fluorite has particular resonance with our closest relationships. It encourages us to show and voice love, even when we are beset by self-doubt, anger, or resentment. When used externally, it is said to ease stomach upsets caused by food poisoning, although medical advice should always be sought.

HEALING ACTION If you are struggling with conflict, distrust, or recrimination in a close relationship, meditate with green fluorite. Position at the heart chakra to ease negative feelings about loved ones, replacing them with empathy, compassion, and forgiveness. Place green fluorite in the family corner of the home, which is midway through the house on the left, if you enter by the front door.

CARE Fluorite scores just 4 on the Mohs' scale, so it is more suitable for display or for jewelry. Fluorite is not water-safe, so clean with a dry cloth if necessary. It is toxic and may react dangerously with stomach acid, so do not use in gem elixirs and do not ingest. Do not expose to acids.

*Meditate with green jade for calmness
and fresh insight.*

GREEN JADE

APPEARANCE Green jade may be one of two
minerals, jadeite and nephrite, which share a similar
appearance and properties. It ranges from pale apple-
green to bright emerald, from translucent to opaque.
RARITY Green is the most common color of both
nephrite and jadeite. Jadeite is the rarer and more
highly priced of the two minerals. Both forms of jade
have been used for statues and carvings for millennia,
in cultures from China to New Zealand, Mexico to
India.
FORMATION Both nephrite and jadeite form during
the metamorphism of rocks, particularly where two
tectonic plates are converging. Much jade is found as
pebbles and boulders in stream valleys, with a brown,
weathered rind hiding its beauty.
ATTRIBUTES While all colors of jade bring harmony,
green jade has particular resonance with relationships.
It offers insight into why conflict has arisen and how
we can best move forward, without anger, blame, or
denial. It is said to calm the nervous system.
HEALING ACTION Green jade helps to balance the
chakras, so position over any chakra that is blocked
or overstimulated. If you are encountering conflict,
with anyone from a teenager to a work colleague,
meditate with green jade for calmness and fresh
insight. Place a jade carving in the relationships
corner of the house, which is at the back right
if you enter by the front door.
CARE Jade is durable and easy to carve. It scores 6–7
on the Mohs' scale. Wipe jade clean with a soft, soapy
cloth, then rinse with clean water and dry carefully.
Do not soak. Keep jade out of direct sunlight.

GREEN PREHNITE

APPEARANCE This translucent, grass-green or
dusty-green mineral is usually found as globular
masses or stalactites.
RARITY Crystals are easily bought from specialty
suppliers, while cabochons or faceted gems can be
purchased from jewelers. Most gem-quality prehnite
is mined in South Africa and Australia.
FORMATION This mineral, first identified by Colonel
Hendrik von Prehn in South Africa, contains calcium,
aluminum, silicon, and oxygen. It is often found in
basalt and gneiss. Crystals often have a brown ferrous
coating, which is chemically removed.
ATTRIBUTES A crystal that frees the powers of
the mind, aiding memory, intuition, and prophecy.
In addition, it links our emotions with our intellect,
helping decision-making and conflict resolution.
Prehnite may be helpful for treating bladder
infections, although there is no scientific proof.
HEALING ACTION At the heart chakra, green
prehnite helps us to make decisions with a
combination of head and heart, reasoning, and gut
feeling. If you are studying for exams or working
toward a challenging goal at work, place this crystal
on the crown chakra. Place on the table when
undertaking tarot reading, scrying, or any form
of prophecy.
CARE Prehnite may react dangerously to stomach
acid, so do not use in gem elixirs. It scores 6–6.5
on the Mohs' scale. Wipe clean with a soft cloth
and warm, soapy water. Never use acidic cleaning
products as they will dissolve this mineral. Prehnite
will fade gradually over time if it is on display.

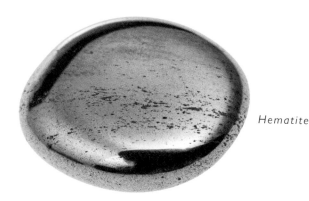

Hematite

HEMATITE

APPEARANCE Hematite is gray to rust-red with a steely luster. Its crystals take many forms, from plates, columns, and radiating fibers to rosettes. Hematite is opaque.

RARITY This ubiquitous mineral can be bought as tumbled stones or fine crystal rosettes, often called iron roses. It is occasionally used as a decorative stone. Hematite is frequently sourced from Brazil, England, Italy, or Canada.

FORMATION An iron oxide, hematite is found widely in rock and soils. It usually precipitates from sea water or standing fresh water, but can also crystallize in hot magma.

ATTRIBUTES Hematite is a strongly grounding crystal, tethering the spirit when we are spaced out or emotionally lost. It is highly beneficial for concentration. Hematite helps us to focus on the here and now, breaking free from the past and viewing the future with equanimity. Some say that hematite helps with blood disorders, but there is no scientific proof of this claim.

HEALING ACTION Meditate with hematite when feeling emotionally lost or confused. Place a hematite crystal on the desk to benefit study or work. Position on the earth chakra to ground a wandering or yearning spirit.

CARE Hematite scores 5.5–6.5 on the Mohs' scale, but is brittle. Clean in warm, soapy water with a soft cloth. Hematite will rust if left damp. Due to its iron content, hematite should not be ingested or used in gem elixirs. It is soluble in acids, so may react dangerously with stomach acid.

HONEY CALCITE

APPEARANCE As its name suggests, this variety of calcite is the color of honey. Calcite often forms pyramid-shaped crystals or grains, as well as complex forms such as "flowers." It is transparent to translucent.

RARITY Much of the world's honey calcite is sourced from Mexico. It may also be called golden or amber calcite.

FORMATION Calcite is calcium carbonate, which is colorless. It is the presence of impurities including iron that give it a golden tint. Calcite is a major ingredient of sedimentary rocks such as limestone and chalk, as it formed the shells and skeletons of the tiny sea creatures from which these rocks formed.

ATTRIBUTES All varieties of calcite stimulate the mind. This kindly stone teaches us to use our intellectual gifts wisely, never to score points against others. It also encourages us to use our skills for more than pure financial gain, whether that means finding a better balance between work and home life or devising a complete career change. Some say that honey calcite improves dexterity and hand–eye coordination.

HEALING ACTION Place honey calcite in the career area of the home, which is immediately as you enter the front door. Meditate with this mineral if you are feeling burned out from overwork.

CARE Calcite is brittle and soft, scoring just 3 on the Mohs' scale. It should not be handled excessively. Calcite is not soluble in pure water but is soluble in rain water, which is slightly acidic. Do not use in gem elixirs. If cleaning is necessary, wipe with a soft cloth.

HOWLITE

APPEARANCE Well-formed crystals of howlite are rare: This mineral is usually found as irregular white nodules covered by dark veins resembling spider's webs. Howlite is translucent to opaque.

RARITY Widely available, howlite is usually bought as tumbled and polished stones, but is also dyed and used as inlays and cabochons in jewelry. Sources include Canada and the southwestern United States.

FORMATION This calcium borosilicate hydroxide is found in evaporite deposits in dried-out lakes.

ATTRIBUTES Howlite is famed as the mineral that can give insomniacs a good night's sleep. It eases stress, repetitive thoughts, and compulsions. It also guards against mood swings that result in anger, tetchiness, or prickliness. Some say that howlite can ease back and neck pain caused by tension.

HEALING ACTION Place howlite under the pillow or beside the bed for an unbroken and refreshing night's sleep. Meditate with howlite to cool the temper and ease tension. Wear howlite jewelry to combat stress and intrusive thoughts.

CARE Howlite scores 3.5 on the Mohs' scale. It is soluble in acids, so should not be used in gem elixirs as it may react dangerously with stomach acid. Undyed howlite can be cleaned in lukewarm, soapy water. Dyed howlite should not be immersed.

IOLITE

APPEARANCE Iolite is the transparent, gem-quality variety of the mineral cordierite. The name iolite comes from the ancient Greek for "violet." It ranges from lilac to blue to gray and appears to change shade when viewed from different angles.

RARITY Although much softer than sapphire, iolite is often used as a less-expensive substitute for the precious gem. Iolite is found in Australia, Brazil, Canada, India, Madagascar, Myanmar, Namibia, Sri Lanka, Tanzania, and the United States.

FORMATION A magnesium iron aluminum silicate, iolite forms as fine-grained sedimentary rocks, which are metamorphosed by great heat and pressure.

ATTRIBUTES This crystal defuses conflict. Its effect can be felt in interpersonal conflicts as well as internal battles, between head and heart, reason and intuition, optimism and pessimism. Some crystal therapists say that iolite eases problems of the sinuses and respiratory system.

HEALING ACTION For frequent familial conflict, place iolite in the dining room or family room, where its calming vibrations can soothe anger. When you are torn by two conflicting courses of action, meditate with iolite.

CARE Iolite may react dangerously with stomach acid, so it should not be used in gem elixirs. Scoring 7–7.5 on the Mohs' scale, it is suitable for jewelry. Iolite can be cleaned in warm, soapy water with a soft cloth.

KUNZITE

APPEARANCE This transparent to translucent crystal is usually pink to purple. It exhibits an effect called pleochroism, or appearing as different colors in changing lights and from different angles. Kunzite is striated, which means that many parallel hairline grooves can be seen.

RARITY Discovered in 1902, kunzite was named after George Kunz, Tiffany & Co.'s chief jeweler. This crystal

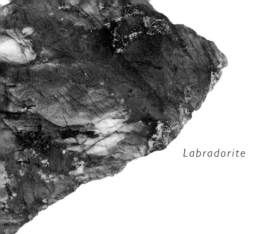

Labradorite

is more widely available than in the past. It is now mined in the United States, Canada, Mexico, Brazil, Myanmar, Afghanistan, and Pakistan.

FORMATION Kunzite is a form of the mineral spodumene, which grows in intrusive igneous rocks, such as granite, that are rich in lithium. It is a lithium aluminum silicate. The pink to purple tint is given by the presence of small quantities of manganese.

ATTRIBUTES Kunzite activates the heart chakras, helping to bring them into balance and cooperation with the other chakras, particularly those of the throat and third eye. In this way, kunzite awakens love and chases away negativity, but also encourages the expression of creativity and frees intuition. It is said to strengthen the cardiovascular system.

HEALING ACTION Place over the higher heart or heart chakra to boost mood and alleviate mild depression. Wear as a pendant to heal heartache, particularly the pain caused by intrusive memories of past events. Some call kunzite the "mother's stone" because, when placed under the pillow, it can help new mothers to get a good night's sleep while calming and rejuvenating the heart—ready to start the new day with compassion and unconditional love.

CARE Keep out of sunlight, which causes fading. Clean only in warm, soapy water. Do not use in gem elixirs as it contains lithium. Kunzite scores 6.5–7 on the Mohs' scale.

LABRADORITE

APPEARANCE The mineral labradorite has a background color of gray, brown, green, blue, or yellow, but is known for its particular iridescence, known as labradorescence, usually in shades of blue, purple, turquoise, and gold. Labradorite is found as plates and masses.

RARITY Labradorite is named after Labrador, in Canada, where it was first identified. It is also sourced from Australia, China, Madagascar, Slovakia, and the United States. The mineral is often cut as a cabochon to show off its labradorescence.

FORMATION Formed in igneous rocks such as basalt and gabbro, labradorite is a member of the feldspar group of minerals. It contains atoms of calcium, sodium, aluminum, silicon, and oxygen. Its labradorescence results from the reflection of light between layers of crystals that all face in one direction. These crystals are too small to be seen under an ordinary microscope.

ATTRIBUTES Labradorite is a powerful crystal that heightens perception, intuition, and clairvoyance. It opens our consciousness, leading us one step closer to true understanding. It brings messages from the spirit world and our unconscious, allowing them to surface in dreams. Some say that labradorite also helps disorders of the eyes and brain.

HEALING ACTION Hold labradorite at the third eye to awaken clairvoyance. Use it to open the higher chakras (first working on the lower chakras in turn) to widen consciousness. Place labradorite by the bedside for wonderfully lucid dreams.

CARE Labradorite scores 6–6.5 on the Mohs' scale. Do not soak labradorite in water as it will dissolve. Do not use it in gem elixirs. It can be cleaned by wiping with a damp, soft cloth, then drying thoroughly.

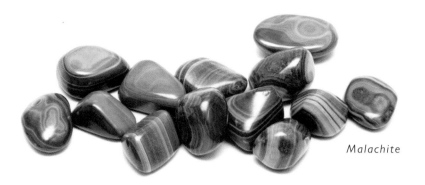

Malachite

LAPIS LAZULI

APPEARANCE A rock rather than a mineral, lapis lazuli is an intense blue, flecked with white calcite or golden pyrite.

RARITY Lapis lazuli is commonly available but expensive, particularly for top-quality stones. The foremost mines are in Afghanistan and Pakistan, but the rock is also sourced in Russia, Mongolia, Italy, Chile, the United States, and Canada.

FORMATION Lapis lazuli is a metamorphic rock that contains large quantities of the mineral lazurite, with smaller quantities of calcite, pyrite, and sodalite, among other minerals.

ATTRIBUTES As with all blue minerals and stones, lapis lazuli facilitates contact with the spirit world, enhances psychic abilities, and benefits dream work. In addition, this is a strongly protective stone that blocks psychic attack and helps the user to withstand emotional bondage. It works against repression, depression, and purposelessness, while working toward enlightenment and clarity. Lapis lazuli is also said to clear headaches caused by eyestrain and overwork.

HEALING ACTION Wear or place at the throat chakra to encourage honesty and openness in communication. Wear or place at the third eye chakra to enhance psychic abilities, stimulate the mind, encourage positivity, and overcome insomnia. Wear as earrings or pendants for protection, but to avoid over-stimulation do so only for short periods at first.

CARE Depending on its exact composition, lapis lazuli scores 5–6 on the Mohs' scale. If cleaning is necessary, briefly dip in room-temperature water with a very mild soap. Use a soft cloth to avoid scratching. Do not use in gem elixirs, as some lapis lazuli inclusions are toxic and may react dangerously with stomach acid.

MAHOGANY OBSIDIAN

APPEARANCE Streaked or speckled in red-brown and black, this variety of obsidian often displays a pattern like the grain of rich mahogany wood. Its texture is smooth and glass-like.

RARITY This shade of obsidian is less common than the jet-black variety. Much commercially available mahogany obsidian comes from Mexico.

FORMATION Obsidian forms when lava rich in lighter elements—such as silicon, oxygen, aluminum, sodium, and potassium—cools quickly, giving little time for crystal growth. Mahogany obsidian's reddish shade is caused by traces of elements such as iron.

ATTRIBUTES Mahogany obsidian is gentler than its jet-black sister. While it aids searchers for emotional and mental clarity, it also offers the support and nurturing that discovering the truth often requires. It allows us to balance acknowledgment of the past with future growth. It is said to ease headaches.

HEALING ACTION Worn as a pendant or bracelet, mahogany obsidian offers direction, as well as nurturing the courage to pursue those goals. Meditate with mahogany obsidian to sow the seeds of resourcefulness. Place on the root chakra to encourage honest but forgiving self-confidence.

CARE With a score of 5–6 on the Mohs' scale, obsidian is relatively easy to fracture and scratch. Clean only with warm, soapy water and a soft cloth. Do not breathe in obsidian dust.

Moonstone is powerfully attuned to the female reproductive system.

MALACHITE

APPEARANCE This mineral displays bands of bright green, dark green, and blackish-green. Usually opaque, it grows as stalactites, masses, and plates. After cutting, the sawed faces exhibit the hallmark banding.

RARITY Malachite is widely available from mineral suppliers, who should also offer advice on its toxicity, safe storage, and care. It may also be bought as polished cabochons and beads. Gem-quality malachite is sourced from the Democratic Republic of the Congo, Australia, France, or the United States.

FORMATION This copper carbonate hydroxide mineral forms underground, when carbonated water interacts with copper minerals or when a copper solution interacts with limestone.

ATTRIBUTES Malachite is a crystal of empathy. It encourages us to understand and forgive the mistakes and weaknesses of others. It also allows us to journey beyond ourselves, into other lives and other worlds. While under the influence of malachite, dreamers may receive messages from spirit guides and angelic entities.

HEALING ACTION This stone must be used only in its polished form and under the direction of a qualified crystal therapist.

CARE Keep away from children and pets. The high copper content of malachite makes it toxic, so do not inhale its dust or use in gem elixirs. It is heat-sensitive and reacts dangerously with weak acids, including possibly stomach acid. This mineral is soft, with a Mohs' hardness of 3.5–4, so avoid excessive handling. Clean with lukewarm water and a gentle soap.

MOONSTONE

APPEARANCE Also known as hecatolite, moonstone displays an effect called adularescence or schiller. This is a milky, usually bluish glow that looks like moonlight on water. Although moonstone is usually white, it can be brown, gray, pink, blue, and green.

RARITY Moonstone can be sourced worldwide, including from Armenia, Australia, Mexico, Madagascar, Myanmar, India, Sri Lanka, and the United States. Jewelry inlaid with moonstone, often in the style of René Lalique, is widely available.

FORMATION Moonstone is a combination of two closely related minerals in the feldspar group, orthoclase and albite. The intergrown minerals stack in alternating layers, which create this gemstone's adularescence as light bounces off these microstructures. Moonstone forms from hydrothermal deposits.

ATTRIBUTES Moonstone is powerfully attuned to the female reproductive system and is said to ease premenstrual syndrome and menopausal mood changes. This is a calming crystal that can also ease stress and insomnia. It encourages emotional healing and serenity.

HEALING ACTION Meditate daily with moonstone if you are experiencing menopause. Place moonstone under the pillow or by the bedside for a deep and refreshing night's sleep. Wear moonstone jewelry during times of emotional stress.

CARE Moonstone scores 6–6.5 on the Mohs' scale. It is quite easy to fracture, so it is best suited to pendants or earrings than rings. Clean by dipping in warm, soapy water.

Place morganite at the higher heart chakra to truly know you are worthy of achieving success.

MORGANITE

APPEARANCE Morganite is a pink variety of the mineral beryl. It grows in pale-pink to salmon-colored crystals that are transparent to translucent. It often forms hexagonal columns, but may also be found as plates, grains, and chunks.

RARITY Morganite is a fairly rare, semiprecious stone. Sources include Brazil, the United States, Madagascar, and Myanmar.

FORMATION Pure, colorless beryl is composed of beryllium, aluminum, silicon, and oxygen. Pink beryl is tinted by traces of manganese. It is often found in granitic pegmatites, which are igneous rocks studded with enlarged crystals. This variety of beryl was named after the American banker J.P. Morgan.

ATTRIBUTES All varieties of beryl help us to meet our potential. Pink beryl is particularly useful for freeing ourselves from the negative feelings that hold us back from achieving our goals. With its warm, encouraging energy, beryl removes the will to fail. It is also said to strengthen the bones and joints.

HEALING ACTION Place morganite at the higher heart chakra to truly know you are worthy of achieving success. Meditate with this beryl when you fear failure. To feel constantly encouraged and supported, wear a morganite pendant close to the heart.

CARE Morganite scores 7.5–8 on the Mohs' scale. Use warm, soapy water and a soft cloth for cleaning. Beryl contains beryllium, a known carcinogen, so do not inhale its dust.

MOSS AGATE

APPEARANCE This variety of agate has swirling green markings that resemble moss. The matrix is usually colorless and translucent.

RARITY Moss agate is often sourced from Australia, India, or the United States.

FORMATION Agate is a translucent form of quartz and chalcedony, itself composed of fine intergrowths of quartz and moganite. Both these minerals are forms of silicon dioxide, with different molecular frameworks. Agate often grows as nodules inside igneous rock. Cavities are filled with silica-rich fluid, which slowly crystallizes. The moss-like forms are inclusions of oxidized iron hornblende.

ATTRIBUTES Moss agate is a nurturing crystal, encouraging us to care for our gardens, homes, families, and friends. Like other forms of agate, it heightens our vision, allowing us to see clearly how and why others need our help. It has particular resonance with the bond between parents and their children. Some say that it eases headaches caused by eyestrain or spending too long staring at a screen.

HEALING ACTION Moss agate is the ideal gift for a new mother. If a loved one has recently given birth, meditate with moss agate to understand how best to show her support without overwhelming or dictating. Position moss agate in the health and family area of the home, which is on the left and midway through the house if you enter by the front door.

CARE With a rating of 6.5–7 on the Mohs' scale, agate is suitable for jewelry and frequent gentle handling. Clean in warm, soapy water. Avoid extremes of temperature. Do not inhale agate dust, which can cause silicosis.

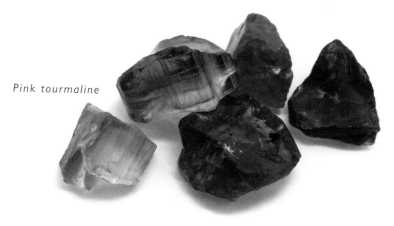

Pink tourmaline

PERIDOT

APPEARANCE Peridot is the name for gem-quality olivine. It may also be known as chrysolite. Peridot ranges from yellow, through yellow-green and olive, to lime. Crystals are orthorhombic and translucent to transparent.

RARITY This popular semiprecious stone is often sourced from Afghanistan, Pakistan, Myanmar, Vietnam, China, Egypt, and the United States.

FORMATION A magnesium iron silicate, olivine is found in igneous rocks, such as basalt and gabbro, which are rich in magnesium and iron. Occasionally it is found in volcanic areas in nodules called bombs. Olivine has also been discovered in meteorites, as well as on the Moon and on Mars.

ATTRIBUTES Since the days of ancient Egypt, peridot has been used to ward off evil spirits and drive away nightmares. This is a crystal that guards the heart, protecting us from thoughtlessly hurtful words and deeds while giving us the emotional strength to face loss and separation. Some say that it helps with palpitations, but medical advice should always be sought first.

HEALING ACTION If you have a tendency to fall in love too easily, wear a peridot pendant so you do not give your heart away to those who do not deserve it. Sleep with peridot under the pillow if you are prone to nightmares or night terrors. When struggling with separation from a loved one, meditate with peridot.

CARE Peridot scores 6.5–7 on the Mohs' scale, making it suitable for jewelry. However, peridot is sensitive to sweat, so avoid frequent wearing against the skin. Clean in warm, soapy water. Avoid dry dusting, which can cause scratches.

PINK TOURMALINE

APPEARANCE Pink to red tourmaline is sometimes called rubellite. A translucent to opaque crystal, pink tourmaline is often found in columnar, radiating, or needle-shaped forms that are triangular in cross section.

RARITY This semiprecious gem is available from jewelers and specialty stores. Some specimens may have been artificially irradiated to deepen their color.

FORMATION Tourmaline is one of the most complicated silicate minerals, containing elements such as aluminum, iron, lithium, magnesium, potassium, and sodium, among others. Pink tourmaline is usually rich in lithium and manganese. Prolonged natural irradiation deepens the pink to red. Pink tourmaline is found in metamorphic rocks such as schist and marble.

ATTRIBUTES Like all tourmalines, this variety offers spiritual protection. It is a powerful crystal for clearing blockages and dispersing negative energy. Pink tourmaline also encourages trust and generosity in our close relationships. It teaches us to love so that we can be lovable. This tourmaline is also said to treat the endocrine system.

HEALING ACTION Wear a pink tourmaline pendant to open your heart to loving and being loved. Meditate with pink tourmaline when you find it hard to trust yourself and others. Position a pink tourmaline crystal on the higher heart chakra when you know you are guilty of not feeding relationships with your loved ones.

CARE Tourmaline rates 7–7.5 on the Mohs' scale. Clean with warm, soapy water and a soft cloth.

PYRITE

APPEARANCE Also known as fool's gold thanks to its deceptively similar appearance to gold, pyrite is pale yellow and shiny. Its crystals form cubes, often with striated faces. It may also be found as octahedra, stalactites, globes, and masses.

RARITY Pyrite is the most common sulfide mineral. It is widely available from specialty mineral suppliers, who should give advice on its toxicity and storage.

FORMATION Pyrite is composed of iron and sulfur. It is found in metamorphic, igneous, and sedimentary rocks. It forms by a variety of processes, including contact metamorphism (the intrusion of hot magma) and diagenesis (chemical and physical changes) in sediments rich in organic matter.

ATTRIBUTES This crystal is highly motivating. It encourages us to aim high and dream big. It helps us to work hard to achieve our goals, no matter what obstacles we have to overcome. It encourages mental and emotional resilience. Pyrite is also a grounding crystal, helping us to engage closely and positively with reality. It is said to be rejuvenating and energizing.

HEALING ACTION Due to its toxicity, pyrite should be used only under the direction of a qualified crystal therapist.

CARE Keep pyrite specimens away from children and pets. Pyrite may contain the poison arsenic. On no account should it be ingested, inhaled, or used in gem elixirs. Keep specimens dry and in a plastic box to avoid decomposition, which will release hydrochloric acid. Do not wash. It scores 6–6.5 on the Mohs' scale.

RAINBOW FLUORITE

APPEARANCE Transparent to translucent, rainbow fluorite features bands or zones of green, turquoise, blue, and purple. It is found in cubes, octahedrons, columns, and masses. Many crystals fluoresce (a phenomenon named after the mineral) in ultraviolet light.

RARITY Fluorite is an extremely common mineral, but gem-grade specimens of rainbow fluorite may be priced as semiprecious stones. It is popular among mineral collectors.

FORMATION Fluorite commonly forms in felsic igneous rocks, which are rich in lighter elements. It is composed of calcium and fluorine. Pure fluorite is colorless, but impurities—usually caused by variations in hydrothermal fluid—can tint it any shade.

ATTRIBUTES All varieties of fluorite help us to make positive changes in our lives. Rainbow fluorite helps us to find much-needed balance in our hectic lives. It allows us to balance work and home, love and friendship, intellect and senses.

HEALING ACTION If you are feeling burned out by work or caring for loved ones, meditate with rainbow fluorite. Place on the desk as a constant reminder that there is more to life than the next deadline. Place in the center of the home to bring together all its different people and pursuits.

CARE Fluorite scores just 4 on the Mohs' scale, so take care when wearing fluorite jewelry. Fluorite is not water safe, so clean with a dry cloth if necessary. It is toxic too, so do not use in gem elixirs and do not ingest. Do not expose to acids.

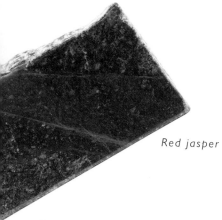

Red jasper

RED JADE

APPEARANCE The decorative stone known as jade is one of two minerals with similar properties and appearance, jadeite and nephrite. Red specimens are jadeite. They range from translucent to opaque.

RARITY Natural red jadeite is extremely rare. Many specimens of "red jade" have been dyed. Some stones marketed as jade may be jasper or other substitutes.

FORMATION Jadeite forms during metamorphism, where two tectonic plates are converging. Much jadeite is found around the rim of the Pacific Ocean, in the Ring of Fire. The mineral is often found as pebbles and boulders in stream valleys, with a dark, weathered rind covering its beauty.

ATTRIBUTES All colors of jade bring harmony. Jade helps to balance the chakras, as well as finding equilibrium between the conflicting demands of body and mind. Red jade has particular resonance with the emotions, helping to reduce mood swings, irritability, and angry outbursts. It is said to regulate the hormones and the metabolism.

HEALING ACTION Hold red jade over any chakra that is blocked or overstimulated. If you are experiencing mood swings, use this mineral for meditation. If you feel that justified anger is building inside you, position red jade over the throat chakra so that you can voice your feelings calmly and kindly.

CARE Jadeite scores 6.5–7 on the Mohs' scale. Wipe jadeite clean with a soft, soapy cloth, then rinse with clean water and dry carefully. Jadeite should not be soaked. Keep out of direct sunlight.

RED JASPER

APPEARANCE Jasper is an opaque stone, with red its most common color. It breaks with a smooth surface and takes a high polish.

RARITY Red jasper is common worldwide. Note that "jasper" is sometimes used as a descriptive term for a colorful, shiny stone rather than as a scientific term.

FORMATION Jasper is an opaque variety of quartz, usually combined with chalcedony, which is itself composed of very fine intergrowths of quartz and moganite. Both these minerals are composed of silicon and oxygen atoms, but have different molecular structures. Jasper often forms where fine, soft sediments are cemented together by silicon dioxide. It is the included particles of sediment that make jasper both opaque and colorful. Red jasper is tinted by iron inclusions.

ATTRIBUTES All varieties of jasper are supportive and protective. Red jasper also helps us bring to light intangible truths: the meanings of dreams, the genuine nature of our own desires, and the best path to take at times of indecision. It is said to strengthen bones, joints, and ligaments.

HEALING ACTION Place red jasper under your pillow to access the spiritual truths of your dreams. Wear a red jasper pendant or bracelet as a guide through difficult decisions, from buying a home to business negotiations.

CARE Jasper is fairly hard, scoring 6.5–7 on the Mohs' scale. Clean with warm, soapy water and a soft cloth. Do not inhale quartz dust, which can cause silicosis.

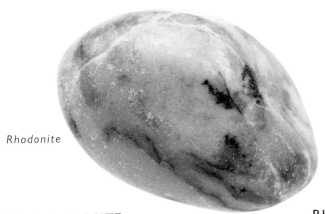

Rhodonite

RHODOCHROSITE

APPEARANCE Ranging from cherry red to pale pink, rhodochrosite forms columns, blades, and rhombohedrons. Its name comes from the ancient Greek for "rose-colored." Rhodochrosite is transparent to translucent.

RARITY Easily obtained, rhodochrosite is a key ore of manganese. However, faceted stones are rarely available due to this mineral's softness. Attractive, banded rhodochrosite is mined from Argentina.

FORMATION This mineral grows in hydrothermal veins, where it is often found in association with silver.

ATTRIBUTES While many red stones inspire personal and particular love, rhodochrosite inspires a selfless love—for humankind, for other species, and for our planet itself. It allows us to balance our own needs and self-respect with the desire to help others.

HEALING ACTION Those who devote their time to caring, whether for young children or adults, may find it useful to meditate with rhodochrosite. When placed at the root chakra, rhodochrosite helps us find balance between selfless love and self-care. Place this mineral at the higher heart chakra if your goal is to raise money for charity or to maintain planet-friendly resolutions, such as cycling to work or planting seedlings.

CARE This mineral is very soft, just 3.5–4 on the Mohs' scale. Always remove jewelry before exercise or chores. Do not wipe or rub when dry, as even household dust could scratch. Clean only with warm, soapy water and a soft cloth. It is soluble in acids, so may react dangerously with stomach acid. Do not use in gem elixirs as it contains manganese.

RHODONITE

APPEARANCE Rhodonite is usually fuchsia to rose-pink. It is commonly found as grains and irregular chunks, but may also form plate-shaped crystals. It is transparent to translucent.

RARITY This relatively rare mineral is sourced in Argentina, Australia, Brazil, Canada, India, Russia, and the United States. Large, well-formed crystals are highly sought after.

FORMATION Alongside other minerals rich in manganese, rhodonite forms in rocks that are altered by contact metamorphism (baking by nearby magma) and hydrothermal fluids.

ATTRIBUTES Rhodonite is a crystal that brings balance, between the heart and head, between jealousy and coldness, between generosity and self-denial. It soothes and harmonizes energy flow between the chakras. Rhodonite is also said to balance the metabolism and the action of the body's glands.

HEALING ACTION Meditate with rhodonite if you are prone to extremes of emotion or find yourself alternating between acting out and guilt. Place on the higher heart chakra to encourage a love that is suffused with kindness, friendship, and respect. To encourage supportive, nurturing relationships, position a rhodonite crystal in the love corner of the home, which is in the back right if you enter by the front door.

CARE Rhodonite scores 5.5–6.5 on the Mohs' scale. Do not expose rhodonite to dramatic changes in temperature. Clean with lukewarm, soapy water and a soft cloth. Do not use in gem elixirs as it contains manganese and is soluble in acids, so may also react dangerously with stomach acid.

Uncut, cloudy rubies are distinctly more affordable than high-quality, faceted gems.

ROSE QUARTZ

APPEARANCE This variety of quartz ranges from pale pink to rose red. Quartz crystals often grow as six-sided prisms ending in pyramids. Rose quartz may display diasterism, a star-shaped pattern of light when lit from behind.

RARITY Rose quartz is common worldwide. Sources include the United States, Brazil, and India.

FORMATION Quartz is a ubiquitous rock-forming mineral, often found in felsic rocks such as granite. Colorless quartz is made of silicon and oxygen atoms, but traces of manganese, titanium, or iron can tint it pink.

ATTRIBUTES Rose quartz is a crystal of love, kindness, and forgiveness. It is the ideal stone for someone who has loved and lost, and is now finding it hard to move forward and welcome new relationships. Rose quartz also helps us to truly understand others, opening the door to selfless nurturing. It is said to aid the regeneration of the body's cells.

HEALING ACTION To welcome love into your life, wear a rose quartz pendant close to the heart. To nurture your existing relationships, both romantic and familial, place a rose quartz twin (two conjoined crystals) or cluster in the relationship corner of your home, which is in the back right if you enter by the main door.

CARE Quartz scores 7 on the Mohs' scale. Clean using warm, soapy water and a soft cloth. Do not inhale quartz dust, which can cause silicosis.

RUBY

APPEARANCE This variety of the mineral corundum is named for the Latin for red (*ruber*). Rubies range from orange-red to purple-red. Gem-quality corundums of other shades are known as sapphires. Rubies are translucent to transparent. When crystals have enough materials, space, and time to grow, they form hexagonal prisms.

RARITY Rare and desirable, rubies are considered to be precious stones. Along with diamonds, sapphires, emeralds, and amethysts, they are among the traditional cardinal stones, priced above all others. Rubies are priced by their color, cut, clarity, and carat weight. Uncut, cloudy rubies are distinctly more affordable than high-quality, faceted gems.

FORMATION It is composed of aluminum and oxygen. Chromium tints the mineral red. Rubies form underground under extreme heat and pressure.

ATTRIBUTES Ruby encourages us to be extroverted, sociable, loving, and passionate. It supports dynamic leadership and go-getting. Ruby should be used with wisdom, so that the raw power of this stone does not encourage selfishness or narrow-minded thinking in the pursuit of goals. Some say that ruby is beneficial for the heart and cardiovascular system.

HEALING ACTION To boost confidence in social or professional situations, wear a ruby pendant. Place at the root chakra during meditation to encourage positive and loving feelings. Position ruby in the bedroom to keep sensuality alive.

CARE Ruby is hard, scoring 9 on the Mohs' scale. Clean only with warm, soapy water and a soft cloth. Take fine jewelry to a jeweler for cleaning.

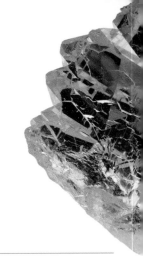

RUTILE QUARTZ

APPEARANCE This variety of quartz contains needle-like inclusions of the mineral rutile. The needles may appear randomly scattered, aligned, or starlike. The rutile may be red, gold, silver, or black. The quartz crystals themselves usually grow as six-sided prisms ending in pyramids, as single wands, twins, or clusters.

RARITY While rutile quartz is fairly common, a good-quality crystal with attractively arranged needles is priced as a semiprecious gemstone.

FORMATION Rutile is titanium dioxide. It forms easily in high-temperature and high-pressure metamorphic and igneous rocks. Quartz is a common silicate mineral that often encloses other minerals without significantly altering their structure.

ATTRIBUTES This gem allows us to overcome difficulties and challenges, ranging from physical feats such as mountain climbs and marathons to emotional endeavors such as surmounting our own fears and failings. Some crystal therapists say that rutile quartz is helpful for impotence, although there is no scientific proof of this claim.

HEALING ACTION Meditate with rutile quartz to enhance motivation during times of low energy and lethargy. Wear a rutile quartz pendant or earrings when courage is needed, whether that is when challenging phobias or facing up to mistakes.

CARE This is a tough and durable stone, scoring 7 on the Mohs' scale. Do not inhale quartz dust. Wash in warm, soapy water with a soft cloth.

SELENITE

APPEARANCE Pure selenite crystals are colorless or white. Transparent specimens are known as selenite. Those that are pearly, silky, and display chatoyance (a cat's-eye effect caused by light reflecting in a fibrous internal structure) are called satin spar. Common crystal forms are plates, prisms, and columns, which are often twinned. Crystals that form curved rosettes may be called gypsum flowers.

RARITY Selenite is a very common mineral. Delicate and transparent crystals may take a slightly higher price.

FORMATION Selenite and satin spar are varieties of gypsum. They are calcium sulfate dihydrate, which means they contain molecules of water. Selenite is an evaporite mineral, forming as water evaporates from salt flats, seas, caves, and mud or clay beds.

ATTRIBUTES Selenite helps us to learn the lessons that life gives us. If we are unhappy, it helps us to pinpoint what is troubling us so that we can make changes. When we are working toward a goal, selenite helps us to see clearly the steps that we must take to get there. This mineral also heightens clairvoyance and telepathy. Some crystal therapists say that selenite is useful for treating joint and muscle pain.

HEALING ACTION To avoid complacency and to keep nourishing a long-term relationship, meditate with a twinned selenite crystal. For extraordinary insights, use satin spar during scrying. Position selenite at the third eye to heighten awareness of ourselves, others, and the spiritual realm.

CARE Selenite dissolves in acids and water, so do not use in gem elixirs. It scores just 2 on the Mohs' scale,

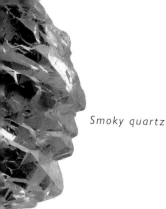
Smoky quartz

which makes it soft enough to be scratched by a fingernail. If necessary, clean very gently with a soft cloth.

SMOKY QUARTZ

APPEARANCE Smoky quartz is gray to black, sometimes with yellowish tints, and ranges from transparent to almost opaque. Quartz crystals often grow as six-sided prisms ending in pyramids.

RARITY Smoky quartz is common worldwide. Ensure that you buy from a reputable source that does not sell quartz that has been artificially irradiated.

FORMATION Pure quartz is made of silicon and oxygen atoms. Smoky quartz gets its appearance from natural irradiation of traces of aluminum in the crystal structure. Quartz is a common rock-forming mineral, found in felsic rocks such as granite.

ATTRIBUTES Smoky quartz offers strength in the face of difficulty, as well as practical solutions to nebulous problems and fears. This crystal helps us to accept ourselves as we truly are, both physically and mentally. Some crystal therapists say this variety of quartz helps with ailments of the legs, including nighttime cramps.

HEALING ACTION Positioned at the earth or root chakra, smoky quartz is grounding, helping us to turn ideas and dreams into workable reality. This crystal is an ideal gift for anyone who struggles with body image or is overly self-critical. A wand of smoky quartz is particularly effective at dispelling negative energy.

CARE Quartz, which is named for the old Germanic word for "hard," scores 7 on the Mohs' scale. Do not inhale quartz dust, which can cause silicosis. Clean in warm, soapy water with a soft cloth.

SODALITE

APPEARANCE Usually royal blue, sodalite may occasionally be sourced in violet, green, or yellow. Although individual crystals are translucent, it is commonly found as opaque masses in which white veins can be seen. It fluoresces in ultraviolet light.

RARITY Sodalite is a fairly rare rock-forming mineral. Royal blue sodalite is often used as cabochons and inlays in jewelry. Sources of good-quality sodalite include Canada and the United States.

FORMATION Composed of sodium, aluminum, silicon, oxygen, and chlorine, sodalite forms in magma that is rich in sodium.

ATTRIBUTES Sodalite is a crystal that directs us to the truth. It helps us to perceive practical, financial, emotional, and spiritual truths. It allows us to speak those truths without fear. It helps us to see the meanings and motivations of others clearly. Some crystal healers say that sodalite helps to balance the metabolism.

HEALING ACTION Place on the throat chakra to allow honest and courageous speech. Meditate with sodalite if you are in need of emotional or spiritual direction. Place in the knowledge corner of the home, which is to the left if you enter by the front door.

CARE Sodalite scores 5.5–6 on the Mohs' scale, so is better suited to earrings and pendants than to frequently knocked rings and bracelets. Do not soak this crystal, as this could splinter a crack. Do not use in gem elixirs as it is soluble in acids and may react dangerously with stomach acid. Wipe clean with a damp, soft cloth.

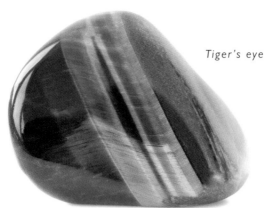

Tiger's eye

SUNSTONE

APPEARANCE This transparent to translucent mineral is often found in shades of yellow, orange, and red. It has a spangled appearance, as if it contains glitter, caused by light reflecting from small copper or hematite inclusions.

RARITY Sunstone is found in the United States, Australia, Norway, and Sweden. Gem-quality specimens are often Norwegian.

FORMATION Sunstone is a form of oligoclase, a member of the feldspar group of rock-forming minerals. Oligoclase is found in igneous and metamorphic rocks.

ATTRIBUTES Sunstone helps us to offer those small acts of human kindness that make everyday life joyful. It also encourages us to recognize and accept the kindness of others. This stone brings happiness, not through great change or drama, but through pleasure in the ordinary, from a walk in the park to a cake shared with a friend. Sunstone is said to regulate the metabolism and ease aches and pains.

HEALING ACTION Meditate with sunstone to experience joy in the moment, to focus on the here and now, not the troubled past or the doubtful future. If you find your workplace fraught or stressful, carry sunstone or place it on your desk. Place sunstone on the sacral chakra to combat feelings of dissatisfaction and irritability with others.

CARE This mineral scores 6–6.5 on the Mohs' scale. Remove sunstone jewelry before exercise or chores. Clean with warm, soapy water and a soft cloth. Do not use in gem elixirs as its inclusions may be toxic.

TIGER'S EYE

APPEARANCE Tiger's eye is red-brown to gold and displays chatoyancy, often called a cat's-eye effect. It has a silky luster.

RARITY Tiger's eye is usually cut into cabochons to show off its chatoyancy. Jewelers who cut and grind tiger's eye must take precautions as its amphibole fibers include asbestos. Tiger's eye is sourced around the world, including from Australia, Myanmar, Namibia, South Africa, and the United States.

FORMATION Tiger's eye is formed of chalcedony (a combination of the silica minerals quartz and moganite), with embedded fibers of amphibole minerals that have mostly turned to limonite, an iron ore. It is these fibers that create the cat's-eye effect as they reflect the light.

ATTRIBUTES In many parts of the world, tiger's eye is believed to ward off the evil eye. It is a strongly protective crystal, keeping dark entities and curses at bay. It also gives us the strength to withstand temptation, as well as the self-confidence to weather confrontation and criticism. Tiger's eye is said to speed the mending of broken bones.

HEALING ACTION This stone should be used under the direction of a qualified crystal therapist.

CARE Keep tiger's eye away from children and pets. Tiger's eye contains silicon and asbestos. Asbestos fibers cause lung cancer and asbestosis. Cut and finished cabochons of tiger's eye are considered low risk to display. However, do not ingest, do not use in gem elixirs, and do not breathe in tiger's eye dust if it shatters. Handle infrequently and wash hands afterward. Tiger's eye scores 6.5–7 on the Mohs' scale. Clean in warm, soapy water with a soft cloth.

Turquoise has been prized as a gem since the days of ancient Egypt.

TURQUOISE

APPEARANCE This blue-green, opaque mineral is found as chunks and nodes. The dark, spidery lines of limonite veining (iron ore) can often be seen.

RARITY There are only a few large deposits of turquoise in the world, the best known in Iran, Egypt, Turkey, China, Mexico, and the United States. More affordable stones may be brittle and crumbly.

FORMATION Turquoise is composed of copper, aluminum, phosphorus, oxygen, and hydrogen. The mineral gets its color from its copper. Typically, the mineral forms underground in a two-step process. First, hydrothermal fluid leaches copper from the host rock, filling veins and fractures with copper ore. Next, groundwater reacts with the copper ore as well as aluminum and phosphorus in the rock, slowly forming turquoise.

ATTRIBUTES Turquoise has been prized as a gem since the days of ancient Egypt, when it was used for grave furnishings as well as in amulets that brought good luck and protection for the wearer. This is a stone that both heals and strengthens, helping us to overcome past trauma, emotional turmoil or anxiety, and to move forward with optimism. It is also said to speed the healing of physical wounds and injuries.

HEALING ACTION When placed or worn close to the higher heart chakra, turquoise helps us to overcome anxiety, shyness, or low self-esteem. At times of emotional stress, meditate with turquoise to engender calm and hope for the future.

CARE Turquoise scores 5–6 on the Mohs' scale, so protect it from drops and knocks. If soaked, turquoise will absorb the water and any chemicals it contains. If cleaning is necessary, wipe with a soft, clean, and untreated cloth. Do not use in gem elixirs as turquoise contains copper.

ZOISITE

APPEARANCE Brown zoisite may be pleochroic, exhibiting different colors from different angles and in different lights. It is transparent to translucent. Zoisite is found as chunks, striated prisms, and columns. Different shades of zoisite are known as tanzanite (blue to violet), thulite (pink), and anyolite (green zoisite combined with ruby).

RARITY Translucent zoisite is fairly common. High-quality transparent zoisite is priced as a semiprecious stone.

FORMATION Zoisite is found in metamorphic rocks or igneous rocks that formed at high temperature and pressure deep underground. It contains atoms of silicon, aluminum, calcium, oxygen, and hydrogen.

ATTRIBUTES Zoisite can help the user turn sadness to hope, anger to acceptance, and anxiety to calm. It is an ideal crystal for those looking for a fresh start, either practically or emotionally. Where relationships have gone astray, it may help with rebuilding trust. It is said to strengthen the joints, particularly the hips, although medical advice should always be sought.

HEALING ACTION For those suffering from writer's block or anxiety about a new creative project, place zoisite on your desk as a paperweight. Meditate with zoisite to help find your way toward positive change.

CARE Zoisite scores 6–7 on the Mohs' scale. Do not use in gem elixirs. Clean in warm, soapy water with a soft cloth.

CRYSTALS FOR COMMON AILMENTS

Eyestrain

Eyestrain occurs when you've been doing activities that involve using your eyes intensely for a long period of time without a break, such as using a computer, reading, sewing, or driving. It can also occur if you've been straining your eyes in dim light or have been in very bright light. Eyestrain can make your eyes feel tired, sore, watery, dry, or itchy. You may experience blurred or double vision, have a headache, and be sensitive to light. Sometimes your back, neck, or shoulders might feel sore and achy too. It can sometimes be caused by underlying eye issues, such as changes in your eyesight or conditions such as a dry eye syndrome. Most eyestrain is temporary and not serious, but if you experience prolonged or severe symptoms, always see a qualified medical practitioner.

Key crystals
• Blue lace agate—use the gentle, calming energy of a blue lace agate stone to ease eyestrain, by placing it on the third eye chakra on your forehead.
• Emerald—place an emerald on the third eye chakra, or around the outside of your head, to soothe eyestrain and tired eyes.

You may also like to make an indirect crystal elixir and gently dab the mixture above your eyes (don't put it directly on the eyes).

Additional therapies

If eyestrain has been caused by extended periods of driving, reading, sewing, or using a computer or tablet screen, try to cut back and have regular breaks when doing so. Make sure you have your eyes tested regularly to see if you need glasses or new prescription lenses. Improve lighting, rather than straining to see in dim light, and make sure you get plenty of sleep, to avoid eyestrain due to being tired or stressed. Gentle yoga or adjusting your posture while seated may be beneficial if you also have related back, neck, or shoulder problems.

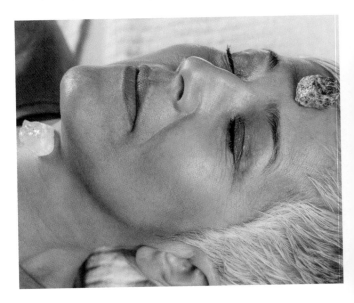

Earache

Earache can have various causes, such as a buildup of wax in the ear, referred pain from toothache, a perforated eardrum, or a sore throat or cold. If you also have a fever with earache, it could be caused by an ear infection or flu. Always avoid putting cotton buds in your ear to try to clean them, as it can compress and push earwax further into your ear, rather than removing it. If you think you could have something stuck in your ear, have ear swelling, have a lot of fluid coming out of your ear, experience a change in hearing, or a very high temperature and shivering, always seek the advice of a medical practitioner.

Key crystals
• Celestite—place celestite on or near the ear, as its cleansing energies may help to ease the discomfort of earache and encourage the dissipation of any toxins or infections.
• Blue chalcedony—place a blue chalcedony stone on or near the source of the pain, or hold it in the palm of your hand. The cleansing and balancing may help to ease discomfort.
• Rhodonite—wear rhodonite crystal earrings to gently ease earache caused by blocked ears. Rhodonite is also said to help fine-tune hearing.

Additional therapies
Alongside any treatments prescribed by a medical practitioner, placing a warm flannel on the ear could help to relieve some discomfort. If you have a fever with your earache, you may benefit from a cooling flannel instead. A few drops of olive oil can soften hard earwax. Some people suggest specially designed Hopi ear candles can help, but it's best to go to a trained holistic therapist for an ear candling session.

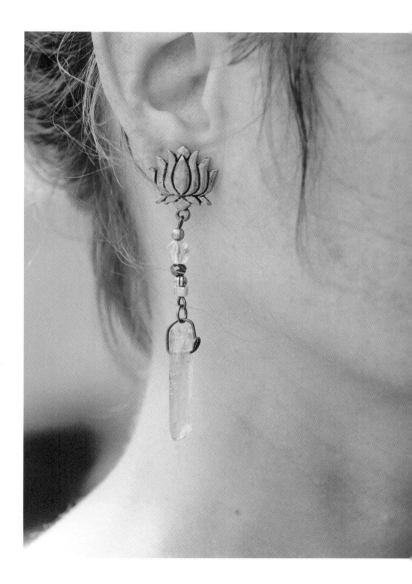

Indigestion

Indigestion is a feeling of discomfort in your upper abdomen. Mild indigestion is common and may occur after you've eaten a big meal, fatty foods, or rushed through eating a meal. Symptoms of indigestion include bloating, a warm or burning sensation in your upper abdomen, burping, flatulence, and nausea. Sometimes indigestion can be linked to other health conditions. If you have regular bouts of indigestion, or it's severe, consult your health practitioner.

Key crystals
• Citrine—hold, wear, or place on your body to detoxify, balance, and reenergize the digestive system.
• Jasper—jasper may help support the digestive system, so pop a piece in your pocket, or place on your stomach, to help aid digestive problems.
• Peridot—place on the throat chakra to relieve hiccups, burping, or general indigestion problems. Wear on a necklace to aid ongoing issues.
• Tourmaline—place tourmaline on the solar plexus chakra to cleanse and purify the body and remove blockages, helping energy to follow through in a normal manner.

Additional therapies
Take care of what you eat and drink and watch out for spicy, greasy, or fatty foods that may trigger symptoms. If you rush food, try to slow down and become more mindful about slowly chewing each mouthful. Cut down on sparkling drinks, caffeine, and alcohol, and avoid smoking. Peppermint can ease digestive complaints, so drink a cup of peppermint tea after eating.

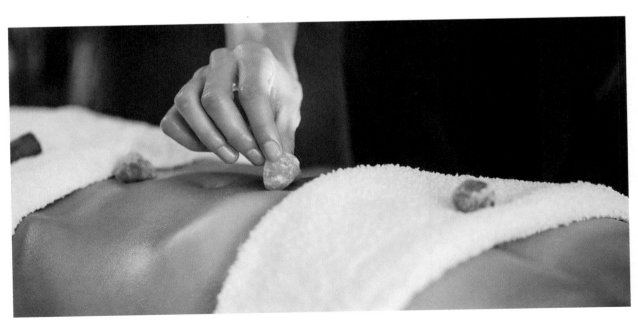

Constipation

Constipation is a bowel condition where you have infrequent bowel movements of three or less per week or find it difficult to pass stools. Symptoms include having hard or lumpy stools, straining to open your bowels, feeling that you can't completely empty your bowels, and the sensation of a bowel blockage. Constipation is common and it's not unusual to experience it at some point in your life, but for some people the symptoms can be chronic and ongoing. The most common causes of constipation include not eating enough fiber in your diet, not drinking enough water, taking prescribed medications that change your bowel movements, spending long periods sitting or lying down, not exercising enough, stress, or ignoring the urge to go to the toilet. It's also common to experience constipation when pregnant or in the weeks after you've given birth. If you frequently have constipation, see a medical practitioner.

Key crystals
• Amber—amber is a good crystal to use to help support a healthy colon and digestive system.
• Calcite—place a piece of calcite on your stomach or solar plexus chakra to encourage bowel movements.
• Sodalite—place sodalite on or around your abdomen to help ease stomach cramps associated with bad constipation. Make a crystal gem elixir and add it to a spray bottle. Spray it onto your abdomen and massage it in.

Additional therapies
Regular exercise can help the digestive system and reduce the risk of constipation.

Diet can play a big role in constipation, particularly if you don't eat enough fiber. Aim to include more fruits, vegetables, and healthy whole grains in your diet and drink plenty of water to aid digestion. Massaging your stomach might help get things moving, as can exercising regularly. If you're stressed, try meditation or yoga to aid relaxation.

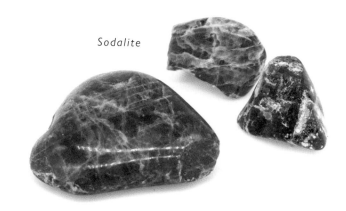

Sodalite

Stress

A certain amount of stress is stimulating, but prolonged stress can cause mental and physical damage. When stress is encountered, hormones stream into the blood, the pulse quickens, the lungs take in more oxygen, blood sugar increases to supply energy, and perspiration breaks out. If the stressful situation ends, the body begins to repair the damage caused. However, if the situation does not resolve, the body runs out of energy. Common causes of stress include work issues, relationship problems, financial worries, life changes, and illness. Symptoms of long-term stress include insomnia, depression, digestive problems, ulcers, palpitations, high blood pressure, heart disease, and impotence.

Key crystals

• Charoite—place on the third eye, heart, or solar plexus chakras to help with overcoming emotional turmoil, dealing with change, and living in the present moment. Charoite encourages calm and may help with short-lived obsessions and compulsions.
• Green aventurine—place on the heart or solar plexus to comfort, protect, heal the heart, and settle mild digestive disorders. It may also help to dispel negative thoughts and restore well-being.

Additional therapies

During brief periods of stress, practicing breathing techniques and positive visualizations may help to calm the mind. In the longer term, regular exercise, meditation, yoga, and talking therapies may all be beneficial. Take a B-vitamin supplement, as this essential vitamin is often depleted by stress.

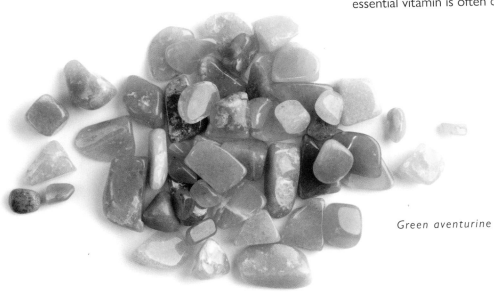

Green aventurine

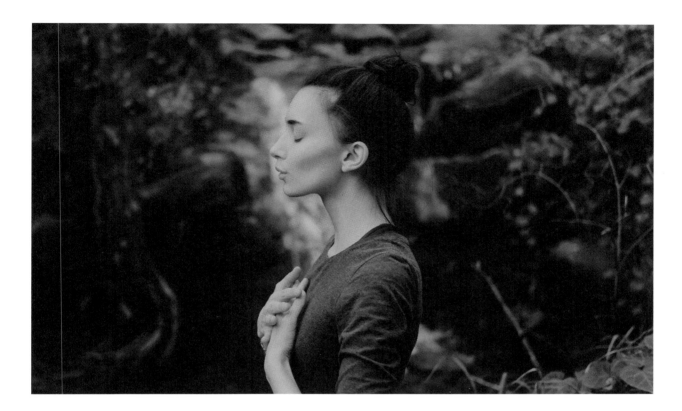

Anxiety

It's normal to feel anxious from time to time, but some people are plagued with constant anxiety, worries, and fears. Feelings of anxiety can range in severity from mild to severe. When anxiety is constant, it can take over and affect your home, work, and social life. The symptoms may start off as psychological, but constant anxiety can lead to physical symptoms such as restlessness, insomnia, dizziness, palpitations, irritability, fatigue, and difficulty concentrating. See your doctor if you're experiencing signs of anxiety, as sometimes it can be caused by an underlying health condition.

Key crystals
• Green calcite—make a crystal elixir using the indirect method and spray directly onto your body or add to bathwater when you're feeling anxious. Green calcite is a comforting crystal that could help to restore balance in your mind and help you let go of negativity and worries.

• Black tourmaline—place black tourmaline on the root chakra to help ground you and release tension. If your crystal has a point, place it with the point facing away from you, to draw off negative thoughts.
• Amethyst—wear an amethyst crystal pendant on a necklace to help calm your body and mind. It may help with decision-making if you're feeling anxious about making the right choices.

Additional therapies
When you're feeling anxious, breathing exercises where you simply focus on your breath, and breathing slowly on a count from one to ten, could help to calm feelings of anxiety. Flower remedies that you take under your tongue may help with mild anxiety, and creative visualizations, where you mentally imagine the best outcome of a situation or event, could be useful.

RESOURCES AND FURTHER READING

Here are some relevant organizations that you might find useful for further information.

Academic Consortium for Integrative Medicine & Health
imconsortium.org

Academy of Nutrition and Dietetics
www.eatright.org

Alliance of International Aromatherapists
www.alliance-aromatherapists.org

American Herbalists Guild
www.americanherbalistsguild.com

American Holistic Health Association
www.ahha.org

American Holistic Nurses Association
www.ahna.org

American Society for Nutrition
nutrition.org

American Society of Alternative Therapists
asat.org

Bach Centre
www.bachcentre.com

Canadian College of Holistic Health
cchh.org

Foundation for Alternative and Integrative Medicine
faim.org

National Association for Holistic Aromatherapy
naha.org

National Association of Holistic Health Practitioners
nahhp.com

National Center for Complementary and Integrative Health
nccih.nih.gov

Natural Health Practitioners of Canada
nhpcanada.org

Natural Medicines
naturalmedicines.therapeuticresearch.com

The Herb Society of America
www.herbsociety.org

Further reading ideas

For more ideas on the topics covered in this book, you might like to read these titles.

Allotment Month by Month
Alan Buckingham
DK, 2019

Aromatherapy for Self-Care: Your Complete Guide to Relax, Re-balance, and Restore with Essential Oils
Sarah Swanberg
Rockridge Press, 2020

Complete Massage
Neal's Yard Remedies, Victoria Plum
DK, 2019

Encyclopedia of Herbal Medicine
Andrew Chevalier
DK, 2016

Healing with Whole Foods
Paul Pitchford
North Atlantic Books, 2002

Meditation with Intention
Anusha Wijeyakumar
Llewellyn Publications, 2021

Mindfulness: An Eight-Week Plan to Finding Peace in a Frantic World
Mark Williams, Dr. Danny Penman
Rodale Books, 2012

Plant-Based Nutrition
Julieanna Hever, Raymond J. Cronise
Alpha, 2018

Plant-Powered Beauty
Amy Galper and Christina Daigneault
BenBella Books, 2020

RHS Grow Your Own Veg & Fruit Bible
Carol Klein
Mitchell Beazley, 2020

The Book of Crystal Grids
Philip Permutt
CICO Books, 2017

The Crystal Code
Tamara Driessen
Ballantine Books, 2018

The Complete Juicing Recipe Book
Stephanie Leach
Rockridge Press, 2020

The Encyclopedia of Essential Oils
Julia Lawless
Red Wheel, 2013

The Healthy Smoothie Bible
Farnoosh Brock
Skyhorse, 2014

The Holistic Home
Laura Benko
Skyhorse, 2016

The Little Book of Chakras
Patricia Mericier
Gaia, 2017

The New Optimum Nutrition Bible
Patrick Holford
Crossing Press, 2005

INDEX